W9-BYP-713

BINOCULAR VISION

FOUNDATIONS AND APPLICATIONS

R.W. Reading, M.O., Ph.D.
School of Optometry
Indiana University
Bloomington, Indiana

BUTTERWORTHS

Boston • London

Sydney • Wellington • Durban • Toronto

Copyright © 1983 Butterworth Publishers
All rights reserved.

No part of this publication may be reproduced, stored
in a retrieval system, or transmitted, in any form or by
any means, electronic, mechanical, photocopying, recording, or otherwise, without the prior written permission of the publisher.

*Every effort has been made to ensure that the drug dosage
schedules within this text are accurate and conform to standards accepted at time of publication. However, as treatment
recommendations vary in light of continuing research and
clinical experience, the reader is advised to verify drug dosage
schedules herein with information found on product information sheets. This is especially true in cases of new or in-
frequently used drugs.*

Library of Congress Cataloging in Publication Data

Reading, R. W.
  Binocular vision.

  Includes bibliographies and index.
  1. Binocular vision. I. Title. [DNLM: 1. Vision—
Physiology. WW 103 R287b]
QP487.R37 1983   612'.84   82-14615
ISBN 0–409–95033–5

Butterworth Publishers
10 Tower Office Park
Woburn, MA 01801

10 9 8 7 6 5 4 3 2 1

Printed in the United States of America.

To Shirley Anne
and
Rogers Edwin

About the Author

R.W. Reading is Professor of Optometry and former Chairman of the Department of Visual Sciences at Indiana University, where he also received his Ph.D. in Physiological Optics with minors in Astronomical Photometry and Sensory Psychology, and his B.S. and M.O. degrees in Optometry. He is the author of numerous articles dealing with aspects of vision and is currently serving as Vice-President of the National Board of Examiners in Optometry.

CONTENTS

Foreword

The fact that we have two eyes instead of one, and that they normally function in a kind of collimation, gives rise to a host of problems, phenomena, and scientific data. These problems, phenomena, and data justify a categorical subdivision of physiological optics most conveniently identified as binocular sensory aspects of vision; or, more briefly, binocular vision. As a topic it involves numerous concepts, analyses, sensations, and experimental techniques that are neither a part of the monocularly considered aspects of vision nor of the complex motility mechanisms making continuous binocular vision possible; though often treated as incidental to one or the other. This is not to suggest that binocular sensory vision is independent of other subdivisions of the broad discipline of physiological optics; rather it is to explain the need for a textbook compilation of available scientific information pertinent to our understanding of binocular vision as a sensory function. Professor Reading has undertaken to provide such a compilation with this book.

Dr. Reading is regarded by his immediate colleagues as a most comfortable blend of teacher and researcher. A firm respecter of, but not a slave to the classics, he dares to pursue the increasingly crucial role of the teaching professor as an interpreter and organizer of our overwhelming glut of science information. He is keenly aware of the role of physiological optics, by whatever name, as the foundation science of optometry, and especially of the relationship of binocular sensory vision to the practitioner's clinical challenges.

A subdivision of visual science in greater need of textbook presentation, especially for the optometry curriculum, could hardly have been selected. If I may indulge a bit lightheartedly in a quotation, as Dr. Reading has done so effectively at the opening of each chapter, let me repeat from Erasmus, "Homer wrote of no more weighty a subject than of a war between the frogs and mice; Virgil of a gnat and a pudding cake; and Ovid of a nut." May this book be a reasonably analogous literary venture.

Henry W Hofstetter
Rudy Professor Emeritus
of Optometry
Indiana University

Preface

The problems of seeing both *depth* and *direction* from the standpoint of the sensory cooperation of two eyes are explored in this text. Its topic is binocular vision and its scope necessitates discussion of perception and eye movements and their influence on our sense of sight.

Binocular Vision: Foundations and Applications brings together under one cover information scattered across the literature of numerous disciplines. For this reason, it is hoped that the work will serve as a standard reference for this field. It is designed for use as a text for courses in Physiological Optics (also called Visual Science). Such courses are typically offered to students with backgrounds in the fundamentals of ocular anatomy and neural physiology. Readers familiar with visual optics, ocular motility, and monocular aspects of vision will recognize the application of many of the principles of these disciplines to the issue of seeing with both eyes. Yet, in general, the material in this text stands alone and should be understandable to any reader with three or four years of undergraduate training.

The chapters in this text have been written to facilitate almost any order of presentation befitting the individual teaching style of the instructor. At some institutions, chapters that deal with applications will be useful background material for clinical courses. These particular sections should be of general interest to clinicians. Graduate students and researchers will find the text a useful starting point for their own investigations into many of the specific aspects of cyclopean seeing.

While every attempt has been made to define terminology in the text proper, readers unfamiliar with this area may wish to consult *The Dictionary of Visual Science* by Drs. Cline, Hofstetter, and Griffin for complete and authoritative definitions. In addition, a good medical dictionary will prove helpful for detailed definitions of general terms associated with the purely biological aspects of binocular vision.

One of the real challenges in writing this book is that the information on binocular vision continues to appear in so many different places, which suggests that the topic has broad appeal to workers from many separate areas. It is my hope that those interested in this topic will benefit from this attempt to collect information and will contact me with additional topics and materials for inclusion in future revisions. Certainly optometry students are deserving of the very best that can be produced. For too long they have been asked to master material that does not exist in any single reference source.

Another problematic aspect of binocular vision is the unevenness of available information. While it was my intention to present the best available evidence, this was frequently less than complete, and suggests that the study of the binocular process might well benefit from more systematic development. Still, recent advances in our understanding of vision have occurred at such an incredible rate that this text, or any other, represents no more than a single assessment of the field at a given point in time. After reading this text, the serious student will naturally want to refer to recent issues of the vision journals to remain apprised of the latest developments and findings.

A textbook is only one of many learning resources. No written word can substitute for the motivation communicated by an enthusiastic and knowledgable instructor. Nor can it totally replace the experience gained from well-chosen laboratory demonstrations or actual clinical encounters. Nevertheless, written compilations, such as this one, provide the thoughtful reader with material needed to begin to turn "ideas over in the mind." This process is an individual one, and it is at the foundation of all forms of learning.

Each chapter starts with a short quotation. This was done to interject a change of pace, not to make light of the subject matter. Scientists are sometimes criticized for taking their work too seriously. It is important to all of us not to lose sight of our common roots in humanity.

R.W. Reading

Acknowledgments

I wish to acknowledge the people who have helped me without attempting to delegate any of the responsibility for errors that may have been committed. To my wife, Shirley, who challenged me to begin this undertaking and has sustained me throughout its development, my never ending gratitude and affection. She also provided much needed editorial and translation services. Dr. George Woo has read an earlier version of the manuscript and made most astutue and timely suggestions. Various sections have been reviewed in an earlier form by Drs. Arthur Afanador, Merrill Allen, Richard Aslin, Clifford Brooks, Freddy Chang, Ronald Everson, Gary Hafner, Henry Hofstetter, Edwin Marshall, Ingeborg Schmidt, and William Somers.

The style of presentation depends heavily upon good illustrations. Here, Jacque Kubley's skills in graphic matters as an accomplished biomedical illustrator and Diane Jung's talents as an artist have helped to produce not only useful drawings, but frequently works of genuine beauty. Elizabeth Egan has been a great help in providing literature search suggestions and has opened the full extent of the Optometry Library facilities to the author.

It is also appropriate to thank those students who have made helpful suggestions and offered enthusiastic encouragement. Finally, I would like to express my abiding appreciation to Dr. Ingeborg Schmidt, the instructor who first introduced me to the study of binocular vision, Dr. Henry Hofstetter, who directed my graduate studies in this area, and to Dr. Gordon Heath, whose good offices supported many of the activities necessary to produce this monograph.

R. W. Reading

1

SPATIAL SENSE

Helmholtz—the physiologist who learned
physics for the sake of his physiology, and
mathematics for the sake of his physics, and
is now first rank in all three.

William Kingdon Clifford

NATURE AND SCOPE OF PHYSIOLOGICAL OPTICS

Physiological optics is a term describing a series of courses in the optometry curriculum that cover virtually all aspects of vision. Its name was
created by Herman Helmholtz, the great scientist of the 1800s who
made substantial contributions to astonomy, thermodynamics, acous-
tics, hearing, and vision (Warren and Warren, 1968).

Previously the word *optics* stood alone without such modifiers as
physiological, physical, or *geometric* and was at least partially equivalent
in meaning to the modern term *vision.* Therefore, the antecedents of
physiological optics can be traced through the contributions of scientists
such as Hering, Donders, Young, Newton, Alhazen, and Aristotle,
among others (Boring, 1942; Hofstetter, 1948).

The study of vision is usually considered a hybrid discipline because it draws heavily on the principles and contributions of other
sciences. It is unique in the sense that both synthetic and analytic
methods are employed to answer variations of the question, How is it
that I see? (Levene, 1977).

The subject matter usually is classified into five major topics, each
of which supports or provides the foundation for a particular clinical
area: visual optics, ocular motility, monocular visual function, binocular
visual function, and ocular physiology. These areas also contain fundamental information on the physiology of seeing (*Transactions*, 1959).

While the study of visual science is not the only means of understanding and advancing clinical practice, it is certainly the most reliable and steadfast way because it is founded on rather solid methodology (Hofstetter, 1950).

COMPONENTS OF SENSORY ASPECTS OF VISION

As with any science, some classification is necessary so that we can fit specific information into a larger framework. In particular, the sensory aspects of vision can be divided into a series of subsenses (Walls, 1953). We can speak of the light sense, the color sense, the form sense, and the spatial sense. Examples of topics included under each heading are shown in Table 1–1.

The subdivisions not only allow for an orderly presentation of the subject matter of physiological optics, but also seem to reflect basic and usually different specialized functions of the visual system. Certainly, there is some overlap because the function of one sense can alter the function of another. Nevertheless, many attributes of how we see color, for example, are virtually independent of how we perceive brightness or darkness. Visual science has advanced most rapidly by first considering these topics in isolation and then studying their interrelationships. Finally, the task is completed when the attributes of vision can be related to the behavior of the organism as a whole (Walls, 1953).

VISION AND ITS RELATION TO HUMAN BEHAVIOR

Certainly our knowledge of the visual system has been impressively advanced in recent times. Anyone, who has spent some time studying the biological sciences must have acquired some convictions about the nature of humanity and how behavior can be shaped by the internal

Table 1–1. Sensory Aspects of Vision with Examples

Heading	Sample Topic
Light sense (intensive vision)	Brightness thresholds
Color sense (color vision)	Hue discrimination
Form sense (form vision)	Visual acuity
Spatial sense (spatial vision)	Stereopsis

Source: Walls (1953).

as well as the external environment. Nevertheless, it is a mistake to overemphasize the functions of *one* sensory system, namely vision, and consider it the sole determinant of human behavior or performance. For example, to say that the quality of visual performance is an absolute determinant of human performance is to invite disaster. The adaptability of behavior is an impressive attribute of being human. Frequently other attributes such as motivation, intellect, and emotions can help compensate for certain sensory defects (see, for example, Seefelt, 1962).

Actually, the greater sin of confusion and ignorance usually is committed in reverse: observations of human behavior are translated to laws of physiological optics, and otherwise clear waters are muddied by false information and false hopes, which can lead only to frustration. For example, young children frequently copy b when presented with the letter d. Does this mean that they are seeing backward or that the complex processes of learning a language have yet to be completed? Let us discuss some facts now, and let such philosophical relations develop as a natural fruit of our labors.

MONOCULAR SENSORY FUNCTION REVISITED

You may notice that discussion of form, color, and light seems most appropriate in a text on the monocular sensory functions of vision. However, because of the overlap of these topics, we will have reason to revisit each when we look at the sensory aspects that are (or are not) unique to binocular vision. We talk about eye movements often, but here we emphasize their perceptual consequences.

Sometimes scientists seem very proud of the purity of their fields. If one chooses to study some seemingly obscure topic just for the sake of interest, she or he is said to have the attitude of a true scientist. While there is nothing wrong with study motivated only by simple intellectual curiosity, most clinically oriented students would like to investigate something related to the problems of their patients. In binocular vision, the clinically related problem of the greatest importance is strabismus, or squint. While not all the answers about this important anomaly are known, we present the most important information on the sensory aspects of both normal and abnormal binocular vision.

SPATIAL ORIENTATION

To accomplish these goals, we have to explore the spatial sense in two parts: the orientation aspect and the localization aspect. *Orientation,* as we use it here, refers to the means by which the organism establishes a stable, constant relationship with its surroundings. The organism accomplishes this by referring to the position of objects with regard to a reference point. This point is the self, or ego. In turn, the organism relates the ego to the surroundings mainly through the activity of the static and kinetic equilibrium mechanisms. These mechanisms are discussed in greater detail in texts on ocular motility (see, for example, Alpern, 1969). More generally, the "sense of gravity" keeps us informed of our body orientation with respect to the terrestrial surroundings for the purpose of stabilizing our visual perceptions and, to a very large extent, fixing a consistent relationship between ourselves and the immediate environment (Howard and Templeton, 1966).

We can see a somewhat humorous effect of these stabilizers not working if we view a home movie in which an inexperienced camera operator has walked along while shooting a scene. The picture bounces up and down in a very distracting way because the camera is not equipped with a stabilizing device and the operator was unaware of this outcome because his or her stabilizing apparatus was working normally.

EGOCENTRIC LOCALIZATION

The localization aspects of the spatial sense consist of the means of detecting the positions of individual objects or points in the visible surroundings. Again, the locating process is based on the ego as the center of the visual world. For precise specification of the visual stimulus, a coordinate system can be constructed with the egocenter as its origin. Given this, to localize requires two things: the distance between the point or object and the egocenter and the direction of the point or object with respect to the egocenter (Walls, 1952). For example, direction can be specified by applying a set of polar coordinates in which the ego center is at the origin. Distance can be specified by making the coordinates three-dimensional. Therefore, a meridian-eccentricity-distance system can be used to uniquely specify the location of any point in the visual field (Fry et al., 1945).

The perception of direction is mediated by processes identified as local sign and corresponding points, as discussed in Chapter 5. Distance is mediated by a process known as *stereopsis* and a series of perceptions called *empirical cues to depth* (see Chapter 6). Processes associated with eye movements also may be involved in both distance and direction perceptions (see Chapters 5, 11, and 14).

All five major senses can contribute to a sense of position. Thus, for objects in contact with the skin, we receive sensory inputs to the brain via the tactile sense. We can localize sounds by using auditory information. To a significantly lesser degree, olfaction and taste information can help create a pattern of sensory inputs that result in an egocentric localization of certain objects (Walls, 1952). Finally, the senses associated with muscle activity, the innervational sense and the proprioceptive sense, may contribute to the egocentric localization process. In Table 1–2 we summarize these sensory inputs.

OCULOCENTRIC VERSUS EGOCENTRIC LOCALIZATION

In the study of vision, we make a distinction between oculocentric and egocentric localization. *Oculocentric* localization is a limited but impor-

Table 1–2. Egocentric Localization System

Sensory Input	Comment
Static and kinetic equilibrium mechanisms*	Orientation—compensatory eye movements and sensory information about head position from the vestibular mechanism
Local sign, corresponding points, stereopsis, and empirical cues	Perception of distance and direction of remote objects
Tactile	Perception of location of touching objects only
Auditory	Perception of location of a sound source; cruder than vision but enjoyable for listening to stereophonic music
Olfactory	Crude localizing ability—must assume that the stronger.the well-known odor, the closer the source of the odor, but an unusually strong odor can produce an error in localization
Taste	Extremely crude—"If you can taste something, it must be located in your mouth"
Innervational*	Commands to move the extraocular muscles result in neural signals that tend to stabilize perception
Proprioceptive*	Skeletal muscles provide information about contractility of the muscle

*May be considered an orientation aspect also.

tant concept. Here the coordinate system is centered on the point of fixation, which is, of course, imaged on the center of the fovea. An object or a point is localized in this system by saying that it is, for example, 1° to the right and 0.5° above the object of regard. Changing this point's oculocentric localization requires only a change in fixation. Direct fixation of the object itself now puts it at the origin of this system because the eye movements involved have produced a change in the oculocentric position of the object. In general, during and after this refixation, no large or permanent change has occurred in the egocentric localization of the point, and therein lies the need for the distinction between the two systems of localization.

Consider the analogy offered by television (Rubin and Walls, 1969). The oculocentric system is represented by the TV camera that swings about to bring various aspects of the surroundings into view, and the egocentric system is represented by the TV viewing screen that provides a stable assessment of the relationships of the scene regardless of any regular movements of the camera. That is, the egocentric system is centered within the body and thus is fixed with regard to an environmental reference, while the oculocentric system swings about as the eye moves.

ECCENTRIC FIXATION

There is an important clinical anomaly that further illustrates the need for this distinction between oculocentric and egocentric localizations. In eccentric fixation, patients point their eyes by using retinal points other than the center of the fovea (Burian and von Noorden, 1974). This means that the eye movements may be organized around an eccentric area. Normal eye movements are performed on the basis of a positional signal whose origin is at the foveal center. Does the eccentric fixater represent a shift in oculocentric space values of points on the retina? To find an answer, some precautions must be observed.

The simplest way to study this phenomenon is to shine a narrow beam of light from an ophthalmoscope into the eye from a vantage point that is physically straight ahead of the patient. In this position, responses based on egocentric localization are identical to the oculocentric ones when the patient is asked to look directly at the center of the beam.

When asked to fixate, such patients position the beam's image off the fovea, but nevertheless report that it is located "in a straight-ahead position." Furthermore, the eye movement that positions the beam on this eccentric point is simple and direct. Burian and von Noorden (1974) called such a pattern *true* eccentric fixation. They also find off-fovea fixation of another kind. In these patients no directional shift has occurred, and eye movements are made up of two components, a movement to the fovea and then a movement to the eccentric area used for peripheral viewing. They called this behavior *eccentric viewing*.

INFLUENCE OF FORM

One other point about localization needs to be made. The perception of form can influence the perception of both distance and direction. An example of this influence on direction perception is shown in Figure 1–1, which is one of many visual illusions whose study has generated volumes of speculations, theories, and even art forms (Boring, 1942). These influences are mentioned throughout the text (see Chapters 5 to 7, 9, and 12 to 14).

LOCALIZATION RELATED TO ORIENTATION

In a sense, localization plays a role in orientation because it establishes the position of points or objects in the surroundings of the observer

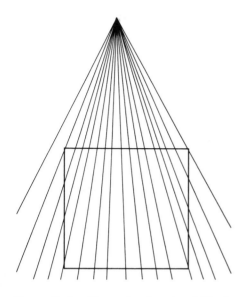

Figure 1–1. Example of a visual illusion.

and tells that person which are stationary and which are moving, and in what direction. To operate, or locomote, in the given environment and manipulate certain objects, the observer must have a fixed reference and a stable perception of the relationship of objects.

We have classified those mechanisms that mainly contribute to establishing a reference as belonging to orientation. Those having to do with the perception of the relationship of points or objects and their movement are classified here as having localization or spatial functions. While this way of treating the information is useful, it is by no means the only way of viewing the functions of the various sensory inputs.

Egocentric localization probably involves even more than just co-ordination, integration, or selection of sensory inputs. Certainly, the part of memory that is identified with visual imagery plays an important role in sustaining the sense of body location and its relationship to objects in the surroundings (Howard and Templeton, 1966).

REFERENCES

Alpern, M. (1969), "Types of eye movement," *The Eye*, vol. 3, Academic, New York, 65–174.

Boring, E. G. (1942), *Sensation and Perception in the History of Experimental Psychology*, Appleton, New York, 236–245.

Burian, H., and von Noorden, G. (1974), *Binocular Vison and Ocular Motility*, St. Louis, Mosby, 233, 228–234.

Fry, G. A., Treleaven, C. L., and Baxter, R. C. (1945), "Specification of the direction of regard," *American Journal of Optometry*, 22, 351–360.

Hofstetter, H. W. (1948), *Optometry: Professional, Economic, and Legal Aspects*, Mosby, St. Louis, 17–35.

Hofstetter, H. W. (1950), "Aims in modern optometric education," *Journal of the American Optometric Association*, 22, 270–275.

Howard, I. P., and Templeton, W. B. (1966), *Human Spatial Orientation*, Wiley, New York, 1–11.

Levene, J. R. (1977), *Clinical Refraction and Visual Science*, Butterworth, London.

Ogle, K. N. (1962), "The spatial sense," *The Eye*, vol. 4, Academic, New York, 215–407.

Rubin, M. L., and Walls, G. L. (1969), *Fundamentals of Visual Science*, Charles C Thomas, Springfield, Ill., 359–367.

Seefelt, E. R. (1962), "Effects of initial spectacle wearing on subsequent high school scholastic grade scores," *American Journal of Optometry*, 39, 477–493.

Transactions and Reports of the Conference on Training in Physiological Optics (1959), Indiana University, Bloomington, National Science Foundation, 11–13.

Walls, G. L. (1952), "The common sense horopter," *American Journal of Optometry*, 29, 460–477.

Walls, G. L. (1953), *Optometry 105B Notes*, University of California, Berkeley, 1–2.

Warren, R., and Warren, R. P. (1968), *Helmholtz on Perception: Its Physiology and Development*, Wiley, New York, 1–15.

2

EVOLUTION OF BINOCULAR VISION

> Much we know about man is derived from the study of sweet peas and a species of vinegar fly.
>
> *Author unknown*

EYE PLACEMENT

Some rather dramatic differences exist in the visual systems of various species. By just looking at different kinds of animals we can see that eye position changes from a lateral location in some animals to a frontal position in others. Thus the field in which objects are visible for any given position of the head is larger in the animal with laterally placed eyes (Walls, 1942). Certainly if an animal needed an early warning of approaching danger, it would be advantageous to be able to see a large panoramic section of the surroundings without having to move the head. Positioning the eyes in a frontal location so that the visual fields of the two eyes overlap creates a blind region in the surroundings in which something can approach undetected. However, frontal eyes must be good for something. A look at such differences will help to elucidate the nature of binocular vision. Here we consider only some of these changes that seem to be associated with binocular vision in humans primarily. For more detailed discussions of the evolution of vision, see Walls (1942), Hughes (1977), and Masterton and Glendenning (1978).

MONOCULAR VISUAL FIELD

Early estimates of the size of the static monocular visual field were made by clamping the specimen's head to a firm support positioned before a perimeter arc, dissecting away the tissue behind the eye, and moving a light along the arc while noting its image through the sclera (Walls, 1942). The resulting field is called the *trans-scleral field* (Hughes, 1977). In another approach, the field was estimated by determining the solid angular subtense that is admitted through the entrance pupil (Walls, 1942). This is sometimes called the *optical field* (Hughes, 1977). Perhaps the best approach is to locate the forward limits of the functional retina and then project this out through the exit pupil to determine the field size (Hughes, 1977). This field is sometimes referred to as the *retinal field*, and it is determined by projection ophthalmoscopy.

Projection ophthalmoscopy is accomplished by mounting an ophthalmoscope on a firm support that allows it to be rotated through an angle of exactly 180°. Positioning the support close to the eye under examination and looking through an aperture, the investigator centers the field of view on a particular feature of the fundus. Then the investigator flips the ophthalmoscope through an angle of 180° so that now its illuminating system acts as a projector. This allows the location of the fundus feature to be translated to a suitable surface such as a tangent screen or perimeter arc (Bishop et al., 1962). To determine the size of the visual field, the edge of the retina, the ora serrata, would be the feature used in working with the primate retina. A histological examination is required to confirm that these fundus limits do contain neural structures capable of supporting vision.

Behavioral methods might apply also to visual field measurements in animals. These methods, which involve training and rewards, have been used successfully to measure visual acuity in the falcon (Fox et al., 1976) and stereopsis in the monkey (Bough, 1970). They are also useful in examining nonverbal humans (see, for example, Courtney and Heath, 1971).

Hughes (1977) reported that the lateral extent of the retinal field for the cat was only 143° as compared with an optical field of 181°. In rabbits and rats the optic field is the same size as the retinal field, but in humans the retinal field is only about 179° while the optical field is some 200° in lateral extent. The human monocular visual field, measured with the eye fixating straight ahead, is about 160° wide.

BINOCULAR VISUAL FIELD

When the eyes are in the primary position, regarding objects at infinity, the binocular visual field can be considered as simply the amount of overlap of the two monocular fields. Figure 2–1 shows how the eye position varies in three species of birds. With this difference in eye position, there is a difference in the degree to which the two fields overlap. This may be a slight simplification since the degree of overlap, and therefore presumably binocular function, is best described in terms

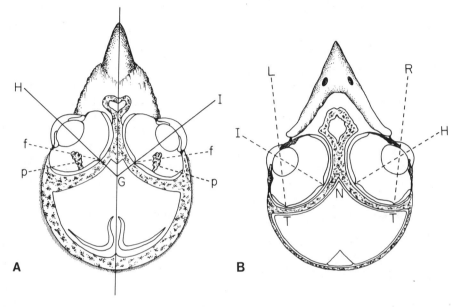

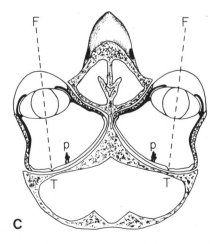

Figure 2–1.   Eye position in *(A)* the titmouse, *(B)* the swallow, and *(C)* the owl. Lines through the fovea represent the fixation axes. *P* is the pecten (Reprinted by permission from Duke-Elder, 1958).

of the angle formed by extending the visual axes of the two eyes until the axes intersect. For frontal eyes, of course, the visual axes are virtually parallel. As illustrated in Figure 2–1 for the titmouse, this angle is about 90°; for the swallow, the angle is about 120° for the nasal visual axes and about 22° for the temporal visual axes. However, in most primates the more nearly frontal the eyes, the smaller the angle. For the owl, with eyes more nearly frontal than those of the swallow, the angle is still about 26°. Figure 2–2 shows the degree of overlap, or the size of the binocular optical field, for a rabbit and a cat (Hughes, 1977). Figure 2–3 shows the binocular visual field for humans (White, 1964).

Authors say that panoramic vision is possessed by those animals that are preyed on by others and that frontal eyes and overlapping fields are possessed by hunters who have less to fear from a blind-side attack. In humans, the fineness of spatial judgment required to manipulate tools and other objects in the immediate surroundings is cited as the advantage of having the eyes in a frontal position (Walls, 1942). However, Hughes (1977) pointed out that by considering only the static visual field one ignores the role of eye and head movements in the behavior of some animals. These movements would tend to reduce the significance of this shift in eye position as it relates to static and dynamic field size.

EYE MOVEMENTS AND THE EVOLUTION OF BINOCULAR VISION

Some animals such as certain fish, birds, reptiles, and mammals have rather prominent snouts, bills, or other facial protuberances that set a

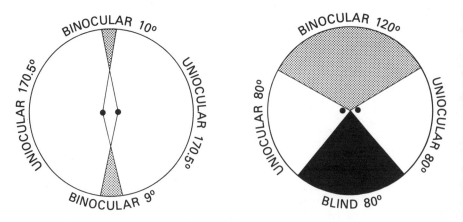

Figure 2–2.   Optical fields of a rabbit and a cat (Modified, and reprinted by permission from Duke-Elder, 1958).

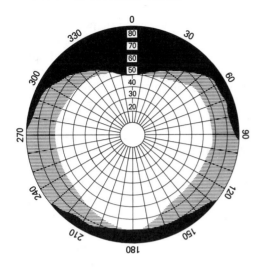

Figure 2–3.   The human binocular visual field as determined by perimetry
            (Webb, 1964).

limit on how close an object can be and still be imaged in both fields.
Figure 2–3 shows that this prominence limits the near range of binocular
overlap for the rabbit. In humans, the nose and brow impose limits that
make the measured field slightly smaller in the nasal and superior
meridians than is the retinal field.

   Only simians and humans appear to have developed an ability to
converge the eyes so as to bifixate objects as close as a few centimeters
from the bridge of the nose. Cats and dogs also can demonstrate convergence, but to a restricted degree. Other animals sometimes show a
reflex convergence associated with fright or other forms of excitement
(Walls, 1942).

   The evolution of voluntary eye movements is associated with the
evolution of the area centralis. In monkeys as in humans, the center
of the fovea mediates the finest discriminations of color, form, and
space. All such eye movements are coupled or yoked in order to accomplish bifixation and maintain images of common features of the
environment on homologous retinal positions (Walls, 1942). In humans,
the lateral extent of the field through which bifixation can be achieved
is about 95° (Cline et al., 1980).

PARTIAL DECUSSATION

Another dramatic change in the visual system involves decussation of
the optic nerve fibers at the chiasma. For laterally placed eyes, where

the fields do not overlap, there is total decussation, or total crossing over. All optic nerve fibers from the left eye cross over to course in the right optic tract, and vice versa. In the visual system of mammals possessing frontal eyes, there exists a so-called partial decussation: some of the optic nerve fibers pass to the ipsilateral optic tract instead of to the contralateral tract (Bishop, 1975). Figure 2–4 shows the arrangement in humans. The ratio of crossed to uncrossed fibers in a given visual system is sometimes related to the amount of overlap or to the size of the binocular visual field. Table 2–1 illustrates this relationship.

Partial decussation allows the two messages generated in the eyes by an object on one side of the straight-ahead position to be received in the opposite visual cortex. Total decussation does not permit this direct convergence of pathways from the two eyes to one cortical hemisphere. If these two pieces of information are to be combined, the result has to be mediated by some connection between the two hemispheres.

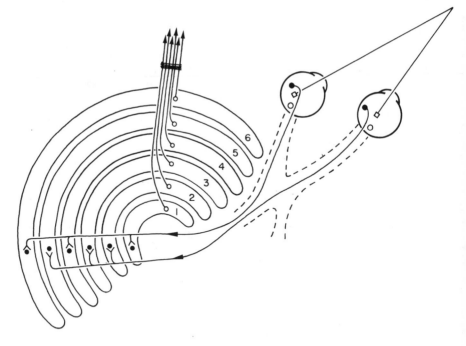

Figure 2–4.   Schematic diagram shows how corresponding points synapse with the cells of the lateral geniculate nucleus. A second set of corresponding points is shown with their axons leaving the nucleus.

Table 2–2. Comparison of Percentage of Uncrossed Optic Nerve
Fibers with Size of Binocular Visual Field

Animal	Approximate Percentage of Uncrossed Fibers	Size of Binocular Visual Field
Horse	13	65°
Dog	33	98°
Primate	50	124° to 200°

Since total decussation usually implies no overlap of the two fields, the
convergence of the two messages at one central location most likely
subserves the need to coordinate the two independent visual information inputs by selecting which image is to receive the attention of
the animal.

A potential advantage of partial decussation is that the two messages from overlapping areas can be put together at an early stage of
information processing that takes place in the cortex. From this convergence point, for example, commands to move the eyes could be sent
out quickly and the eyes moved to track an object even before it is
identified in conscious perception as a result of additional information
processing (Walls, 1942). Note that the signal to move the eyes to change
fixation is based on the oculocentric localization mechanism.

Also partial decussation could permit early combination of the two
visual inputs into one perception without which all objects in the binocular visual field would appear double. This unification process is called
fusion. Furthermore, as we will see, the percentage of optic nerve fibers
that decussate or fail to decussate in humans can be related to the
differences in the visual capabilities of the nasal retina and of the temporal retina, and this fact has implications that apply directly to the
nature of binocular vision (Bishop, 1975).

Of course, even in a system with partial decussation, the two
hemispheres have to be interconnected. Otherwise there would be no
binocular function or fusion along the midline that is imaged on the
vertical meridian through the fovea of each eye (Bishop, 1975).

AN EVOLUTIONARY HYPOTHESIS

Nature is full of exceptions. For example, the owl has frontally placed
eyes, total decussation at the chiasma, and only static and statokinetic

reflex eye movements (Walls, 1942). Here the projections from the geniculate to the telencephalon are the bilateral ones (Pettigrew and Konishi, 1976). Furthermore, some birds possess two foveae in each eye. One is placed so as to overlap the field of its counterpart in the other eye (see Figure 2–2).

Walls (1942) suggested that the evolution of many visual attributes was an independent process. For example, he considered that color vision evolved at least three different times and suggested that the processes of seeing color might be quite different among fishes, birds, reptiles, and mammals. Since we gather information where we find it, we should be cautious of these differences and aware of the limitations of directly extrapolating information from animal studies to surmise exactly how things work in the human visual system. Nevertheless, certain basic principles and mechanisms are invariant throughout the animal kingdom. For these, studies of the visual systems of various animals are invaluable.

There is a tendency to consider that the human visual system can be described as a perfection of visual attributes such as greater visual acuity, more perfect color vision, and finer stereopsis (Duke-Elder, 1958). However, the development of superb visual performances and highly differentiated visual centers seems to be related to the degree of "selective pressure," or the importance of vision in the life of the animal, which is not exclusively at its best in humans (Masterton and Glendenning, 1978).

For mammals, perhaps the reason for the development of the retinogeniculate-telencephalic pathway is best explained by Polyak (1957). Polyak's theory noted that mammals emerged in an environment dominated by large predatory reptiles. This forced mammals to be nocturnal, or cave dwellers, and the result was a reduction in the up-to-then dominant retinotectal pathway. As these reptiles became extinct, the mammals emerged into the diurnal world and the selective pressure for good vision returned. At this point, because of the concurrent development of the neocortex and its greater potential for adaptation to environmental changes, the system expanded into this telencephalic region rather than redeveloping into the tectum. This theory is said to explain the evolutionary development of the visual system in birds and reptiles. Both systems simply show retinotectal expansions because neither passed through a reduction phase.

The unique development of the primate visual system has been described by Masterton and Glendenning (1978) as the expansion and elaboration of the dorsal lateral geniculate nucleus and striate cortex and subsequent elaboration of a tectopulvinar extrastriate system. Apparently the latter is concerned with eye movement control and visually guided behavior (see Chapter 12).

GROWTH OF THE VISUAL SYSTEM

In the embryological development of the human visual system, the position of the eyes moves from lateral to frontal placement in the head. According to Keeney (1951), the angle between the orbital axes is approximately 50° at birth. In adults this angle is about 45° (Duke-Elder, 1958). A part of the functional significance of this small difference might be associated with the total amount of convergence needed to bifixate near objects. However, during this maturation period, there is an increase in interocular separation from 45 to 65 mm (Alpern, 1969), which would tend to offset this. Furthermore, the relative position of the two eyes is determined mainly by the nature and amount of orbital-tissue contents, as well as the amount of tonic innervation to the extraocular muscles (Alpern, 1969).

In its simplest form, neural growth can be considered as taking place in three stages. First, embryogenesis and subsequent differentiation of the brain occur. At this stage, neuronal and glial cells first appear. Second, there is a period of maximum brain growth in which axons and dendrites grow longer, cells enlarge in size, and consequencely the brain size increases. In addition, cells migrate and some misdirected pathways are resorbed. Third, the brain reaches adult size and maturity of structure and undergoes dramatically less change until senescence (Rapporort and Fritz, 1972). For a more detailed description of neural development, see Cowan (1979).

In general, the development of the brain parallels that of the eye, except that the development of neuronal connections in both the lateral geniculate nucleus and the visual cortex occurs sequentially. Ganglion cells grow into the optic stalk by week 6 of embryonic development. By week 8, formation of the chiasma is well along, and the optic tracts begin to appear. By inference, since myelination, starting centrally, proceeds peripherally to the tracts by week 28, these higher centers are well elaborated at this time (Keeney, 1951). Certainly the cortex is well formed at birth (Conel, 1939).

As the size of the brain continues to increase during postnatal development, cells grow in size and the dendritic fields of the neurons increase, as does the number of glial cells. The system continues to undergo a progressive process of myelination and vascularization. Postnatal cell proliferation is confined to microneurons (Altman, 1967). Figure 2–5 illustrates some of these growth patterns. Hickey (1977) showed that the postnatal development of the lateral geniculate nucleus undergoes a period of rapid increase in cell size. This occurs during the first 6 to 12 months. He considered that at least 2 years after birth is required before all cells reach maturity.

There is a strong correlation between the progression of myelin

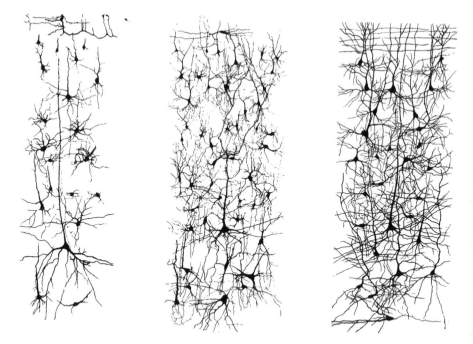

Figure 2–5.   Golgi stains of the human occipital cortex: *left*, at birth; *center*, at
1 month of age; *right*, at 6 months of age (Conel, 1939, 1941, and
1951).

formation and the functional aspects of the nervous system (Altman,
1967). Because the human visual system is partially myelinated at birth
and fully so in the early months of life, the newborn has a functional
but immature visual system. Nevertheless, Hubel and Wiesel (1963)
found that the cortical cells in newborn kittens showed responses "strikingly similar to those in the adult." This suggests that the substrate for
vision is in place at birth and requires only elaboration or growth to
reach maturity. Significant postnatal structural elaboration occurs as
illustrated in Figure 2–5, and this correlates with the development of
visual functions. For binocular vision, this correlation suggests that
structural elaboration should exist in a recognizable form in the early
months of life and reach maturity in the early years (see Chaper 10).

SIGNIFICANCE OF BINOCULAR VISION

Overlapping fields provide a basis for the perception of stereopsis.
Stereopsis is commonly believed to be a sign of a highly advanced visual

system. However, recent demonstrations of stereoscopically mediated behavior in toads (Collett, 1977) suggest that this relationship may have some striking exceptions. In humans, stereopsis would appear to be a useful aid for localization without identification and for fine manipulations in the immediate surroundings. However, stereopsis can be supplanted by other information derived from form, position, and movement, which all require only one eye (Guilfoyle, 1938). Bishop (1975) suggested that stereopsis provides a basis for distance judgments prior to acquiring the experience necessary to use the so-called monocular cues in an unambiguous fashion. Certainly, being binocular would make seeing a more simple task and ensure better judgments under the widest range of environmental conditions (see, for example, Reading and Hofstetter, 1965).

Furthermore, the loss of eye coordination as a result of muscle damage or disease in adults leads to the striking disadvantage of persistent diplopia. Total loss of vision in one eye produces a smaller static visual field and forces the adult to compensate with increased eye and head movement. Certain sensory and motor conditions also place a stress on the system. Here binocular viewing can produce fatigue, discomfort, and reduced performance. If such conditions cannot be alleviated, then, in these instances, binocular vision is a distinct disadvantage.

REFERENCES

Alpern, M. (1969), "Types of movement," *The Eye*, vol. 3, Academic, New York, 111–121.

Altman, J. (1967), "Postnatal growth of the mammalian brain," *The Neurosciences*, Rockefeller University, New York, 723–743.

Bishop, P.O. (1975), "Binocular vision," *Adler's Physiology of the Eye*, Mosby, St. Louis, 558–614.

Bishop, P. O., Henry, G. H., and Smith, C. J. (1972), "Binocular interaction fields of single units in the cat striate cortex," *Journal of Physiology*, 216, 466–502.

Bishop, P. O., Kozak, W., Levick, W. R., and Vakkur, G. J. (1962), "The determination of the projection of the visual field on the lateral geniculate nucleus in the cat," *Journal of Physiology*, 163, 503–539.

Bough, E. W. (1970), "Stereoscopic vision in the macaque monkey: A behavioral demonstration," *Nature*, 225, 42–44.

Cline, D., Hofstetter, H. W., and Griffin, J. R. (1980), *Dictionary of Visual Science*, Chilton, Philadelphia, 237.

Collett, T. (1977), "Stereopsis in toads," *Nature*, 267, 349–351.

Conel, J. L. (1939), *The Postnatal Development of the Human Cerebral Cortex*, vol. 1, Harvard University, Cambridge, 61–69 and plates 57 and 58.

Courtney, G. R., and Heath, G. G. (1971), "Color vision deficiency in the mentally retarded: Prevalence and a method of evaluation," *American Journal of Mental Deficiency*, 76, 48–52.

Cowan, W. M. (1979), "The development of the brain," *Scientific American*, 241, 112–133.

Cunningham, T. J., and Murphy, E. H. (1978), "Ontogeny of sensory systems," *Handbook of Behavioral Neurobiology*, vol. 1, Plenum, New York, 39–71.

Duke-Elder, S. (1958), *System of Ophthalmology*, Mosby, St. Louis, vol. 1, 666–705; vol. 2, 391.

Fox, R., Kehmkuhle, S. W., and Westendorf, D. H. (1976), "Falcon visual acuity," *Science*, 192, 263–265.

Guilfoyle, W. J. U. (1938), "Experiences of a uniocular pilot," *Ophthalmological Societies of the United Kingdom, Transactions*, 57, 431–433.

Hickey, T. L. (1977), "Postnatal development of the human lateral geniculate nucleus: Relationship to a critical period for the visual system," *Science*, 198, 836–838.

Hubel, D. H., and Wiesel, T. N. (1963), "Receptive fields of cells in striate cortex of very young, visually experienced kittens," *Journal of Neurophysiology*, 26, 994–1002.

Hughes, A. (1977), "The topography of vision in mammals of contrasting life style: Comparative optics and retinal organization," *Handbook of Sensory Physiology*, vol. VII/5, Springer-Verlag, Berlin, 618–644.

Keeney, A. H. (1951), *Chronology of Ophthalmic Development*, Charles C Thomas, Springfield, Ill., 13.

Masterton, R. B., and Glendenning, K. K. (1978), "Phylogeny of the vertebrate sensory systems," *Handbook of Behavioral Neurobiology*, vol. 1, Plenum, New York, 1–38.

Pettigrew, J. D., and Konishi, M. (1976), "Neurons selective for orientation and binocular disparity in the visual wulst of the barn owl," *Science*, 193, 675–677.

Polyak, S. (1957), *The Vertebrate Visual System*, University of Chicago, 763–1055.

Rapporort, D. A., and Fritz, R. R. (1972), "Molecular biology of developing mammalian brain," *Structure and Function of the Nervous System*, Academic, New York, 273–316.

Reading, R. W., and Hofstetter, H. W. (1965), "Extra horopteral stereopsis in vehicle operator orientation," *Highway Research News*, 17, 84–91.

Walls, G. L. (1942), *The Vertebrate Eye*, Cranbrook, Bloomfield Hills, MI, 288–338.

White, W. J. (1964), *Bioastronautics Data Book*, National Aeronautics and Space Administration, Washington, 17–23.

3

BINOCULAR FUSION, SUPPRESSION, AND RIVALRY

> History repeats itself. That's one of the things wrong with history.
>
> *Clarence Darrow*

FUSION

Characteristics

One of the oldest questions about vision concerns the apparent paradox of seeing singly with two eyes. As the early philosophers explored this issue, they realized that double vision also occurred in the normal binocular visual world. They referred to the fact that one percept could arise from two retinal images as the result of a process known as *fusion*, or *haplopia*, while they referred to the double percept as *diplopia* (Boring, 1942). The word *fusion* means unification, and it has been considered from a number of different viewpoints.

One way to look at fusion is related to motor responses. *Fusional eye movements* are movements performed by the eyes to obtain or maintain binocular single vision (Alpern, 1969). In its simplest form, a motor hypothesis would state that the entire process of fusion consisted of simply moving the eyes to accomplish the superimposition of similar contours (Rubin and Walls, 1969). Naturally eye movements are a necessary component in any fusional activity. However, when we discuss suppression, rivalry, summation, and stereopsis, it becomes clear that fusion involves much more than just eye movements.

Another way to obtain single vision is by alternation. According to this hypothesis, perception occurs as a result of a cyclic process of receiving an impression first from one eye and then reversing it so as to receive information from the other eye. The resulting impression is from one eye at a time, and at no stage is there a simultaneous binocular percept.

The most elaborate version of this hypothesis says that the alternation process occurs on a point-by-point basis. The perception of an object imaged on point a of the left retina and on point a' of the right retina is totally the result of stimulation of point a at time t and totally the result of stimulation of the corresponding point a' at time $t + \Delta t$. By this process, the total percept is made up of a mosaic of points from one or the other eye and is a constantly changing point-by-point sampling of information from various corresponding points of the two eyes.

If this theory is correct, there is no such thing as simultaneous binocular vision (Verhoeff, 1935). However, observations of alternation during rivalry indicate that the rate is rather slow. Dove (Ogle, 1962) has shown that stereoscopic perceptions are possible with extremely short exposures. Since no known biological mechanisms can alternate fast enough to account for stereopsis with brief presentations, it is highly improbable that an alternating process accounts for all the phenomena associated with fusion and binocular vision. Nevertheless, rivalry can occur and must be accounted for in any theory of fusion.

A physiological hypothesis is founded on the structures and functions of the visual pathways and is supported by increasing amounts of neuroanatomical and neurophysiological evidence. It represents the mainstream of thought in physiological optics today (Rubin and Walls, 1969). The phenomenon of fusion is based on a relationship between points on the two retinas. This relationship is known as *corresponding points*. The images that fall on corresponding points are seen in the same place in the binocular field of view. Images on noncorresponding points are projected to different places (see Chapter 5 for a more precise definition of corresponding points).

This hypothesis states that corresponding points are anatomically connected and that these connections form a final common pathway, or fusion center. Where this final common pathway is located and the exact nature of the combining process are two big issues that have received a great deal of attention. Because of early difficulties in measuring the way in which the visual system performs, as well as the relative crudeness of early neuroanatomical information, not only has progress been slow, but also it has led some investigators to abandon the search and conclude that the process of fusion is motor, alternate, or even psychic. We look at some of the more recent evidence for the physiological theory when we take up the neural aspects of binocular vision in Chapters 10 and 12.

Early frustrations with the physiological hypothesis led to the search for another explanation. It was easy to find in the physiology-psychology or mechanistic-vitalistic dichotomy of the 1800s: What seemed inadequately explained by anatomy and physiology was concluded to be psychological in character (Hering, 1977). Since the evidence for a fusion center was not specific and the psychophysical information about the nature of fusion was somewhat ambiguous, fusion was thought to be a psychic process (Rubin and Walls, 1969). Specifically, Helmholtz (1925) first advanced this theory because he felt that the physiological theory could not explain rivalry without some additional hypotheses, and the theory could not operate without incredibly fine alignment and adjustment of the two eyes. Furthermore, a condition seen in certain strabismics, known as anomalous correspondence (see Chapter 14), seemed to indicate that corresponding points could be changed.

What is implied here is that fusion is a part of consciousness and so is far more complex than the processes exclusively associated with the visual sense. Certainly there are examples of perceptions in which visual information is modified or created by higher mental processes. Visual hallucinations and the visual imagery of dreams are two cases. Furthermore, people report seeing a familiar face in a crowd of strangers if their emotions are in a particular state. After all, it is the conscious part of us that does the seeing (Walls 1942).

Again, for emphasis, note that we can consider fusion processes in their simplest form and in relative isolation from other activities, or we can consider the relationships of the visual inputs and subsequent visual processing to everything else associated with life and living. The classical physiological approach is to seek the simplest, earliest, most peripheral structure and mechanism that combine the messages from the two eyes. The next step is to discover whether fusion recurs in more central locations as well as the nature and significance of these recurrences. The endpoint of this line of investigation would relate these processes to other visual attributes and possibly even to skeletal muscle activity. Certainly such information would have its clinical implications, but direct application to a patient's problems might require a good deal more investigation and development of measurement and treatment techniques.

Worth (1903) also considered that fusion was a psychic act. His theory outlined the stages of development in infants and recovery in older individuals who have suffered from binocular anomalies. He classified fusion into three grades. Grade 1 fusion consists of the patient's ability to place two targets directly on top of each other and to see both at the same time. This is known as *superimposition*. Grade 2 fusion, or motor fusion, means that the patient can hold superimposition over a range of forced convergence and divergence of the eyes. Grade 3 fusion consists of the patient being able to appreciate stereopsis. This classification system is widely used to help diagnose and treat binocular anomalies. Note that a part of grade 1 and all grade 2 are motor fusion elements. A refinement of grade 3 is presented in Chapter 8.

Kepler is credited with considering that fusion is accomplished by the projection from the retina of the points stimulated to a locus of intersection at the external object itself (Porterfield, 1759). As a theory it has been rejected because it seems to be too simple or too vague to account for certain perceptual phenomena such as size constancy (Boring, 1942). However, projection is the basis of stereoscopy and is useful in predicting where patients will localize stereographic representations of geometric forms viewed binocularly (see Chapters 5, 7, and 8).

A Composite View

Eye movements are required to produce single percepts, rivalry can occur in the visual system, and projection has a certain predictive function. Perhaps it is best to consider fusion as the result of the coordination of motor and sensory processes that are mediated mainly by mechanisms associated with the visual pathways and are possibly subject to modifications by other processes related to eye movements and higher mental functions. Other characteristics associated with binocular fusion are discussed in Chapters 6, 7, 11, and 15.

Alternatives

In addition to fusion and diplopia, suppression and rivalry occur under certain circumstances. *Binocular suppression* can be defined as the failure of one of the two monocular visual systems to perceive a normally visible object in all or a part of the binocular visual field. For example, if we look at Figure 3–1*a and b* in a stereoscope, we note the configuration represented in Figure 3–1*c*. At least some of the time the center part of the horizontal line appears to be missing or suppressed. However, if we look at Figure 3–1*a* and *b* in a stereoscope, when the left eye is closed, this segment is restored. Rapid alternate occlusion of the two

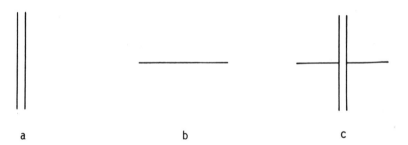

a   b   c

Figure 3–1.   (a) Target presented to left eye. (b) Target presented to right eye.
              (c) Schematic representation of the perception resulting from
              viewing a and b in a stereoscope indicates suppression of a seg-
              ment of the horizontal line between the two parallel lines (Kauf-
              man, 1963).

eyes produces successive perceptions of the two complete monocular
images. As used here, the word *binocular* means simultaneous vision
with both eyes. Suspension of binocular vision eliminates one percept.
Of course another way to suspend binocular vision is to close one eye.

   Rivalry is the periodic or intermittent extinction of brightness,
color, or contour from the perception of one eye as a result of stimulation
of the other eye (Levelt, 1965). For example, Figure 3–2a shows a configuration of stimuli presented separately to the two eyes in a stereoscope, and Figure 3–2b represents the resulting perception at time *t*
after the two targets are fused. Figure 3–2c shows a representation of
the perception at time *t* + Δ*t*. This perception will continue to fluctuate
in a mosaic or patchwork way as long as the targets are held in
superimposition.

   Intuitively, suppression is used to indicate a rather stable state of
nonseeing and rivalry an instable fluctuation between competing components. However, in the literature on binocular vision typically the
terms are used interchangeably. One possible solution to this difficulty
is to treat the instantaneous failure to perceive a binocularly viewed
object by one of the monocular systems as suppression, and the fact
that this perception may change over a rather longer period as rivalry.
With abnormal suppression the process appears to be a more permanent
one, and perhaps the term *suppression* should be reserved for this instance only.

   The phenomenological experience of rivalry is at the foundation
of the alternation theory of binocular vision. The reasoning runs that
a target such as those in Figure 3–2 allows us to see the results of an
ongoing process of rivalry, whereas everyday viewing of essentially
identical contours masks its presence. Furthermore, Verhoeff (1935)

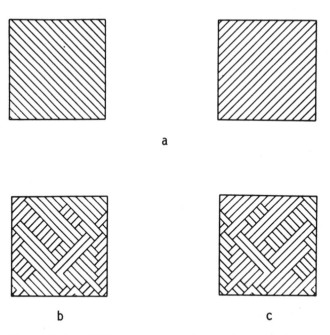

Figure 3–2.   (a) Target presented to right and left eyes in stereoscope. Schematic representations of resulting perception (b) at time X and
(c) at time X + ΔX (Modified from Walls, 1965, and reprinted by
permission of the Cranbrook Institute of Science).

notes that only with special introspective attention can a subject perceive that some objects in a binocular field are diplopic. Verhoeff considers that this lack of awareness of diplopia in the everyday scene
illustrates a normal alternation process at work. As we have seen, the
perception of stereopsis with very short exposures is strong evidence
that the theory is implausible.

MONOCULAR SUPPRESSION

A phenomenon analogous to binocular suppression occurs in monocular viewing. The *Troxler phenomenon* describes the fading of perceptions
that occur in the periphery of the monocular visual field upon prolonged, steady fixation. This phenomenon is thought to be due to the
fact that peripheral objects are neurally encoded by a fixed set of rather
large receptive fields, and that the micromovements of the eyes during
steady fixation are of an insufficient magnitude to sweep the images
onto an adjacent set of receptive fields. In short, the images are effec-

tively stabilized and the perceptions fade away, just as do the perceptions of an image fixed in position on the retina (Davson, 1972).

The Troxler effect can occur in both eyes at the same time, but
simply occluding one eye does not alter the effect in the other eye.
Therefore, the effect is independent of what is happening in the other
eye and can be described as a form of monocular suppression (Levelt,
1965).

Description

The best way to describe the principles of binocular suppression and
rivalry is to illustrate them. For all illustrations in which the two monocular components are presented, fusion can be accomplished without
using a stereoscope by a strategy known as *free fusion*. This is done by
learning to converge the eyes so as to bring the two components into
registry. When this controlled crossing of the eyes is done, the binocular
image will be flanked by two monocular ones. Using a finger positioned
between the plane of the page and the nose at various distances as a
temporary fixation object makes learning this trick rather easy for most
binocular observers (Helmholtz, 1925). Readers with low positive convergence amplitudes will find that small amounts of base-out prism
before the eyes facilitate free fusion, and all binocualr observers will
find such prism useful for relieving any associated stress. Using this
process, you can observe directly the effects produced by fusing Figures
3–1 through 3–5 and thus verify the descriptions presented.

A CONTOUR VERSUS A HOMOGENEOUS FIELD

Figure 3–3a shows a black circle on a plain background as presented
to one eye, and Figure 3–3b shows a structureless field presented to
the other eye. If the background of Figure 3–3a is, for example, red but
of the same luminance as the white background in Figure 3–3b, then
the binocular perception can be represented as in Figure 3–3c. The
contour suppresses the perception of the underlying white background
and is not confined to the area of the circle itself, but spreads over some
distance to create a halo of red around the configuration. Of course,
the effect does not depend on the use of a red color in one of the
backgrounds; red is used here simply to permit easy identification of
the neural image being suppressed.

Studies of the stumulus strength of contours located in different
parts of the binocular field show that if a target is fixated, it has max-

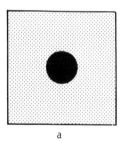 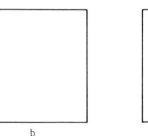 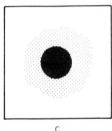

a   b   c

Figure 3–3. Target presented to the left (a) and right (b) eyes in stereoscope. Red background in (a) is indicated by light shading. (c) Schematic representation of the resulting perception (Reprinted by permission from Kaufman, 1963).

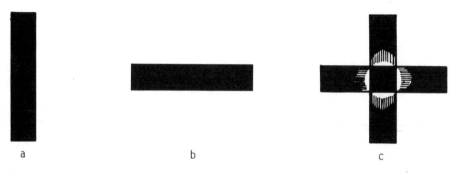

a   b   c

Figure 3–4. Right (a) and left (b) targets presented as in Figure 3–3. (c) Schematic representation of resulting perception (Modified, and reprinted by permission from Kaufman, 1963).

imum ability to suppress homogeneous backgrounds. More peripheral contours have less ability to suppress, but in the periphery the Troxler effect is operative and the situation can be rather more complicated (Levelt, 1965).

ONE CONTOUR VERSUS ANOTHER CONTOUR

If one presents contours that cross at right angles in the binocular view, one has a situation like that in Figure 3–4. When Figure 3–4a and Figure 3–4b are fused, the resulting perception is a center square, reported to be darker than either of the blacks of the separate percepts, and a halo or spread of suppression around the contours. This is represented schematically in Figure 3–4c (Hering, 1942).

A DARK CONTOUR VERSUS A LIGHT CONTOUR

In Figure 3–5 one target has white contours on a black background while the other target has black contours on a white background. Fusion of the configuration produces a stereoscopic impression of depth, while the background appears glossy, a perception called *luster*. It is very much like the monocular perception of a bright, highly polished, metal surface. However, in this instance, it is binocular luster since it depends on the contributions of both monocular percepts (Helmholtz, 1925).

ONE COLOR VERSUS ANOTHER COLOR

Monocular mixtures of red and green appear yellow. If we mix these two colors binocularly by shining a red light into one eye and a green one into the other, a yellow sensation also results. This binocular color mixture is called *binocular color fusion*. However, the mix is a fussy one, and any small alteration in wavelength, luminance, or configuration of one of the two stimuli or of the backgrounds throws the perception into binocular rivalry. Even at its best, the resulting yellow is a desaturated sensation (Walls, 1942). Trick (1978) used this technique recently to study the nature of color perception at the cortical level.

STIMULUS STRENGTH

Levelt (1965) used the term *stimulus strength* to describe the power of a given stimulus to produce contralateral suppression. While most of these assessments are relative and descriptive, the spread of suppres-

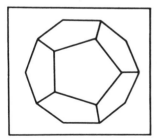 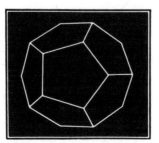

Figure 3–5.   Right *(a)* and left *(b)* targets presented as in Figure 3–1 (Levelt, 1965).

sion has been used to investigate the decrease in strength as a function of increasing distance from contours (Kaufman, 1963).

Using targets like those in Figure 3–1, Kaufman increased the angular distance between two parallel lines. For each angular separation, he measured the time during which the subject reported seeing a gap in a horizontal line and the total number of alternations between seeing and suppressing the gap that occurred over a total viewing time of 30 seconds. Figure 3–6 shows the results for the mean suppression time of 10 subjects as a function of the angular separation in the parallel lines. He also used a configuration in which the parallel lines were positioned in a horizontal plane. Results for this arrangement are presented in Figure 3–6. These data show that suppression decreases as the position from the contours becomes more remote. They also show

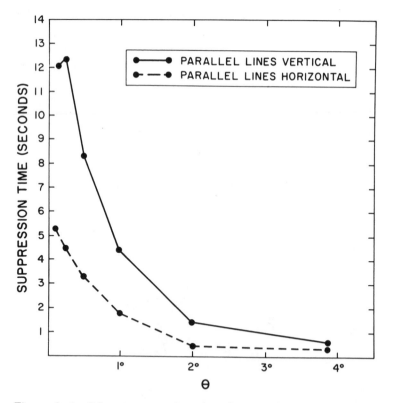

Figure 3–6. Mean suppression time for 10 subjects plotted as a function of angular separation θ of two parallel lines (Reprinted by permission from Kaufman, 1963).

that the effect is much less for observations taken with a horizontal orientation of the parallel lines.

The spread of suppression can be somewhat reduced by short-ening the exposure time to less than about 200 ms, which is about the same as the reaction time for voluntary saccadic eye movements. This fact indicates that voluntary eye movement may increase the spread but does not cause it.

It is not clear what causes the difference in suppression spread in the horizontal and vertical meridians. Kaufman (1963) found more cor-rective eye movements in the horizontal direction than in the vertical. Yet Ditchburn (1973) presented results from a number of studies in which the range of all micromovements was about equal in these two dimensions.

Studies of ocular tremors, drifts, and microsaccades during steady fixation show that the saccadic movements tend to correct eye posi-tioning errors created by tremors and drifts (Ditchburn, 1973). For binoc-ular viewing, these saccades usually are performed in the same direction in the two eyes and often have the same magnitude. However, Ditch-burn (1973) reported that 2 percent of the horizontal components of the saccades were of unequal magnitude, which produces small disparity-correcting movements. No hint of a corrective function has been re-ported for vertical components. Furthermore, St.-Cyr and Fender (1969) found that drifts also can correct horizontal disparity errors.

The fact that horizontal binocular involuntary eye movements may have a corrective function and may be larger than the vertical move-ments could account for the differences in mean suppression time re-ported by Kaufman. Yet this suggests that only corrective micromovements spread suppression, as do the larger voluntary saccades.

Notice that the maximum suppression time for small gaps is less than 50 percent of the total viewing time. Thus the spread of suppres-sion must be subject to statistical fluctuations; in other words, it is a rivalry effect.

Furthermore, an increase in luminance produces an increase in stimulus strength, and an increase in sharpness or contrast produces an increase in stimulus strength, as does motion of a contour. Table 3–1 summarizes the various relationships involving stimulus strength.

Levelt (1965) suggested that an increase in the strength in one eye will increase the predominance of this stimulus, by reducing the time during which the other eye is dominant (the one receiving the stimulus of lower strength). An increase in the stimulus strength of both in-creases the frequency of alternation.

Table 3–1.   Relative Stimulus Strength as a Result of Various
                 Differences in Stimuli to the Two Eyes

Greater Stimulus Strength (Stimulus to One Eye)	Attribute	Lesser Stimulus Strength (Stimulus to the Other Eye)
Brighter	Luminance	Darker
Higher	Contrast	Lower
Clear	Focus	Blurred
Foveal	Retinal locus	Peripheral
Moving	Movement	Stationary

SELECTIVITY IN BINOCULR RIVALRY

It is generally agreed that suppression is somewhat specific in character.
Creed (1935) had subjects view two different postage stamps in a stereoscope. Each stamp had a different background color and a different
form. Subjects reported instances in which the percept consisted of the
form of one stamp superimposed on the color of the other. Thus form
and color suppression can occur independently. Furthermore, Treisman
(1962) reported that the perception of stereopsis survived the suppression of a monocular color. These two investigations indicate that color
is suppressed binocularly by a process independent of that for form
and depth.

Certainly, depth and form suppression are more closely related
and, in most instances, identical. Contrast reversals would seem to
allow for a special intermediate stage of binocular luster, as described
above, and the perception of stereopsis at least under some conditions
(see Figure 3–5) but not when areas of reversed contrast are unbounded
by darker or lighter contours (Treisman, 1962). Ogle and Wakefield
(1967) found that the perception of stereopsis seemed to inhibit rivalry
of adjacent contours.

OBJECTIVE MEASUREMENTS

Barany and Hallden (1948) reported that the direct pupillary light reflex
was diminished during suppression. Richards (1966) also found this.
However, Lowe and Ogle (1966) could not confirm it; but they did
report that when rivalry occurred between targets of uneven luminance,
the pupils constricted at the onset of the phase in which the brighter
target was dominant.

Fox et al. (1975) found that if each eye was stimulated separately by contours moving in opposite directions, an optokinetic nystagmus could be created (see Chapter 10). The direction of these conjugate eye movements correlates with the subject's reports of the perceived direction of motion and therefore with the dominating eye. Each time rivalry causes a change in the direction of the observed motion, there is a reversal in the fast phase of the optokinetic nystagmus.

Riggs (1969) noted phase shifts in the visually evoked response (VER) from the occipital cortex that correlate with suppression of rapidly alternating stripe patterns. Lawwill and Biersdorf (1968) found both reduced amplitude and peak latency of the VER during suppression (see Chapter 12).

While binocular suppression of the pupillary reflex can be accomplished by a central mechanism's sending inhibitory efferent messages to the brainstem, this might also suggest that suppression can occur peripheral to the visual cortex. Even though most experts feel that suppression is mainly a cortical phenomenon, the pupillary pathways and the lateral geniculate body might be involved also (see Chapter 12).

CLINICAL SCALES OF ABNORMAL BINOCULAR SUPPRESSION

In a routine visual examination, abnormal binocular suppression is demonstrated if diplopia does not occur upon dissociation with a prism, as in phoria testing. Furthermore, in the presence of abnormal suppression, the target will appear to move in the direction of the apex of the prism before the nonsuppressed eye during vergence testing (Borish, 1975). Once it is detected, abnormal suppression should be scaled in terms of its severity. This process requires using relative scales for which no absolute physiological baseline has been established. Nevertheless, this ranking can be important in diagnosing and treating binocular anomalies because it indicates a starting point for treatment and says something about how quickly progress can be expected. Several examples illustrate this scaling process.

Some letters on an acuity chart can be presented to one eye while others are presented to the opposite eye only. If a subject reads those letters that are presented to one or the other eye but not all of them, then suppression has been demonstrated. If different-size acuity letters are employed, it is possible to scale the suppression in terms of visual acuity. An example of such a test is the Grolman vectographic projector slide, a portion of which is shown in Figure 3–7 (Grolman, 1966). Figure 3–7a shows the projected chart as seen by the left eye only, while

VO SR	V CS K	$^6/_{12}$	VOCSRK
CH KR N	C OK DN	$^6/_9$	CHOKRDN
NZ SV RH	N DS KR O	$^6/_{7.5}$	NZDSVKRHO

A   **B**   **C**

Figure 3–7. (a) Portion of an acuity chart seen by the left eye. (b) View seen
             by the right eye. (c) Binocular view in the absence of binocular
             suppression (American Optical Co.).

Figure 3–7b shows the right-eye view and Figure 3–7c shows the view
seen by both eyes in the absence of suppression. For example, if the
left eye is suppressed, the patient will read the top line as v-c-s-k,
skipping o and r, which are exclusively channeled to the left eye by the
use of polarized light and analyzers. In this particular test, note that
several letters on each line are presented so as to be visible to both
eyes. For example, a particular response would be recorded as, say,
O.S. suppression at 6/9 (metric Snellen notation).

Figure 3–8 illustrates a neutral density (N.D.) step table or filter
bar that can be utilized to measure the depth of suppression. The patient
looks through striated lenses, known as Bagolini lenses (Burian and von
Noorden, 1974), which are similar to extremely coarse diffraction gratings. The axes of the striations are placed at the 135° meridian before
the right eye and the 45° meridian before the left eye, as seen in the
figure. This illustration also shows the binocular view of a point source
of light when it is seen through these lenses in the absence of suppression and when the left eye is totally suppressed (von Noorden and
Maumenee, 1973). Next the filter bar is introduced before the left eye
and moved from the zero-density position to positions of increasing
density until the subject reports suppression. Then the bar is switched
to the right eye, and the procedure is repeated. It can be recorded as
suppression with striated lenses and step table, for example, O.D.,
N.D. = 2.5, O.S., N.D. = 1.0. That is, it is recorded in terms of the
neutral density filter through which the patient first reports suppression
for each eye. When the difference is as great as in this example, the
suppression is considered abnormal.

It is also possible to use the amount of defocus required before
the nonsuppressed eye that just breaks down or eliminates the suppression. Unfortunately, these sorts of findings are subject to great variability and so are generally considered to have little clinical value.

However, Humphriss (1969) reported that when a red filter is
placed before one eye and a green filter before the other, the addition

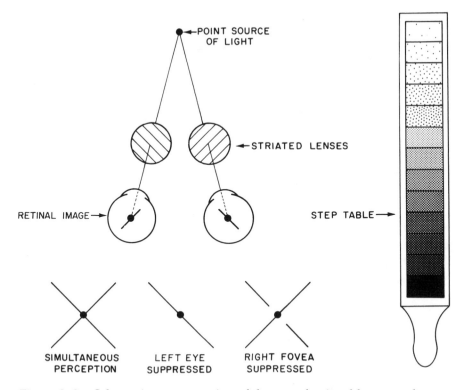

Figure 3–8. Schematic representation of the use of striated lenses and a step table.

of defocusing lenses to each eye in turn produces a reliable way of making relative measurements of binocular suppression. In this instance, the subject reported that a white object appears white or yellowish when it is seen binocularly and either red or green at the onset of suppression (see Chapter 13).

SUPPRESSION FIELDS

Another important feature of suppression associated with binocular anomalies is that usually it is confined to certain regions of the binocular visual field. For example, Figure 3–8 shows a view of a point source of light through a pair of striated lenses in which only the right foveal area is suppressed.

Figure 3–9 shows a schematic representation of the position of the eyes for a patient with esotropia. In the figure, the right eye fails to

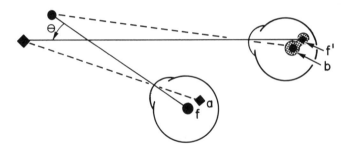

Figure 3–9.   Relative position of the eyes in right esotropia and associated
               binocular suppression fields.

achieve foveal fixation and is designated the deviating eye. The amount
of this deviation is referred to as the *objective angle of squint* and is labeled
θ (theta). With a deviating eye two different objects are imaged on the
two foveae, and the patient usually sees these in the same visual direction. This is known as *confusion*. This figure also shows that the
object fixated by the left eye, called the *fixating eye*, is imaged extrafo-
veally in the right eye, so the patient sees any given object as appearing
to be in two locations. This constitutes diplopia (Burian and von Noorden, 1974).

Binocular perimetry on such a patient reveals two relative scoto-
matous areas: one centered on the fovea of the deviating eye, effectively
eliminating confusion, and the other centered on the extra foveal point
receiving the same image as the fovea of the fixating eye, counteracting
diplopia. Figure 3–9 shows the retinal positions of these two suppression fields (Burian and von Noorden, 1974).

One technique for performing binocular perimetry consists of using polarizing material so that test and fixation objects are seen separately by the two eyes. This method allows the areas of binocular
suppression to be located and mapped. Figure 3–10 is a diagram of a
stereocampimeter that uses a mirror before the fixating eye to provide
for separate stimulation of the two eyes. The nonfixating eye views a
tangential surface over which different-size test objects can be moved
or introduced to explore the areas of suppression. These two areas are
always found in the habitually deviating eye. The mapping of these
relative scotomas can require some care. For dynamic perimetry (Harrington, 1976), the test object must be moved very slowly so as not to
disrupt the suppression process. For static perimetry (Enoch et al.,
1970), the test light should be introduced gradually at the lowest available increment of luminance.

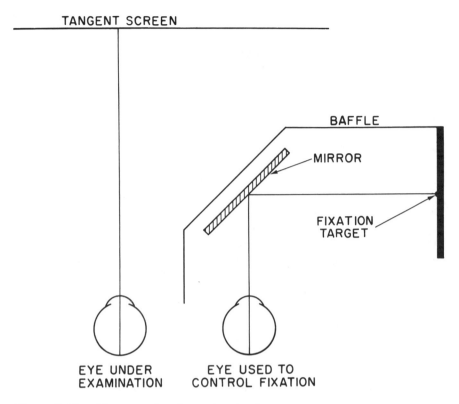

Figure 3–10. Diagram of a stereocampimeter.

NORMAL AND ABNORMAL SUPPRESSION

It is widely held that the suppression found in strabismus is an adaptive process that starts with the simple voluntary suppression of the variety discussed previously and proceeds through an ever-deepening development until it becomes obligatory. This viewpoint considers that amblyopia can come along as part of the development of a pattern of habitual suppression, and amblyopia encourages further deepening of suppression by reducing the stimulus strength of the foveal image in the deviating eye. Eccentric fixation would produce a similar result by moving the effective point of fixation off the foveal center (Duke-Elder, 1949).

Given the prinicples of suppression and rivalry discussed earlier, we might predict that in esotropia, suppression to avoid diplopia would be greatest at points *a* and *b* in figure 3–9, since foveal stimuli should have a greater strength than peripheral ones. The prediction is only half right since, from all reports, point a in the fixating eye functions normally. Certainly nothing in our previous study of normal suppression would suggest that point f' should be suppressed. Of course, if a patient is to avoid confusion, either f or f' has to be eliminated from consciousness (Burian and von Noorden, 1974). Therefore, the relative abilities of retinal loci to affect binocular suppression are different for normal and abnormal patients. The principal difference involves the suppression of the fovea in the deviating eye. In other words, normal suppression occurs only for corresponding regions whereas abnormal suppression can apply to noncorresponding regions.

Jampolsky (1955) reported that the suppression associated with strabismus has a rather long latent period. This is confirmed by the repeated clinical observation that slow alternate occlusion followed by uninterrupted binocular viewing produces simultaneous binocular perception for as long as a minute or two in patients demonstrating abnormal suppression. This brief period of binocularity is followed by the return of abnormal suppression. Contrast this fact with the report of Kaufman (1963) that for exposures shorter than about 200 ms, contour pitted against contour produces suppression and rivalry in the normal subject. In fact, suppression can be observed at exposure times as short as 5 ms (Reading, 1972).

Binocular masking is a term used to describe the elevation of the detection threshold caused by flashing a bright, long-duration masking light into one eye at various times before and after the presentation of a brief test light of adjustable luminance to the other eye. The masking light elevates the detection threshold of the test flash over a period commencing some 50 ms before onset to well over 100 ms following it. Therefore, suppression can be induced by such a masking paradigm. Reading (1970) found that the masking effect for a subject with abnormal suppression was elevated almost one full logarithmic unit of luminance above that for a normal subject. This tends to confirm the unique nature of abnormal suppression.

These differences in location, reaction time, and detection threshold indicate that the suppression experienced in normal subjects may be quite different from that experienced in subjects with binocular anomalies. Perhaps the suppression associated with strabismus is related to eye movements or their innervations in a different way. At any rate, it does not appear to be one and the same as that form experienced in normal subjects. A survey of the literature on binocular anomalies indicates that this distinction usually is not made. Nevertheless, it is important since we might be tempted to conclude that what can be observed in the normal subject leads directly and simply to a sensory anomaly that goes by the same name.

CLINICAL TESTING

In clinical practice the optometrist must be continually on the lookout for suppression. Once it is detected, it should be measured for depth or severity because this factor is important in choosing an efficient course of treatment.

The presence of suppression does not preclude performing measurements, such as phorias (or subjective angles of squint) at different fixation distances which yield important information about the patient's oculomotor system. Usually it is only necessary to alternately occlude the two eyes to obtain information about the relative position of the two targets as viewed through disassociating prisms, in order to quite accurately measure oculomotor imbalances. Table 3–2 summarizes some facts about suppression detection during horizontal vergence testing, and Table 3–3 outlines some of the clinical procedures for the detection and measurement of abnormal suppression.

ANTISUPPRESSION TREATMENT

The concept of stimulus strength forms the basis for the elimination of abnormal suppression. However, since abnormal suppression frequently is encountered as only one of a series of anomalous sensorimotor conditions, its treatment is confounded into the regimes designed to eliminate the oculomotor deviation, amblyopia, eccentric fixation, and anomalous correspondence (Griffin, 1976).

The eradication of abnormal suppression begins with careful attention to the correction of ametropia. Following this, sometimes its

Table 3–2. Image Movement Caused by Suppression

Patient Reports Object Is Moving:	*Direction of Prism*	
	Base in	*Base out*
To the left	O.D. suppressing	O.S. suppressing
To the right	O.S. suppressing	O.D. suppressing

Table 3–3.   Some Clinical Procedures Associated with Abnormal Suppression

---

1. Case history
   A. Patient reports seeing out of one eye only or out of one eye at a time.
   B. Patient reports manifest oculomotor deviation.
   C. Patient reports asthenopia.
2. Refractive procedures: Binocular balance testing
   A. Patient fails to perceive diplopia when usual amount of vertical dissociating prism is introduced before the eyes. (Increase the amount of prism.)
   B. Patient reports disappearance of one of the two targets during dissociated balance test. (Alternately occlude.)
3. Oculomotor imbalance procedures
   A. Diplopia is absent when dissociating prisms are introduced for phoria testing. (Increase the amount of prism or alternately occlude.)
   B. Object moves to side during duction testing (see Table 3–1).
4. Measurement of suppression
   A. Vectographic acuity.
   B. Blur using red and green filters.
   C. Striated lenses and step table.
   D. Binocular perimetry.

---

persistence can be diminished by temporarily fogging the usually dominant eye or by reducing the retinal illuminance to this eye. More extreme cases are treated by special methods in which image motion is utilized to break down the suppression. Or alternate stimulation of the two eyes is performed, either at a slow rate that causes brightness enhancement (Allen, 1969) or at an ever-increasing rate until a binocular view persists upon simultaneous presentation.

Colored filters have been used to emphasize perceptions based on foveal function. It has been suggested that a red filter, that is a filter that transmits maximally in the longer-wavelength region of the visual spectrum, produces maximal stimulation of the foveola and thus encourages simultaneous perception. A detailed discussion of this method can be found in Griffin (1976).

The principle of successful treatment of abnormal suppression is to eliminate its cause. Since it can be caused by ametropia, anisometropia, and aniseikonia, careful correction of these conditions is usually the first step. Abnormal suppression can be associated also with oculomotor imbalances, tropias, amblyopia, eccentric fixation, and anomalous correspondence. Here final success depends on the ability to alleviate these other problems. However, most experts feel that suppression elimination is the first step in these cases also (Worth, 1903).

Another complication in the treatment of abnormal suppression is associated with the retinal locus of the suppressive effect. Foveal suppression is believed to be either signifying a deep-seated process in the presence of oculomotor deviations or easily amenable to direct treatment in the absence of other sensorimotor anomalies (Griffin, 1976). In either case, the rationale for sequential treatment starts with eliminating extrafoveal suppression and progresses to an attack on the foveal variety by using smaller and smaller targets which are to be directly fixated during treatment (Borish, 1975).

REFERENCES

Allen, M. J. (1969), "Shock treatment for visual rehabilitation," *Optical Journal and Review of Optometry*, 106, 27–29.

Alpern, M. (1969), "Types of movement," *The Eye*, vol. 3, Academic, New York, 65–174.

Barany, E. H., and Hallden, U. (1948), "Phasic inhibition of the light reflex of the pupil during retinal rivalry," *Journal of Neurophysiology*, 11, 25–30.

Boring, E. G. (1942), *A History of Experimental Psychology*, Appleton, New York, 104–105.

Borish, I. (1975), *Clinical Refraction*, Professional, Chicago, 822–828.

Burian, H., and von Noorden, G. (1974), *Binocular Vision and Ocular Motility*, Mosby, St. Louis, 214–219.

Creed, R. S. (1935), "Observations on binocular fusion and rivalry," *Journal of Physiology*, 84, 381–392.

Davson, H. (1972), *Physiology of the Eye*, Academic, New York, 251–252.

Ditchburn, R. W. (1973), *Eye Movements and Visual Perception*, Clarendon Press, Oxford, 103–105, 353–355.

Duke-Elder, W. S. (1949), *Textbook of Ophthalmology*, Mosby, St. Louis, 4001–4008.

Enoch, J. W., Berger, R., and Birns, R. (1970), "A static perimetric technique believed to test receptive field properties," *Documenta Ophthalmologica*, 29, 127–153.

Fox, R., Todd, S., and Bettinger. L. A. (1975), "Optokinetic nystagmus as an objective indicator of binocular rivalry," *Vision Research*, 15, 849–853.

Griffin, J. R. (1976), *Binocular Anomalies—Procedures for Vison Therapy*, Professional, Chicago, 43–86, 261–273.

Grolman, B. (1966), "Binocular refraction, A new system," *New England Journal of Optometry*, 17, 118–130.

Harrington, D. O. (1976), *The Visual Fields*, Mosby, St. Louis, 1–65.

Helmholtz, H. (1925), *Handbook of Physiological Optics*, vol. 3, Optical Society of America, New York, 539–541.

Hering, E. (1942), *Spatial Sense and Movement of the Eyes*, American Academy of Optometry, Baltimore, 35.

Hering, E. (1977), *The Theory of Binocular Vision*, Plenum, New York, 1–13.

Humphriss, D. (1969), "The measurement of sensory ocular dominance and its relation to personality," *American Journal of Optometry*, 46, 603–614.

Jampolsky, A. (1955), "Characteristics of suppression in strabismus," *Archives of Ophthalmology*, 54, 683–696.

Kaufmàn, L. (1963), "On the spread of suppression and binocular rivalry," *Vision Research*, 3, 401–415.

Lawwill, T., and Biersdorf, W. R. (1968), "Binocular rivalry and visually evoked responses," *Investigative Ophthalmology*, 7, 738.

Levelt, W. J. M. (1965), *On Binocular Rivalry*, Institute for Perception, Soesterberg, The Netherlands, 31, 75–84.

Lowe, S. W., and Ogle, K. N. (1966), "Dynamics of the pupil during binocular rivalry," *Archives of Ophthalmology*, 75, 395–403.

Ogle, K. N. (1962), "Spatial localization through binocular vision," *The Eye*, vol. 4, Academic, New York, 271–320.

Ogle, K. N., and Wakefield, J. M. (1967), "Stereoscopic depth and binocular rivalry," *Vision Research*, 7, 89–98.

Porterfield, W. (1759), *A Treatise on the Eye, the Manner and Phenomena of Vision*, Hamilton and Balfour, Edinburgh.

Reading, R. W. (1970), "Binocular masking effect in a normal subject and an anomalous subject," *Journal of the American Optometric Association*, 43, 174–178.

Reading, R. W. (1972), "Suppression during brief exposures," unpublished research.

Richards, W. (1966), "Attenuation of the pupil response during binocular rivalry," *Vision Research*, 6, 239–240.

Riggs, L. A. (1969), "Progress in recording of human retinal and occipital potentials," *Journal of the Optical Society of America*, 59, 1558–1566.

Rubin, M. L., and Walls, G. L. (1969), *Fundamentals of Visual Science*, Charles C Thomas, Springfield, Ill., 348, 358.

St.-Cyr, G. J., and Fender, D. H. (1969), "The interplay of flicks and drifts in binocular fixation," *Vision Research*, 9, 245–265.

Treisman, A. (1962), "Binocular rivalry and stereoscopic depth perception," *Quarterly Journal of Experimental Psychology*, 14, 23–37.

Trick, G. L. (1978), "The effect of wavelength or binocular summation," Ph.D. thesis, Indiana University, Bloomington.

Verhoeff, F. H. (1935), "A new theory of binocular vision," *Archives of Ophthalmology*, 13, 151–175.

von Noorden, G., and Maumenee, A. (1973), *Atlas of Strabismus*, Mosby, St. Louis, 92–93.

Walls, G. L. (1942), *The Vertebrate Eye*, Cranbrook, Bloomfield Hills, MI, 336.

Worth, C. (1903), *Squint: Its Causes, Pathology, and Treatment*, Blakiston, Philadelphia, 12–14.

4

BINOCULAR SUMMATION AND INTERACTION

> If things were left to chance, they'd be better.
>
> *Author unknown*

BINOCULAR SUMMATION

Sensory fusion includes the study of the perception of diplopia, haplopia, suppression, rivalry, luster, stereopsis, and the effects known as *binocular summation* (Sherrington, 1904). Summation might better be called interaction, for what is at issue here is simply how the perceptions from the two eyes combine or interact to form a binocular perception (Brown and Mueller, 1965). Historically, the term *summation* has been used owing to the influence of Sherrington, who first worked on the physiology of the spinal nerves and found evidence for summation of neural impulses. Then he turned his attention to a search for similar forms of activity in the visual system.

Among other things, summation can be complete, partial, or negative, as summarized in Table 4–1. The data from binocular experiments can be compared with those from monocular experiments for the absolute threshold, brightness matching, reaction time, critical flicker frequency, and visual acuity (Blake and Fox, 1973). The general expression for all forms of summation involving thresholds is

$$B' = a(R) + b(L) \qquad (4\text{--}1)$$

43

Table 4–1. Examples of Various Forms of Summation

Form of Summation	Weighting Coefficients	$B' = a(R) + b(L)$ Predicted Results $(R = L)$
Complete	$a = b = 0.25$	$B' = 0.5$
Partial	$0.5 > a > 0$ $0.5 > b > 0$, for example, $a = b = 0.35$	$B' = 0.70$
Negative	Either a or b is less than 0, and the other is greater than 1; for example, $a = 2.00$, $b = -0.60$	$B' = 1.40$

where R and L are the magnitudes of the physical stimuli to the right and left eye, respectively, necessary to produce a monocular threshold response and a and b are the weighting coefficients given to these values when performance is binocular. Then B' is the magnitude of the physical stimulus to both eyes that is equivalent to the sum of the weighted monocular components. It is the binocular threshold predicted by the nature of the summative process. For simplicity, Table 4–1 presents examples in which the two monocular thresholds are assumed equal, that is, $R = L$. By convention, threshold conditions have been met when detection is at the 50 percent level.

At Absolute Threshold

Early measurements of the absolute threshold for light detection indicated that the binocular threshold was about 0.70 times smaller than the monocular threshold, or that the binocular sensitivity was about 0.10 log unit more sensitive. This is not complete summation, but rather partial summation and not a particularly large amount. Nevertheless, the increase in sensitivity under binocular conditions could be important behaviorally, for example, in night driving situations. Furthermore, Weale (1955) suggested that it is important to certain deep-sea fish.

PROBABILITY SUMMATION

Does this gain represent evidence for a physiological mechanism of fusion that combines the two monocular perceptions so as to produce a greater sensitivity, or simply has some other factor not related to sensitivity produced the difference? Pirenne (1943) was the first to suggest that the later consideration be applied to a comparison of binocular and monocular threshold data. He assumed that subjects of binocular threshold experiments could not distinguish detection with the right eye, with the left eye, or with both. If this is the case, then the binocular probability of detection is altered.

For example, if the intensity of the light is adjusted so that the probability of detecting the presence of a light on a number of trials for the left eye, P_L, is 0.5 and the probability of detecting for the right eye P_R is also 0.5, then the predicted probability of detecting with both eyes (P_b') is given by

$$P_b' = P_R + P_L - (P_R \times P_L) \tag{4-2}$$

When P_R and P_L are both equal to 0.5, this expression becomes

$$P_b' = 0.5 + 0.5 - (0.5 \times 0.5) = 1 - 0.25 = 0.75 \tag{4-3}$$

This expression says that by having the subject open the second eye, the detection level rises owing to probability summation.[1] To return to the threshold level, the 0.5 level of probability of seeing, a dimmer stimulus must be utilized. This increase in the probability of detection that occurs when both eyes are used is called *probability summation*, and it is assumed that the two eyes act independently of each other (Pirenne, 1943).

PIRENNE'S EXPERIMENT

Pirenne's experimental results are shown in Figure 4–1. The smooth curve marked B represents the predicted frequency of seeing (or probability of detection), and the circles represent the result of experimental measurements. For these results, probability summation predicts binocular thresholds very well (Pirenne, 1943). This implies that the partial summation which occurred was not the result of the workings of any physiological fusion mechanism, but simply the result of probability summation.

A SIMPLE MODEL OF BINOCULAR SUMMATION

Pirenne's experimental methods have been improved on. Nevertheless, his argument survives and yields a simple, useful means for judging the significance of some binocular interactions. As a result of his work,

CARL F. SHEPARD MEMORIAL LIBRARY
ILLINOIS COLLEGE OF OPTOMETRY
3241 S. MICHIGAN AVE.
CHICAGO ILL. 60616

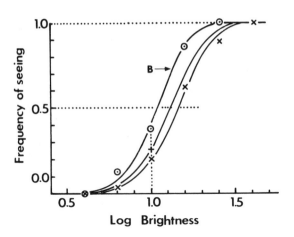

Figure 4–1.   The results of Pirenne (1943). The curve marked *B* is the binocular
             frequency-of-seeing curve predicted from the monocular data.
             The circles are the actual binocular data.

not only must binocular summation be demonstrated for threshold
measurements, but also the resulting difference must exceed the
amount due to probability in order to be used as evidence of the activity
of a fusion center.

   This concept leads to a simple summation model which indicates
that the amount of binocular summation resulting from a comparison
of binocular and monocular performances is the result of two components: that due to the increase in probability resulting from involving
a second independent detector and that due to the activity of a physiological summating mechanism. In this context, binocular summation
equals probability summation plus physiological summation. But, is
there any physiological summation?

SOME COMMENTS ON PIRENNE'S RESULTS

Van de Geer and Moraal (1963) reported that subjects can tell which
eye is being stimulated. They found that subjects were correct in this
kind of judgment at a level that is much greater than chance. Pickersgill
(1961) had reported previously the same ability. These studies suggest
that Pirenne's assumption that the two eyes act independently may not
be entirely true.

   Another problem with Pirenne's experiment was the apparent lack
of precise control of binocular fixation. We now know that summation

is maximum for corresponding points. As the stimuli are moved away from these loci, summation decreases and eventually drops to a level predicted by probability summation (Thorn and Boynton, 1974).

MATIN'S EXPERIMENT

A direct indication that summation occurred in excess of that predicted by probability was presented by Matin (1962). He reasoned that if he carefully controlled binocular fixation so as to deliver two flashes of light to corresponding points at the same time, the summation should be maximum. If the two lights were presented at different times, summation should decrease. As the time between the flashing of the two lights increased, a point should be reached at which the gap in time between their presentation exceeds the temporal limits of any interactive process. Beyond this point, for greater and greater time gaps, summation should be no more than that predicted by probability.

Figure 4–2 shows the results of one of Matin's experiments, which

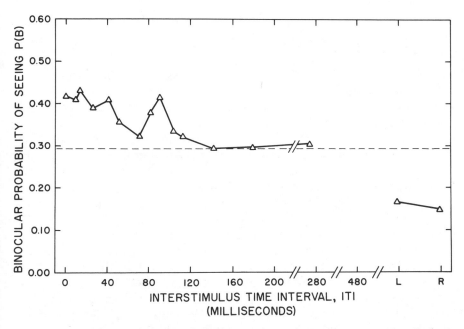

Figure 4–2.   The probability-of-detection data of Matin (1962). The dashed horizontal line is the probability summation level predicted from the monocular data L and R (Reprinted by permission).

indicate summation in excess of probability for interstimulus time intervals (ITIs) of 0 to about 140 ms and only probability summation for intervals greater than the latter value. The horizontal line in this figure is the level predicted by probability summation. Matin found a decrease in summation from 0 to about 60-ms ITI and a secondary peak between about 60 and 120 ms. Matin correlated the time of occurrence of this peak with alterations in the amplitude of the VER (see Chapter 12) with time as reported by other authors and found that the timing was very nearly the same.

This binocular improvement is considered evidence for a physiological fusion mechanism that operates at the absolute detection threshold level to increase binocular sensitivity for corresponding points to a greater degree than is available monocularly, or by having two independent monocular detectors and pooling their responses.

Notice that Matin's experiment tests summation at only one brightness level while Pirenne's study covers five luminance levels over a range of one logarithmic unit. Despite this fundamental difference in method, Thorn and Boynton (1974) confirmed that significant summation takes place when the two stimuli are delivered to corresponding points simultaneously.

AREAL SUMMATION

For monocular detection thresholds, doubling the area produces a lower threshold. Spatial summation in the monocular visual system results in a threshold value that represents less energy per unit area and less total energy (Brown and Mueller, 1965).

Since we know that the binocular threshold is less than the monocular threshold by a factor of about 0.72, we might conclude that this represents a form of areal summation like that stated in Piper's law (Brindley, 1970). Such an effect occuring between areas in the two separate eyes would seem to indicate that some physiological process is at work. Of course, the same effect could occur without any summation in two independent areas if the inclusion of the second allowed more sensitive elements to do the detecting. However, then we would expect the binocular thresholds to be no better than the lower of the two monocular thresholds (Brown and Mueller, 1965). Furthermore, two independent samples also reduce the variance, homologous to the threshold, by this same amount. If independence can be separately established, then this advantage must be attributed to a refinement that results from the additional sampling of information on a purely statistical basis.[2] Note that probability summation, areal summation, and reduced variance with increasing sample size all predict about the same gain in sensitivity for binocular viewing.

BINOCULAR BRIGHTNESS MATCHING

At suprathreshold levels, several studies indicated some slight summative effects (Blake and Fox, 1973). That these effects are small can be observed by closing one eye and then reopening it to compare the impression of brightness in the monocular view with that in the binocular view (LeGrand, 1967).

Some of the results of an experiment by Fry and Bartley (1933) are presented in Figure 4–3. For this figure A was seen monocularly and B binocularly. If the results of their study are plotted along the line $B = A$, no summation has occurred. Similarly, if the results are plotted along the line $B = A/2$ complete summation is indicated. A best-fitting straight line drawn through the actual data points has a slope of about 0.7. This means that binocular brightness is about 1.43 times the monocular brightness, or about 0.15 logarithmic units brighter. The authors concluded that this difference represented the results of physiological summation.

Pirenne had not yet developed the concept of probability summation, and even if he had, it is almost impossible to apply this concept to a suprathreshold brightness-matching situation. Nevertheless, the difference that Fry and Bartley found is close to that predicted by areal summation, and it could mean that a mechanism for fusion operates

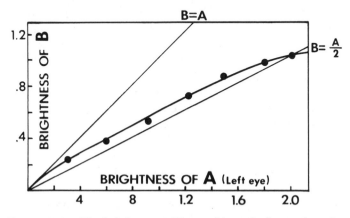

Figure 4–3.   The brightness of B seen binocularly as a function of the brightness of A seen monocularly (Reprinted by permission from Fry and Bartley, 1933).

under conditions in which a binocular object is matched in brightness with a monocular one.

Levelt (1965) presented data which seem to indicate that the nature of the interaction is an averaging process. If R is the luminance of one monocular sensory channel and L the luminance of the other needed to match a given binocular luminance, then the binocular luminance will be $aR + bL$, where a and b are weighting coefficients which together equal 1. Since these coefficients usually have values around 0.5, this is equivalent to a straightforward average. Levelt found that small differences in a and b existed among his subjects and designated the differences as a form of dominance. These coefficients could be altered by changing the contrast or amount of contour information sent to one eye or the other.

Figure 4–4 presents some of Levelt's results. Note that he plots variations in right luminance and left luminance to match a given binocular luminance. While this method of presenting data is quite different from that used by Fry and Bartley, for zero luminance in one eye, the luminance to the other has to be greater than the binocular luminance to produce a match. This is what Fry and Bartley found.

FECHNER'S PARADOX

That the binocular system averages luminance under some conditions is demonstrable. If a neutral density filter is placed before one eye during binocular viewing and the binocular impression of brightness is compared with that obtained by using the unfiltered eye, the scene will appear brighter when it is viewed monocularly. For this situation, the binocular brightness is less than the brighter of the two unequal monocular brightnesses (LeGrand, 1967). This observation is paradoxical in the sense that a simple summation model of binocular brightness predicts that the binocular brightness will always be greater than either of the two monocular brightnesses. If the binocular brightness is less than the brighter monocular brightness, then something like an averaging process has taken place (Blake and Fox, 1973).

SOME COMMENTS ON BINOCULAR BRIGHTNESS

Levelt used successive contrast matches. The subjects adjusted one of the two monocular luminances so that they matched a set amount of luminance seen binocularly, presented in alternation. Fry and Bartley use a simultaneous matching technique in which the monocular field

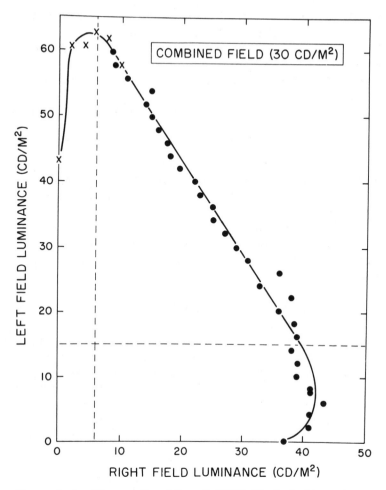

Figure 4–4.   The results of Levelt (1965) illustrate binocular averaging of all
               luminances greater than the levels indicated by the dashed lines
               (Reprinted by permission).

was about 2° away from the binocular one. They suggested that the
system is capable of both summation and averaging because the interaction includes both summative and inhibitory processes. The relative
strengths of these antagonistic activities can produce either summation
or averaging, depending on the stimulus conditions.

Development of this idea has lead to binocular brightness models
involving a cross-correlation process between the brightness of each
point in one eye and a subset of points in the other eye (Engel, 1967,
1969), as well as a vector-sum model (Curtis and Rule, 1978) which

considers that there is no interaction between the stimulated and the unstimulated eye for monocular brightness perception. Both models are based on brightness magnitude estimations and predict averaging and summation quite well. Brightness estimation consists of having a group of subjects view a series of targets of varying luminance and assign a numerical rank to the appearances. According to Stevens (1961), brightness and luminance are related by the power function

$$B = kL^{0.33} \tag{4-4}$$

where B is the brightness magnitude estimation, L the luminance in candelas per square meter, and k is the constant of proportionality whose value depends on the untis of L. For L measured in candelas per square meter, k is equal to 37.3 (Engel, 1967).

While subjects can rank luminance reliably, not everyone is satisfied that the method is valid or, even if it is, that it has the necessary precision to be a fair test of the nature of binocular brightness (Blake and Fox, 1973).

Fechner's paradox is reported to disappear in an empty, borderless field, and further studies have implied that boundaries or borders between light and dark areas are important in determining how the binocular system responds to brightness. Apparently, in a highly structured surrounding with plenty of details such as occur in most everyday scenes, the system averages; but in nearly empty fields summation can be demonstrated. The effect of borders on the binocular system is far from clear and most likely a very complex process. However, we do know that lateral interactions occur within the retina (LeGrand, 1968), and it is reasonable to suppose that an analogous mechanism operates between the two eyes that is mediated by the binocular visual system.

BINOCULAR REACTION TIME

Another feature of the visual system is the fact that the latency of response is an inverse function of the intensity of the stimulus (LeGrand, 1968). Given that stimulus intensity (luminance) and response magnitude (brightness) usually are directly related, if binocular reaction times are shorter than monocular reaction times, summation must have occurred. Gilliland and Haines (1975) found significantly shorter reaction times for binocular viewing over a range of some 100° of the binocular visual field, and Minucci and Connors (1967) found that this reliable superiority was maintained over a 4 logarithmic unit range of luminances for bifoveal viewing.

BINOCULAR FLICKER

When Sherrington (1904) took up the search for evidence about summation in the visual system, he chose to study binocular interactions using the critical fusion frequency (CFF). He reasoned that if summation was complete, the simultaneous binocular CFF should be substantially higher than the monocular CFF. That is, if the two flashes come on and go off at the same time, also called *in phase*, then they should add to produce a brighter percept and, with this, an elevation of the CFF. If the brightness is doubled, the monocular CFF increases about 1.3 times its original value, according to the Ferry-Porter law (LeGrand, 1968). Certainly, it would be a surprise if the binouclar system operated so as to exceed the predictions of this simple law.

For binocular alternating CFF in which the flashing light to one eye comes on at the instant that the flashing light to the other eye goes off, also called 180° *out of phase*, complete summation predicts that no flicker should be perceived because binocular cells would receive continuous alternating inputs and respond in a fashion identical with their response to a physically steady light. Figure 4–5 illustrates these relationships.

Experimental studies (Blake and Fox, 1973) shown that small but significant differences exist in the CFF for the simultaneous, alternating, and monocular conditions. Here, again, partial summation occurs and to a sufficient degree to exceed that predicted by probability summation (Peckham and Hart, 1960). Table 4–2 summarizes some typical findings (Perrin, 1954).

Furthermore, a significant partial-summation effect occurs even with variations in test field size, test field hue, test field intensity, and retinal regions stimulated. These results demonstrate significant summation and thus suggest that a physiological fusion mechanism is operating (Blake and Fox, 1973).

BINOCULAR TEMPORAL MODULATION TRANSFER FUNCTION

Kintz (1969) studied the temporal modulation transfer function (MTF) for both binocular and monocular test conditions. Some of his results are plotted in Figure 4–6. The ordinate is scaled in terms of the reciprocal of contrast C, where

$$C = \frac{L_{max} - L_{min}}{L_{max} + L_{min}} \tag{4–5}$$

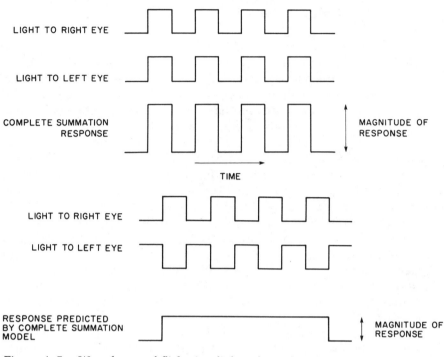

Figure 4–5.   Waveforms of flickering lights show the phase relationship and
response predicted by complete summation: *upper*, binocular simultaneous (in phase); *lower*, binocular alternating (180° out of
phase).

Table 4–2.   Critical Flicker Frequencies Illustrating the Sherrington
Effect

	Typical Photopic CFF Values (Hz)
Binocular simultaneous (in phase)	45
Binocular alternating (180° out of phase)	30
Monocular	40

Condition

Source: Perrin (1954).

Here L_{max} is the maximum luminance of a temporal sine wave, and L_{min}
is the minimum luminance. The abscissa is scaled in hertz (Hz) or cycles
per second.

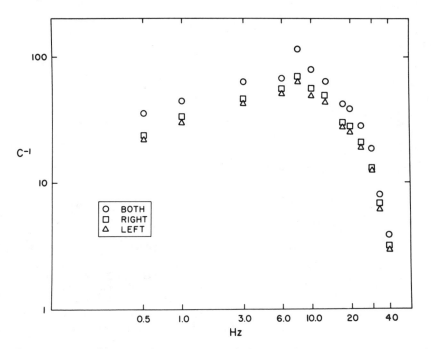

Figure 4–6.   The contrast sensitivity of the visual system to sine wave fluctuations in luminance of a 0.6° circular field on a 7.5° surround
(Kintz, 1969).

Contrast sensitivity is enhanced for binocular viewing of in-phase
temporal sine waves. This enhancement is greater for frequencies from
0.5 to about 20 Hz, and there is a resonant frequency around 8 Hz.
Figure 4–7 presents data pooled from two subjects as a ratio of the
binocular in-phase sensitivity to the best of the monocular sensitivities.
It shows two resonant peaks, one at about 3 Hz and the other at about
8 Hz. By extrapolation we would expect to find no difference in sensitivity above about 45 Hz. Using out-of-phase binocular sine waves
produced a depression in contrast sensitivity below the monocular level.
    Kintz's data tend to confirm the findings of other binocular flicker
studies. In addition, a resonance frequency and a range over which the
binocular system is more sensitive to temporal modulations are revealed. These two facts have both practical and theoretical implications.
They can be interpreted to mean that photic stimulation of a patient
with anomalous binocular vision for the purpose of reestablishing normal function might be accomplished best by using intermittent stimulation at or around the resonance frequency (Mallett and Reading,

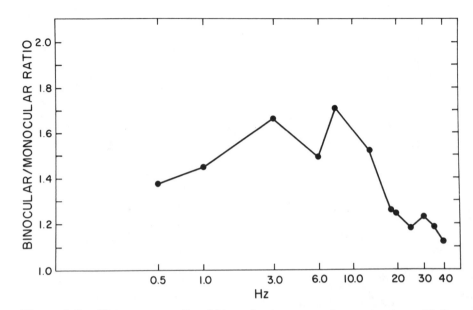

Figure 4–7.   The average ratio of binocular-to-monocular contrast sensitivity
as a function of temporal frequency for two subjects (Kintz, 1969).

1971). Furthermore, they could indicate that the visual system processes information by using a series of analyzers with different temporal frequency spectra and that knocking out one or another of these analyzers could produce different visual anomalies (Ikeda and Wright, 1974). Then binocular anomalies would be created if the lower frequency processors were malfunctioning (see Chapter 12).

Flicker perception could be used to develop a clinical test also. The patient would adjust the flicker rate of a light until it reached the CFF while viewing it with one eye only. Then the patient would view the light with the other eye and make the necessary adjustments in flash rate to eliminate any return of flicker. Finally, the rate would be set at the more sensitive of these two monocular CFFs, and the patient would view it binocularly. An abnormal patient should see a steady, nonflickering light.

Correlation of the results of such a test with those of other tests of sensory and motor function would be needed on a group of patients with binocular anomalies and a group of normal subjects to establish the utility of such a test as a diagnostic aid. Also it would be necessary to establish that flicker rates are determined by the same mechanisms that mediate fusion, stereopsis, and other binocular functions (see Chapters 10 and 12).

BINOCULAR RECOGNITION ACUITY

Barany (1946) analyzed recognition acuity data in the same fashion as Pirenne evaluated absolute detection threshold data. Since he did not know about Pirenne's work until after his paper had been published, he independently developed what we now call probability summation and extended the concept to applications involving visual acuity. He found no summation beyond that predicted by probability summation.

Horowitz (1949) compared monocular acuity to binocular acuity for various test conditions. He concluded that binocular visual acuity was superior to monocular visual acuity, but that the difference could be reduced by certain conditions which improved monocular acuity, including the control of pupil size by exposing the nontested eye to the same luminance as the tested eye.

BINOCULAR SPATIAL MTF

Campbell and Green (1965a) studied binocular visual acuity, using contrast sensitivity with sine wave gratings of varying spatial frequency. Figure 4–8 shows their plot of average contrast sensitivity for two subjects as a function of spatial frequency for the right eye, left eye, and both eyes. The average ratio of binocular-to-monocular contrast sensitivity was not significantly different from $\sqrt{2}$, or a binocular improvement of 42 percent. Campbell and Green used the principles of information theory to explain this difference. If the retinal signals are independent and contain noise, e.g., random events that are unrelated to the retinal images' patterns of light and dark, then combining two such inputs should produce an improvement in binocular acuity equal to 1.41 times the monocular value. This is what they found, and they consider that there is no interaction for acuity beyond that predicted by increasing the sample size.[4]

These investigators chose to make the binocular-monocular MTF comparisons using normal viewing. As they have demonstrated, in another study (Campbell and Green, 1965b) the monocular MTF is limited by the aberrations and diffraction of the eye's optics. If interference fringes could be formed on corresponding points, one might find that the binocular neural system is superior to the monocular system with regard to visual acuity. However, at present we do not have the results of such an experiment.

In addition, using luminance levels much lower than those of Campbell and Green, Home (1978) found that the average binocular-to-monocular contrast sensitivity ratio was about 1.5 when compared

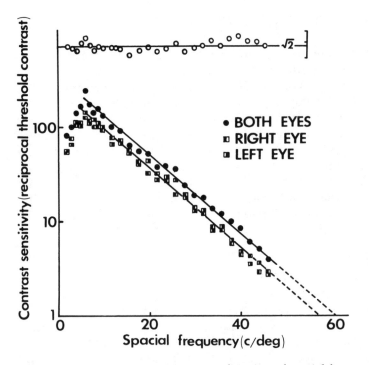

Figure 4–8. Contrast sensitivity as a function of spatial frequency. Upper plot
is the binocular-to-monocular ratio (Campbell and Green, 1965).

with the preferred eye and 1.6 when compared with the nonpreferred
eye. He used 20 subjects. This suggests summation in excess of that
expected by combining independent samples and indicates that the two
signals are neither independent nor equal. Apparently binocular visual
acuity demonstrates a superiority to monocular visual acuity that indicates the workings of a physiological summative process, at least at
moderate luminance levels.

These results have a certain implication for the clinician who frequently compares monocular and binocular visual acuity as an index
of binocular visual performance. Performance should be better binocularly by about one line of letters on a visual acuity chart. If it is not
better by at least this amount, or if it is the same as or worse than the
monocular visual acuity, then the clinician has the right to suspect the
presence of a binocular anomaly. To improve the diagnostic value of
this comparison, monocular visual acuity should be measured while
the nontested eye is covered with a translucent occluder, which tends
to more nearly equalize the luminance to the two eyes.

SIGNAL DETECTION AND BINOCULAR INTERACTION

According to classical threshold theory such as discussed earlier, detectability occurs as a simple probabilistic function over a certain range of stimulus values; according to signal detection theory, however, the subject's bias can be adjusted by changing the frequency of "firing blanks" and altering the "payoff factor." Blanks are fired by pretending to expose the subject to a stimulus and noting the frequency with which she or he reports that something was detected. This "false-alarm rate" can affect responses and thus depress or elevate the true physical stimulus value conventionally designated as the threshold. Furthermore, if detection leads to certain rewards or if failure to detect produces some negative consequences, then the response bias can be altered further (Galanter, 1962).

Signal detection theory is based on information theory, and so the message or signal is embedded in a spectrum of extraneous activity called *noise* (Egan and Clarke, 1966). In this context, detection occurs when the signal plus the noise is sufficiently different from the noise alone to exceed the particular decision criterion set by the subject.

Eriksen (1966) considered that probability summation prediction was too high because it gave double weight to the guessing factor. He divided detection into two parts: trials that are correctly perceived and trials that are not correctly perceived but in which the subject guesses correctly. For binocular viewing, the proportion of trials in which the subject has to resort to guessing would be reduced since a hit in either eye or both eyes would now produce a perception. Since Pirenne did not correct monocular probabilities for this factor, expectations of binocular performance based on these predictions are inflated.

Threshold data can be corrected for guessing, which brings the false-alarm rate under direct control. Further, payoff rates can be set at some nominal level of reward for correct responses, and thus the subject's bias can be brought to a more or less constant level.

If we accept the premises of signal detection and agree to its direct application to the visual sense, then a comparison of thresholds such as presented earlier ceases to be important. What is needed is a comparison of the receiver operating characteristics (ROCs). These are derived by altering the subject's criteria of detection and plotting the hit rate versus the false-alarm rate.

Hake and Rodwan (1966) suggested that using more than two response categories and determining estimated hit rates and false-alarm rates would allow specification of a discrimination index equivalent to that determined by using only two categories and adjusting the decision criterion. This process permits application of these methods to determine ROCs over a range of shifts in hit rates and false-alarm rates.

For example, in Table 4–3 we present hypothetical responses and calculations of hit and false-alarm rates for five categories of responses to stimuli at a given luminance difference between two juxtapositioned targets. These are combined with random presentations in which the two targets are of equal luminance. The response categories used are as follows:

1. Very sure that the stimuli are of different brightnesses
2. Somewhat sure that the stimuli are of different brightnesses
3. Cannot say
4. Somewhat sure that the stimuli are of equal brightness
5. Very sure that the stimuli are of equal brightness

Figure 4–9 shows the receiver operating characteristics for the discrimination of these two luminance differences. A comparison of a few such ROC curves for several luminance steps would elucidate differences in binocular and monocular performance (for further discussion of this issue, see Guth, 1971; Braddick, 1972).[3]

Table 4–3. Hypothetical Responses and Calculations of Hit and False-Alarm Rates for Brightness Discrimination Experiment

Response Category C	Number of Hits h ($\Delta B = 1\%$)	Number of False Alarms f ($\Delta B = 0\%$)
1	20	5
2	50	5
3	20	20
4	5	40
5	5	30
Total	$N_h = 100$	$N_f = 100$

$Hit\ Rate\ (HR) = 1/N_h \sum_{i=1}^{5} h_i$	$False\text{-}Alarm\ Rate\ (FAR) = 1/N_f \sum_{i=1}^{5} f_i$
$HR_1 = 0.20$	$FAR_1 = 0.05$
$HR_2 = 0.70$	$FAR_2 = 0.10$
$HR_3 = 0.90$	$FAR_3 = 0.30$
$HR_4 = 0.95$	$FAR_4 = 0.70$

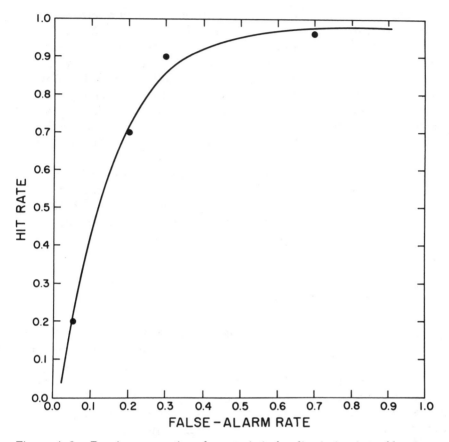

Figure 4–9. Receiver operating characteristic for discrimination of luminance
differences.

Application of these methods is quite useful to clinicians on an
intuitive level, and the experienced practitioner will recognize the operation of these biases in the patients' behavior. For example, many
patients are routinely reluctant to report subtle differences in the quality
of perceptions during successive views through testing lenses lest the
payoff will be a wrong lens prescription. Similarly, certain patients see
identical presentations as different because they are apparently over-
eager to earn the approval of the practitioner.

PHOTOSENSITIVE EPILEPSY

Binocular viewing can have its behavioral disadvantages beyond those
previously discussed. Jeavons and Harding (1975) described patients

for whom flickering lights induce the onset of epileptic seizures. They reported that these attacks could be avoided if the patients would remember to close or cover one eye when they sense flickering lights in the environment. Such situations occur while the patients are watching a poorly adjusted television set, driving through a wooded area when the sun is positioned near the horizon, or viewing an emergency vehicle, such as a police car or an ambulance, with its flashing signal lights operating. Subsequent investigation by these authors indicated that it took twice the intensity of a flickering light to cause a seizure monocularly as it did for binocular viewing. A related observation concerns minimizing the effects of direct disability glare by closing one eye (Mathis and Bourassa, 1968). One experiences this when driving into direct sunlight during the early morning or late afternoon. Indeed, at least one or two effects associated with binocular vision demonstrate complete summation.

OVERVIEW OF BINOCULAR INTERACTION

The comparison of the results of visual performance of binocular and monocular viewing conditions indicates significant but sometimes subtle differences. These differences reflect the uniqueness of the operations of a binocular mechanism and the intrinsic differences between alterations in testing parameters. This intrinsic difference can be evaluated in terms of probability summations, areal summation, decreasing variance with increased sample size, or signal detection.

By using some of these corrections, it can be shown that significant binocular summation takes place at the absolute threshold and for simultaneous binocular critical flicker frequency measurements. Binocular brightness appears to operate on an averaging basis, although test parameters can be manipulated to demonstrate a summative process. Furthermore, binocular reaction times are significantly shorter than the monocular ones. Binocular visual acuity also demonstrates a significant amount of summation, at least at moderate luminance levels.

"Are two eyes better than one?" The answer, based on information from binocular interaction, is yes, but just barely (Blake and Fox, 1973). However, considerations involving stereopsis have not been discussed here. Also the question of the superiority of a normal binocular system to that of an abnormal form needs to be considered. While people who lose one eye sometimes function quite well, they also restrict their activities or replace function with caution, which tends to make their performances appear nearly normal. A person with a binocular anomaly sometimes may be equivalent to a one-eyed observer. In other cases, this may not be so.

NOTES

1. The concept of probability summation also can be developed as follows:
   a. For two monocular threshold levels, by conventional agreement, P_R is equal to 0.5, as is P_L.
   b. Therefore, if independence is assumed, the probability of not seeing either R or L is also 0.5.
   c. The probability of not seeing both R and L is their product, $0.5 \times 0.5 = 0.25$.
   d. The probability of seeing either or both is then $P_b' = 1 - 0.25 = 0.75$ (Pirenne, 1962.)
2. It is also logical to consider that the observer receives twice as much light during binocular stimulation. For total summation, this would produce a binocular threshold energy level that is one-half of the monocular level. By extension of this logic, since the binocular threshold is higher than the predicted value, the system can be considered to demonstrate a lack of summation or even a form of negative summation. However, in such a viewpoint the question of the nature of binocular interaction is ignored instead of addressed.
3. Comparisons of receiver operating characteristics are best made in terms of the index of discrimination d', where

$$d' = \sqrt{2E/N}$$

   Here E is the total energy in the signal, and N is the noise power per unit bandwidth (Egan and Clark, 1966). For vision, noise power must be estimated from dark noise.
4. Note that information theory, areal summation, and increasing accuracy with increasing sample size all predict a similar gain for binocular viewing.

REFERENCES

Barany, E. (1946), "A theory of binocular visual acuity and an analysis of the variability of visual acuity," *Acta Ophthalmologica*, 24, 63–92.

Blake, R., and Fox, R. (1973), "The psychophysical inquiry into binocular summation," *Perception and Psychophysics*, 14, 161–185.

Braddick, O. (1972), "Binocular interaction and signal detection," *Vision Research*, 12, 1435–1437.

Brindley, G. S. (1970), *Physiology of the Retina and Visual Pathway*, Williams and Wilkins, Baltimore, 164–165.

Brown, J. L., and Mueller, C. G. (1965), "Brightness discrimination and brightness contrast," *Vision and Visual Perception.*, Wiley, New York, 208–250.

Campbell, F. W., and Green, D. G. (1965a), "Monocular versus binocular visual acuity," *Nature*, 208, 191–192.

Campbell, F. W., and Green, D. G. (1965b), "Optical and retinal factors affecting visual resolution," *Journal of Physiology*, 181, 576–593.

Curtis, D. W., and Rule, S. J. (1978), "Binocular processing of brightness information: A vector-sum model," *Journal of Experimental Psychology: Human Perception and Performance*, 4, 132–143.

Egan, J. P., and Clarke, F. R. (1966), "Psychophysics and signal detection," *Experimental Method and Instrumentation in Psychology*, McGraw-Hill, New York, 211–246.

Engel, G. R. (1967), "The visual processes underlying binocular brightness summation," *Vision Research*, 7, 753–767.

Engel, G. R. (1969), "The autocorrelation function and binocular brightness," *Vision Research*, 9, 1111–1130.

Eriksen, C. W. (1966), "Independence of successive inputs and uncorrelated error in visual form perception," *Journal of Experimental Psychology*, 72, 26–35.

Fry, G. A., and Bartley, S. H. (1933), "The brillance of an object seen binocularly," *American Journal of Ophthalmology*, 16, 687–693.

Galanter, E. (1962), "Contemporary psychophysics," *New Directions in Psychology*, Holt, New York, 89–156.

Gilliland, K., and Haines, R. F. (1975), "Binocular summation and peripheral visual response time," *American Journal of Optometry and Physiological Optics*, 52, 834–839.

Guth, S. L. (1971), "On probability summation," *Vision Research*, 11, 747–750.

Hake, H. W., and Rodwan, A. S. (1966), "Perception and recognition," *Experimental Methods and Instrumentation in Psychology*, McGraw-Hill, New York, 331–381.

Home, R. (1978), "Binocular summation: A study of contrast sensitivity, visual acuity, and recognition," *Vision Research*, 18, 579–585.

Horowitz, M. W. (1949), "An analysis of the superiority of binocular over monocular visual acuity," *Journal of Experimental Psychology*, 39, 581–596.

Ikeda, H., and Wright, M. J. (1974), "Is amblyopia due to inappropriate stimulation of the 'sustained' pathway during development?" *British Journal of Ophthalmology*, 58, 165–175.

Jeavons, P. M., and Harding, G. F. A. (1975), *Photosensitive Epilepsy*, Heinemann, London, 73–75, 99–102.

Kintz, R. T. (1969), "A comparison of monocular and binocular temporal resolution in human vision," Ph.D. thesis, University of Rochester.

LeGrand, Y. (1967), *Form and Space Vision*, Indiana University, Bloomington, 194–196.

LeGrand, Y. (1968), *Light, Colour, and Vision*, Chapman & Hall, London, 305–307, 423.

Levelt, W. J. M. (1965), *On Binocular Rivalry*, Institute for Perception, Soesterberg, The Netherlands, 34–43.

Lythgoe, R. J., and Phillips, L. R. (1938), "Binocular summation during dark adaptation," *Journal of Physiology*, 91, 427–436.

Mallett, R. F. J., and Reading, R. W. (1971), "Variations in the state of retinal correspondence with intermittent stimuli: A case study," *Ophthalmic Optician*, 11, 847–850.

Mathis, W., and Bourassa, C. M. (1968), "Fusion and nonfusion as factors in aversion to high luminance," *Vision Research*, 8, 1501–1506.

Matin, L. (1962), "Binocular summation at the absolute threshold for peripheral vision," *Journal of the Optical Society of America*, 52, 1276–1286.

Minucci, P. K., and Connors, M. M. (1967), "Reaction time under three viewing conditions: Binocular, dominant eye, and non-dominant eye," *Journal of Experimental Psychology*, 67, 268–275.

Peckham, R. H., and Hart, W. M. (1960), "Binocular summation of subliminal repetitive visual stimulation," *American Journal of Ophthalmology*, 49, 1121–1126.

Perrin, F. H. (1954), "A study in binocular flicker," *Journal of the Optical Society of America*, 44, 60–69.

Pickersgill, M. J. (1961), "On knowing with which eye one is seeing," *Quarterly Journal of Experimental Psychology*, 13, 168–172.

Pirenne, M. H. (1943), "Binocular and uniocular thresholds in vision," *Nature*, 175, 996.

Pirenne, M. H. (1962), "Quantum fluctuation at the absolute threshold, *The Eye*, vol. 2, Academic, New York, 141–158.

Sherrington, C. S. (1904), "On binocular flicker and the correlation of activity of corresponding points," *British Journal of Psychology*, 11, 26–60.

Stevens, S. S. (1961), "The psychophysics of sensory function," *Sensory Communication*, M.I.T., Cambridge, 1–33.

Thorn, F., and Boynton, R. M. (1974), "Binocular summation at absolute threshold," *Vision Research*, 14, 445–455.

van de Geer, J. P., and Moraal, J. (1963), "Discrimination of Which Eye Is Stimulated," Institute for Perception, Soesterberg, The Netherlands, 108.

Weale, R. A., (1955) "Binocular vision and deep-sea fish," *Nature*, 1975, 996.

5

VISUAL DIRECTION: LOCAL SIGN AND CORRESPONDING POINTS

Good too, logic, of course; in itself, but not in fine weather.

Arthur Hugh Clough

DIRECTIONAL SENSE

The discrimination of direction is an important aspect of spatial vision. When it is combined with distance perception, it constitutes the visual basis for much of human behavior. In many situations, the distance and depth mechanisms act completely predictably. In other instances, the perception of form and the mechanisms associated with eye, head, and body movements can modify these impressions.

We first look at the monocular mechanisms and then introduce and elaborate some of the binocular processes. Some of the influences of form and the complications that eye movements introduce are treated also.

The key concepts involved in the directional sense are simple ones: local sign and corresponding points. Nevertheless, both seem to involve rather complicated neural mechanisms whose exposition remains somewhat less than complete.

LOCAL SIGN

Objects in the visual field are imaged across the retina, which is organized to signal differences in visual direction to the higher centers. This is spoken of as a *point-for-point relationship* and can be referred to as a kind of *mapping.* The optical image on the retina is a map of points in the visual field. The sensory information arising from the structures of the retina, including the directional information, can be referred to as a *sensory map* which is closely related to the sensory maps of the geniculate and cortex.

The ability of a series of receptors to signal differences in the directions of stimuli is called *local sign,* or *signature.* It was first worked out by Lotze in 1886 and included an analysis of the attribute for the sense of touch. He enunciated the principle that states that regardless of the mode of stimulation of a point on the skin, if the stimulus is strong enough, it will give rise to a sensation that is unalterably associated with the particular location stimulated (Riggs, 1965).

The concept of local sign also applies to the visual system. Rods and cones or groups of these elements that form receptive fields of ganglion cells have been identified with fixed visual directions. When these units are stimulated by light, electric current, chemical agents, or mechanical force of sufficient strength to exceed a unit's threshold, the response of any individual unit will lead to perception of a point in a fixed visual direction (LeGrand, 1967).

A Demonstration of Local Sign and Projection

The simplest demonstration is the pressure phosphene. By lightly pressing on the sclera of the eye, a ring of light is perceived on the opposite side of the field of view. The pressure on the eye causes a mechanical force that can stimulate the receptors, giving rise to the perception of light. The location of the resulting sensation indicates that retinal stimulation produces an opposite-side perception.

This opposite-side effect frequently is called *projection.* It is said that stimulation of a region of the retina produces a perception of light that is projected out into the surrounding space through a center of projection. More simply, this projection is equivalent to the object-image relationship elaborated in geometric optics. That is, a point-for-point relationship exists between object and image. Insofar as this corresponds to a projection in the geometric sense, the centers of projection for conjugate object and image points are the two nodal points of any optical system. The actual projective aspect arises from the fact that we are aware of the apparent relationship of things external to us. That is, we do not directly sense the image on the retina, but rather sense its projection into surrounding space (see Chapter 3).

Because usually not all points in the field of view are conjugate at any one time, Ogle (1962) and others suggested that it is more realistic to consider the center of the entrance pupil as the object-space location of the center of projection for the eye. It is appropriate to speak of object space because usually the perceptions involving the relationships of objects are measured directly and corresponding image-space relationships inferred from the principles of geometric optics.

MAPS

Retinal, Geniculate, and Cortical

This point-for-point relationship between object and image is only approximately true, however. Aberrations make blurred circles out of object points, and the diameter and density of the individual receptor elements can affect the ability of an optical system to resolve detail. These limitations are implied in the use of the word *mapping*. Maps rarely represent everything. Instead, maps have resolution limits. Usually certain points are selected, or the scale is locally distorted, to emphasize points and areas of special interest.

The relationship among points on a map depends on the shape of the surface where it is formed or projected. The three-dimensional space of the visual field is mapped onto the nearly hemispherical retina. This, in turn, is remapped in the knee-shaped structure of the geniculate and again in the convolutions of the occipital cortex. Figure 5–1 illustrates a map of the various parts of the visual field on the visual cortex. Note that this map emphasizes the foveal area by devoting more cortical space to serve this region (Holmes, 1918). Mapping, as used here, simply implies that the ordering of points remains invariant within the various projections of field to retina, to geniculate, and to cortex. Additional maps involving eye movements in response to stimuli at various positions within the visual field are found in the frontal cortex and the superior colliculus (Masterton and Glendenning, 1978).

Resolution

We can start to map the visual system in humans by determining the threshold for change in visual direction for various points in the visual field, using some kind of resolution acuity task, and constructing a

Thick dark line represents   Upper lip of   F. parieto–
apex of F. calcarina   F. calcarina   occipitalis

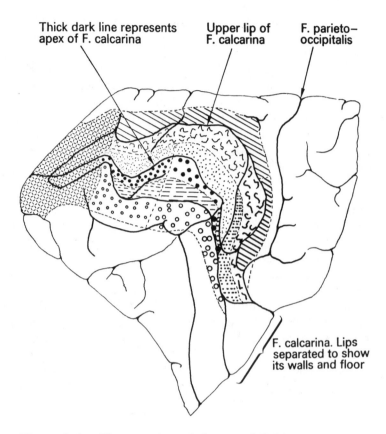

F. calcarina. Lips
separated to show
its walls and floor

Figure 5–1.   The mapping of the visual field onto the visual cortex (from
              Brindley, 1970, modified from Holmes, G. 1918, and reprinted
              by permission).

graph such as that in Figure 5–2 (Mandelbaum and Sloan, 1947). *Visual resolution* is the ability to perceive two target elements as being located in two different visual directions (Cline et al., 1980). While these data represent the start of a mapping procedure and probably are sufficiently complete to illustrate something about horizontal variations, the data are incomplete with regard to the relative sensitivity of the superior and inferior quadrants of the retina. Nevertheless, as we will see, the horizontal differences could form the basis for some important binocular phenomena. Even though fewer points were determined for the nasal eccentricities than for the temporal ones, apparently the temporal hemi-retina has better resolution capabilities than the nasal, for eccentricities smaller than about 10°.

Such maps are difficult to come by because of the arduous task of

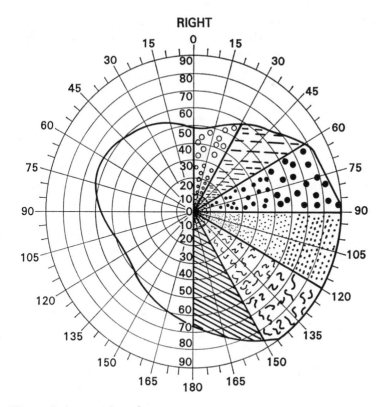

Figure 5–1. continued.

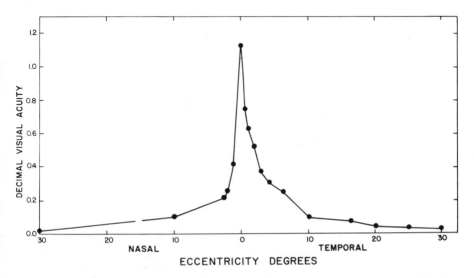

Figure 5–2. Resolution map of the horizontal meridian of the retina (Madelbaum and Sloan, 1947).

making peripheral judgments, the potential contaminations of unintentional shifts in fixation, and the distractions resulting from the Troxler effect. Furthermore, the data of Johnson et al., (1978) indicate very little temporal-nasal differences for both detection and resolution tasks on three subjects.

Vernier

With regard to the spatial sense, the *vernier threshold* can be defined as one in which a displacement of two line segments is detected. That is, the two line segments are seen in different visual directions. Figure 5–3 illustrates the angular nature of measurements of vernier, resolution, and stereoscopic displacements.

   Resolution maps may not represent the best that the visual system can do. Since in psychophysics, we seek to explore the absolute limits

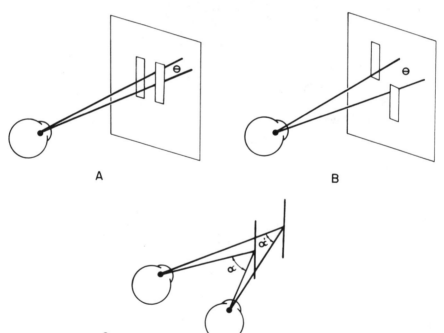

Figure 5–3.   Angular separations involved in *(A)* resolution, *(B)* vernier, and *(C)* stereopsis. Theta is the threshold angle for resolution and vernier. For stereopsis, $\alpha - \alpha'$ specifies the threshold.

of sensory capabilities, perhaps a vernier map is a more desirable one. For central fixation, the resolution threshold is usually between 30 and 60 arcseconds, while the vernier threshold is about 2 to 5 arcseconds (Riggs, 1965). If this difference holds in the periphery, we might expect to be able to map the sensitivity to direction differences at a level that is 6 to 15 times more accurate. However, individual differences may complicate this relationship also. In Figure 5–4 the data of Stockley and Jenkins (1970) are plotted to illustrate the relationship between central vernier thresholds and central resolution thresholds for 30 subjects. This scattergram indicates that the predictability of vernier thresholds from measurements of resolution is not very accurate. Based on this information, we might suspect that an even greater intersubject variability would degrade further the relationship for peripheral thresholds.

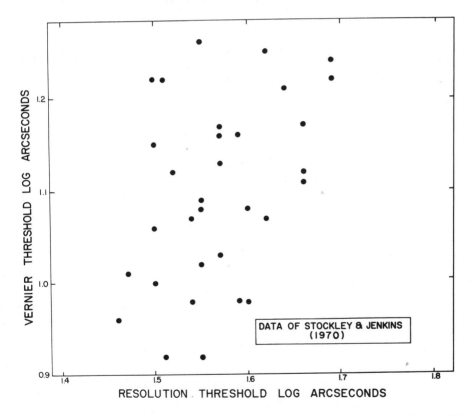

Figure 5–4.   Relationship between resolution and vernier thresholds for 30 subjects (Stockley and Jenkins, 1970).

Figure 5–5 presents the monocular resolution data of Randall et al. (1966) and the monocular vernier data of Bourdon and Hofmann (Legrand, 1967). These data were gathered from three different studies and so are the results with different subjects. The data show that monocular vernier thresholds are smaller than the monocular resolution thresholds out to an eccentricity of about 7°. Freeman (1966), using two subjects, reported that the vernier sensitivity was slightly superior to resolution sensitivity out to about 12° of eccentricity. He found that temporal vernier thresholds were essentially identical to nasal vernier thresholds. Both resolution and vernier tasks provide bases for measurement of the binocular system. Vernier measurements are especially important because of their high precision (see Chapter 11).

STIMULUS PARAMETERS INFLUENCING DIRECTIONAL DISCRIMINATIONS

As with most psychophysical functions, vernier thresholds can be altered by changes in such stimulus parameters as exposure time and target separation. As with other measurements, variability between

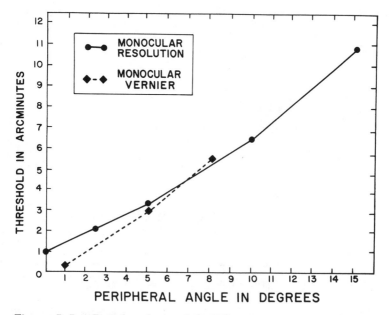

Figure 5–5. Peripheral visual functions comparing resolution and vernier thresholds (LeGrand, 1967).

subjects appears to be significant. Nevertheless, certain relationships or trends can be established. For example, Figure 5–6 shows the threshold angle (in arcseconds) as a function of exposure time (in milliseconds) for two subjects as reported by Keesey (1960). The thresholds were taken under conditions of normal viewing and with the image optically fixed on the retina (Prichard et al., 1960) and show very little difference. Thus involuntary micromovements of the eye have almost nothing to do with vernier thresholds. However, since Barlow (1963) reported that even tight-fitting contact lenses are subject to a slippage, possibly the lack of difference for these two viewing conditions is due to imperfect stabilization.

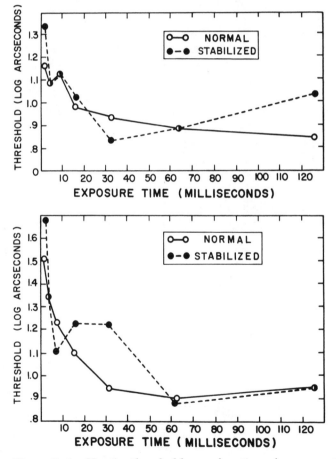

Figure 5–6.   Vernier thresholds as a function of exposure time for two subjects (Replotted from Keesey, 1960, and reprinted by permission).

Figure 5–7 shows the data for two subjects in whom the threshold-of-vernier setting is determined as a function of the angular separation between the ends of the two line segments. The threshold increases as the targets are separated by an increasing angular extent (Fender and Nye, 1962). Here again, both stabilized and normal viewing conditions were used. Perhaps these indicate some small hint of superiority for most thresholds measured under normal viewing conditions.

Figure 5–8 shows the results of a study in which the subject judged the alignment of a three-dot pattern where the center dot was moved until the three appeared to form a perfectly straight line. The two fixed dots were separated by various amounts between 2.5 and 50 arcminutes with the movable dot halfway in between (Ludvigh, 1953). Here the effect of target separation appears to be a complicated pattern that is entirely different from the one noted in Figure 5–7.

Matin (1975) analyzed the vernier task and concluded that it can consist of several entirely different kinds of judgments based on different perceptions of form. In the typical vernier task, the subject judges when a target movement produces a continuous, uninterrupted straight line. Such a task produces data like those in Figure 5–7. Replacing lines with dots is a change in form that produces a different kind of task and a different set of data, like those in Figure 5–8. Matin suggests that dot alignment measures an ability not unlike that of discriminating the orientations of two imaginary lines connecting the three dots. If this is so, it is a judgment closely related to having a subject judge when two real lines are parallel. Figure 5–8 also shows the data of Andrews (1967) (as recalculated by Matin), collected by using real lines set to apparent parallelism, and allows for comparision with the data of Ludvigh.

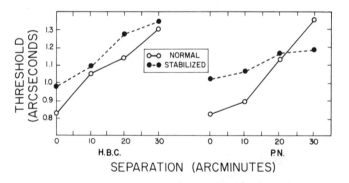

Figure 5–7.   Vernier thresholds as a function of the separation between two line segments (Replotted from Fender and Nye, 1962, and reprinted by permission).

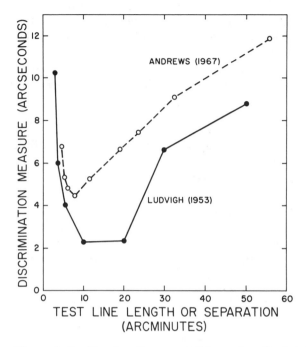

Figure 5–8. Vernier alignment of three dots (Ludvigh, 1953) and parallel alignment of two line segments (Andrews, 1967).

DETERMINING VISUAL DIRECTION BY PARTITION

In other studies, subjects were required to bisect a line segment. In a typical study of this kind, the subjects moved a fixation marker along a rod until they judged that the marker was in the center of a rod. Another way to bisect a line was to fixate a stationary point near the middle and adjust the two endpoints until the right and left portions appeared to be of equal length. It is reported that most observers will set the segment located temporally in the field so that it is physically larger than the nasal segment. This is known as the *Kundt type of partition* (Ogle, 1950). The Munsterberg type is its inverse and is reported by Tschermak (1952) to occur only rarely.

The Kundt type of partition constitutes an overestimation attributable to the temporal hemiretina. That is, since the nasal segment, which is imaged on the temporal retina, is seen larger, in order to make the two portions appear equal, the nasal part of the line must be made smaller. Tschermak considered that this overestimation indicates that the region involved has superior resolution capabilities. Patients suffering from retinal pathologies in which the receptor elements are crowded together do see objects imaged in these regions as magnified. One consequence of this kind of form judgment is that figures such as squares, triangles, and circles, viewed monocularly, will appear distorted, usually enlarged to the nasal side (Helmholtz, 1925).

Apparently, partition is an individual attribute, since both Brown (1953) and Heath (1953) found subjects demonstrating both forms of partition behavior. Furthermore, Brown studied changes in partition settings in a group of subjects over several months. While he found considerable changes, Heath reported that the settings were much more stable.

Studies of the horopter (defined below) attempted to account for the nature of this binocular percept in terms of the nasal-temporal asymmetries of the two eyes. The data presented earlier on resolution, vernier, and partition suggest that there may or may not be a small individual difference. Given that this difference does exist, sometimes

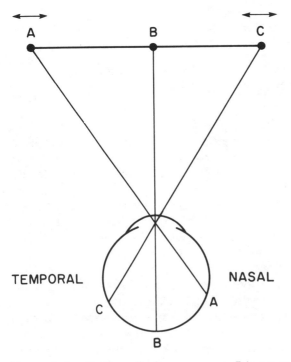

Figure 5–9.   Partion of a line segment. *B* is set so *AB* appears equal to *BC*.

it may be possible to predict the shape of the horopter in at least a qualititative way from such monocular data (see Chapter 11).

DYNAMIC THEORY OF DIRECTION DISCRIMINATION

Vernier thresholds are very fine ones. While Helmholtz (1925) was able to find a basis for resolution thresholds in the size of the retinal mosaic, the diameter of the foveal cones was too large to allow this reasoning to be extended to account for the accuracy of vernier settings. Hering suggested that some kind of averaging of local signs must be involved (Riggs, 1965). Subsequently Andersen and Weymouth (1923) proposed that three kinds of averaging processes were at work: spatial averaging of local signs along the length of lines, temporal averaging among laterally displaced receptors, and binocular averaging between the two monocular inputs.

Figure 5–10 is a schematic illustration of how such averaging processes might work. It shows a vernier misalignment of less than one receptor diameter (A), a group of schematic receptors stimulated at any given moment (B), the resulting individual local signs, and (C), the result of an averaging or best-fit process (D). At the bottom of Figure 5–10B, three receptors are shaded. As the eye scans, it successively images a portion of the line on these receptors. If these individual local signs are averaged also, then the mean is adjusted laterally, as shown

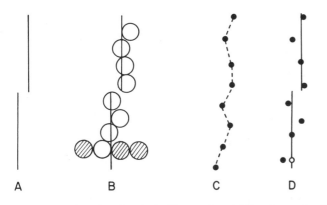

A   B   C   D

Figure 5–10.   A schematic illustration of the dynamic theory of visual acuity.
(A) A vernier target. (B) Receptors stimulated, shading indicates a group stimulated by eye scanning. (C) Resultant individual local signs. (D) Lines indicate the result of averaging. Open circle is result of additional refinement provided by eye movements.

in Figure 5–10D by the open circle. Such a process would occur for all the other clusters laterally displaced from the vertical contour and further refine the directional judgment.

Andersen and Weymouth based their inclusion of spatial averaging on the fact that longer line segments produce lower thresholds. This increase in length would allow more local signs to enter into determining a mean local sign and therefore produce more accuracy. Furthermore, as schematically indicated in Figure 5–10C, a line or an edge would appear broken or irregular without some local averaging process. An alternate explanation of this perceptual smoothing out can be found in the filling-in process reported by Walls (1954) to explain the usual absence of awareness of the blind spot. This mechanism is implicit in the organizational characteristics of some cells of the visual cortex (Hubel and Wiesel, 1962) which respond to lines or to a series of points arranged in configurations of lines (see Chapters 10 and 12).

If the eye performs temporal averaging, then with stabilized images the threshold should be elevated. Data presented in Figures 5–6 and 5–7 show very little evidence of a sensory refinement owing to eye movements. Nevertheless, Ditchburn (1973) considered that such comparisons as these could not prove or disprove the role of scanning in perception. Because typical vernier targets are black lines on a white background, they contain high spatial frequencies (Cornsweet, 1970). A temporal scanning theory predicts a higher spatial cutoff frequency than does a static theory. However, the limiting condition necessary to differentiate between these is obscured by the cutoff frequency of the eye's optical system, which is below both predicted values. This suggests that no difference between normal and stabilized viewing can be found unless the eye's optics are bypassed (Ditchburn, 1973). Increasing exposure time from near zero to about 30 ms for these two theories produces similar results. For longer exposure time and normal viewing, a static system, in which no account of eye movements is available, would suffer a decrease in performance owing to optical smearing. In this same range, an idealized scanning system's performance would continue to improve until it exceeded the performance obtained under stabilized conditions at about 60 to 80 ms (Ditchburn, 1973). Because these kinds of experiments have not been done, Ditchburn concluded that there is no strong evidence for or against temporal scanning.

Even if temporal scanning does exist, Riggs et al. (1954) pointed out that for exposure times of 200 ms, which Keesey showed was needed to maximize sensitivity, the average eye movement would scan an image across only two rows of receptors. Acting alone, temporal averaging could yield only a threshold twice as fine as the angular subtense of a foveal cone, or about 12 arcseconds.

Consider a simple elaboration of the dynamic theory which postulates a series of successive steps to refine local signs. From the data of Fender and Nye, we might reasonably choose a reduction factor equal to 0.5 for spatial scanning. If we started with the angular subtense of a foveal cone of 24 arcseconds, the output of a spatial scanner would be 12 arcseconds. This is the input to a temporal scanner, which, we know, has a reduction factor of no more than about 0.5; so its output might be about 6 arcseconds. If we used the data of Campbell and Green, the binocular reduction factor would be about 0.71, and this final reduction would produce a predicted threshold of about 4 arcseconds. While admittedly this is an oversimplification, it does show how three small scanning processes might be serially combined to produce a good prediction.

Sometimes an annoying characteristic of theories is that they do not indicate the nature of the underlying mechanisms. Walls (1943) suggested that the proliferation between optic nerve fibers and geniculate axons, at least a 1-to-6 increase, is a likely structure to mediate such a process. Fender and Nye (1962) proposed that it is a form of lateral inhibition. The modern viewpoint is that vernier acuity is a form of contour orientation discrimination and is mediated by line-detecting elements in the visual cortex (Matin, 1975). This mean cortical local sign would appear to be the result of interactions among cortical units that sense both spatial and temporal fluctuations in a stimulus (see Chapters 10 and 12). According to Matin, such an explanation also accounts for Ludvigh's three-point alignment data.

VERNIER VERSUS STEREOPSIS

Since both stereopsis and vernier acuity show incredibly fine discriminations, Walls (1943) suggested that they may have a common basis. Figure 5–11 illustrates the geometric similarity. In this figure, displacement in a plane parallel to the observer's face of the upper segment of a test object to position u' produces the perception of a vernier misalignment. Displacement in a plane perpendicular to this, for example, in a direction toward the observer to u produces the perception of stereoscopic displacement. In both cases, the threshold angle would be equal to the difference in the two binocular subtense angles, labeled α and α' here.

Figure 5–11 also shows some of the data of Stigmar (1970) replot-

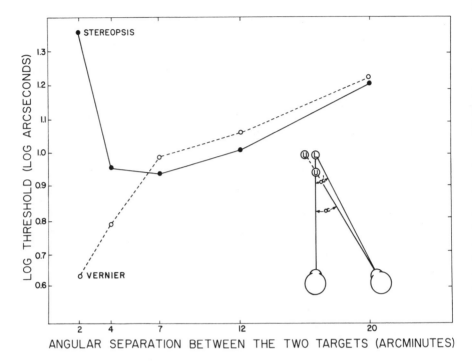

Figure 5–11. The threshold of stereopsis and vernier alignment as a function
of angular separation between the two targets (Stigmar, 1970).
The insert shows their geometric similarity (Reprinted by permission from Walls, 1943).

ted. Between angular separations of the target parts of 4 to 20 arcminutes, the two thresholds are virtually identical. At 2 arcminutes of
separation, stereopsis undergoes a significant elevation. At these small
separations, stereopsis demonstrates something like what Flom et al.
(1963) termed a *crowding phenomenon* for recognition acuity. Here the
crowding of target components seems to provide interference, whereas
in recognition tasks a separate masking contour serves this function.
Except for this effect at small separations, the two perceptions appear
to be mediated by essentially the same mechanism (see Chapter 12).

TRAINING PERIPHERAL FUNCTION

The reports of rather striking individual differences in peripheral visual
performance in a group of subjects may mean that extraneous factors,
physiological capacities, or experience varies. If experience differences

are the cause, then this function may be improved by an appropriate form of training (LeGrand, 1967). Some improvement in athletic ability is believed to result from having the athlete perform some simple task involving peripheral visual judgments. For artistic ability, Sherman (1947) showed the effects of just such an approach.

CORRESPONDING POINTS

The binocular system produces a unique perception of visual direction that is based on the concept of corresponding points. *Corresponding points* are points on the two retinas that give rise to a common visual direction (Cline et al., 1980). If a point on the left retina is selected, then a point on the right retina can be found such that when both are stimulated, a sensation is created of a point-object located in a single position and direction from the observer. Since we will be dealing with points in object space, we should say that one can pick any visual direction or line of sight for the left eye of an observer and then find a visual direction for the right eye that will give rise to a common sensation of direction when both eyes are used. Operationally, corresponding points are determined by finding corresponding lines of sight.

VISUAL SPACE

In this definition, the term *visual* is used to clearly distinguish between how things appear and how they are in the physical world. The distinction is important to an understanding of certain aspects of binocular vision and is far from trivial. *Visual space* is made up of appearances and scaled off in terms of apparent relationships of objects in the field of view. *Physical space* is that form which can be measured with rulers and goniometers. Two examples illustrate the need for this distinction.

Physical measurements of Figure 1–1 show that this four-sided form is indeed a square. Visually the left vertical side seems shorter than the right one, and the top and bottom sides appear slanted. This figure can be seen as a square viewed from an oblique direction (Helmholtz, 1925).

Perhaps an even more dramatic example of these differences is the result of alley experiments. Hillebrand, and later Blumenfeld (Graham, 1965), conducted experiments in which subjects were asked to arrange two rows of point-source lights, as seen in a dark room, parallel to the median plane (e.g., a vertical plane through the perpendicular bisector of the interocular distance). This arrangement of lights was called the *parallel alley.* The subjects were positioned so that their eyes were in a plane located above that of the point-source lights and could judge the position of each set of two points or the whole configuration. They were free to fixate any and all points of light during these determinations. Later the subjects returned to adjust the positions of the points according to the following instructions: "Make an adjustment until the apparent distance between each of your settings and the light point to the left is the same as the distance between each of your settings and the light point to the right." The resulting arrangement was called the *equidistance alley.* Figure 5–12 shows these results (Luneburg, 1950).

Clearly both the equidistance alley and the parallel alley are far from physically parallel. Therefore, the difference between visual space and physical space has been demonstrated again. In the everyday terrestrial world, equidistance is synonymous with parallel. Based on the fact that these two different instructions produce differing results, visual space can be considered as noneuclidean under such measurement circumstances (Luneburg, 1950). However, Fry (1961) presented data for objects in which the eyes remained immobile. He considered this area of visual space quite adequately described by euclidean rules.

Regardless of the exact nature of visual space, what is important for the success of a human operating in physical space is that a fixed relationship be maintained. It is not necessary for the two to match perfectly, because the human is capable of making allowances for any discrepancies. However, the relationship must remain constant. A change in this relationship forces a person to begin again the process of learning to adjust motor responses to what is seen. This adjustment is marked with errors such as stumbling over steps and anxiety about how weird things appear. Patients experience this when they obtain

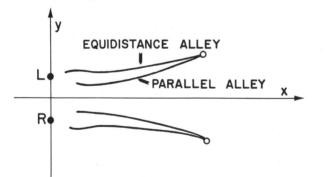

Figure 5–12.   A sketch of a subject's settings of points to the equidistant and parallel criteria, known as alleys (Replotted from Luneburg, 1950, and reprinted by permission).

a new spectacle prescription with some moderate changes in lens power, cylinder axis, base curve, or prism power. However, we should not conclude that such changes are to be avoided or dispensed on a partial basis. Usually counselling of the patient suffices to support rather rapid adjustment to a new pair of glasses. Certainly the improvements in the quality of sensory fusion usually are best accomplished by dispensing the full indicated changes in refractive and oculomotor corrective components (see Chapter 3).

DEFINITIONS

The line passing through the object of regard and the center of the entrance pupil is called the *line of sight* (Alpern, 1969). For clarity, we call this line the *primary* line of sight as Ogle (1950) described it. This allows us to speak of *secondary* lines of sight which are lines from other, nonfixed objects to the center of the entrance pupil. These also can be called *lines of direction* (Cline et al., 1980). The fixation point, or object of regard, is the point of intersection of the two primary lines of sight. The center of rotation is considered a fixed point around which the eyes move.

While the center of the entrance pupil is designated the *monocular center of projection*, the *binocular center of projection* is located at the bisector of the interpupillary line, e.g., the line connecting the two entrance pupils. This binocular center of projection is the egocenter of binocular vision; we discuss its use and measurement in Chapter 13.[1]

We will need to speak of the *plane of regard*, which is the plane formed by the fixation point and the interpupillary line, and the *midsagittal plane*, or *median plane*, which is perpendicular to the plane of regard at the bisector or the interpupillary line (Fry, 1961). Finally, a plane passing through the fixation point and parallel to the face plane is called the *objective frontoparallel plane*, sometimes referred to as the *fixation plane*, whereas the *face plane* itself is that plane formed by the globella and the two superciliary notches (Fry, 1961).

Figure 5–13 illustrates the *circle of equal convergence*, which passes through the fixation point and the centers of rotation of the two eyes. If the object of regard is moved along this circle, the angle formed by the intersection of the two primary lines of sight remains unchanged. Such a movement is termed a *versional eye movement* (Alpern, 1969).

Figure 5–14 shows the Vieth-Mueller circle. It is formed by constructing a circle through the point of fixation and the centers of the two entrance pupils. As shown in the figure, any point on the circle forms the same angle between lines of sight (or lines of direction) at

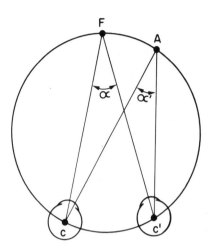

Figure 5–13. The circle of equal convergence constructed through the fixation point F and the centers of rotation c and c' (Fry, 1961).

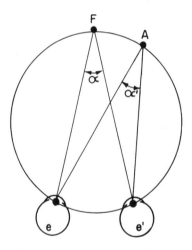

Figure 5–14. The Vieth-Mueller circle constructed through the fixation point F and the entrance pupils e and e' (Fry, 1961).

the two eyes. These angles are sometimes called *binocular subtense angles.* In this figure, the eye remains fixed so that Fe and Fe' are the primary lines of sight. At viewing distances greater than about 1 m, the circle of equal convergence and the Vieth-Mueller circle are practically identical; at closer distances the difference becomes significant (Fry, 1962; see also Chapter 11).

HERING'S LAW OF IDENTICAL VISUAL DIRECTION

Figure 5–15 illustrates an observation originally reported by Hering (1942). If we look at a mark on a windowpane, objects that lie on the primary line of sight of the left eye are seen in the same visual direction as objects that lie on the primary line of sight of the right eye. In the

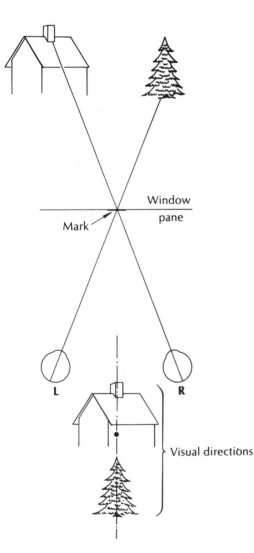

Figure 5–15.   Hering's law of identical visual direction (Ogle, 1950).

illustration, the marker and a chimney seen by the right eye appear in the same visual direction as the marker and a tree, as seen by the left eye. Since two different objects are seen in a common visual direction, this constitutes a condition previously called *confusion*. The two percepts will show some rivalry, but the important fact here is that the observation demonstrates that the centers of the two foveae are one pair of corresponding points. No matter where the two objects are in physical space, if they fall on corresponding lines of sight, they will appear in the same visual direction. Hering called this the *law of identical visual direction*.

HOROPTER

Are there other points that correspond? Early workers assumed that there were because for a fixed point of regard, certain other objects are seen at a common location and so are haplopic, whereas others appear diplopic. These investigators suggested that corresponding points might be spaced out at equal angles from the primary lines of sight. If this is so, then objects that lie on the Vieth-Mueller circle are a unique set of object points that would stimulate corresponding points (Ogle, 1950). For this reason, the Vieth-Mueller circle frequently is referred to as the *geometric horopter*.

The surface in physical space, any point of which produces images in the two eyes that stimulate exactly corresponding points, is called the *horopter*. It is specifically and uniquely identified with the point of intersection of the two primary lines of sight and is the boundary between crossed and uncrossed disparity. That is, the binocular disparity for a point on the horopter is zero (Ogle, 1950). By implication, stimulation of corresponding points produces no stimulus to fusional eye movements and maximum binocular interactions. Later we cite evidence that the empirical horopter does not coincide with the Vieth-Mueller circle and discuss the significance of this departure in Chapter 11.

BINOCULAR DISPARITY

Binocular disparity means that the angle of intersection of the two lines of sight at an object is different from the angle of intersection of two different lines of sight at another object. Figure 5–16 shows this relationship: α is the angle formed at F, and ϕ the angle formed at object B, nearer to the observer than the Vieth-Mueller circle. The binocular

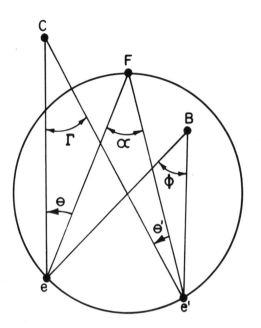

Figure 5–16.   This diagram shows points that are located off the Vieth-Mueller circle.

disparity η between the two is the difference in these two angles: η = α − φ. Because the reference circle here is the Vieth-Mueller circle, the geometric horopter, sometimes this is referred to as *geometric disparity* (Ogle, 1950).

For objects on the Vieth-Mueller circle, η = |α| − |α'| = 0 (see Figure 5–14). For an object on the circle and another farther away (Figure 5–16), η = |α| − |Γ|.

We can diagram the resulting perceptions as shown in Figure 5–17 (Fry, 1961). Figure 5–17A is a physical space diagram showing two objects, one on the Vieth-Mueller circle and the other nearer to the observer and on the midsagittal plane. Figure 5–17B represents a visual space diagram of the directional localizations. This is based on Hering's law of identical visual direction and the Vieth-Mueller circle. The primary lines of sight give rise to one straight-ahead direction of objects located in the midsagittal plane, so the diagram shows one line, c'F'. The visual directions of B are scaled off at visual angles that are equal to the physical angles formed by the intersection of the primary and secondary lines of sight, θ and θ', in Figure 5–17A. Because this object is closer to the observer than the fixation point, they are scaled off in opposite directions. That is, for the left eye it is scaled off to the right and to the left for the right eye. On the visual space diagram, this

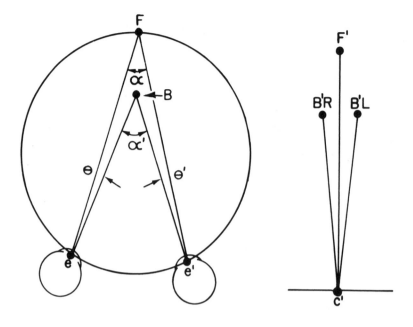

A. PHYSICAL SPACE   B. VISUAL SPACE

Figure 5–17. Diagrams representing *(A)* physical space and *(B)* visual space
that illustrates crossed disparity (Fry, 1961).

results in lines $c'B_R'$ and $c'B_L'$. All lines in this diagram are to originate
at c', which represents the binocular center of projection. For near
objects seen in diplopia, the image seen to the right is due to the left
eye and the image seen to the left is due to the right eye. This is called
crossed diplopia. Uncrossed diplopia is just the opposite, and it is illustrated
in Figure 5–18.

Let us return to the observations about the projection of pressure
phosphenes and extend this to the two eyes. Clearly stimulation of
both nasal retinas will give rise to uncrossed disparity, whereas bitem-
poral stimulation will produce crossed disparity. Off the midsagittal
plane, the situation is only slightly more complicated. Note in Figure
5–16 that for uncrossed disparity of objects to the right, the nasal retinal
angle is larger than the temporal angle. Table 5–1 summarizes these
relationships (see also Chapter 11).

PANUM'S AREA, OR SPACE

Further observation indicates that objects can be located a little way
from the horopter and still be seen as single. Thus precise correspon-

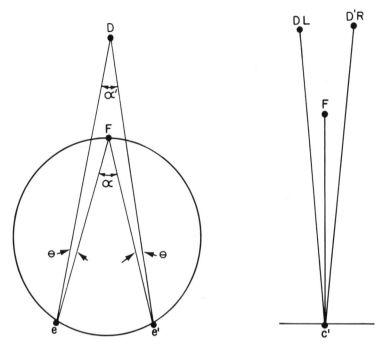

A. PHYSICAL SPACE   B. VISUAL SPACE

Figure 5–18.   A diagram similar to Figure 5–17 that illustrates uncrossed disparity (Fry, 1961).

dence is not required for the perception of haplopia. Furthermore, when an object is located close enough to the horopter to be fused, it also appears in a striking fashion to be at a different distance from another

Table 5–1.   Relationship between Nasal and Temporal Angles at the Eye for Crossed and Uncrossed Disparity

Visual Direction (with Respect to Midsagittal Plane)	Uncrossed Disparity	Crossed Disparity
To the left; N = O.S., T = O.D.	$N > T$	$N < T$
To the right; N = O.D., T = O.S.	$N > T$	$N < T$

N, nasal; T, temporal; O.D., right eye; O.S., left eye.

object located on the horopter locus. This is an example of stereopsis which depends solely on the presence of a sufficient binocular disparity (LeGrand, 1967).

The region that surrounds the horopter in which objects can be seen singly, ruling out suppression, is called *Panum's space*, and it constitutes the spatial area in which sensory fusion is at its best. The region on the retina over which an object can be moved and still be seen as single is known as *Panum's area*. In practice, the terms *area* and *space* are used interchangeably, even though *space* is a better method of describing the region surrounding the horopter in which haplopia occurs (see Chapter 7).

CLINICAL CONNOTATION OF FUSION

In the usual sense, the word *fusion* describes the results of both sensory and motor processes that produce binocular single vision. These sensory processes take place when objects are located at the horopter and in the immediately surrounding space. Note that if we can locate a pair of corresponding positions on the two retinas, by projection we can predict where an object has to be located in space in order to stimulate the retinas (see Chapters 3 and 7).

CORRESPONDING POINTS: A SUMMARY

We can describe corresponding points as those retinal points which, when stimulated, give rise to a common visual direction, produce no stimulus to fusional eye movements, produce maximum binocular interactions, and create an impression of depth in comparison with the apparent depth of almost any other point off the horopter. Some of these statements may need modification later, but, to at least a first approximation, every one of them appears to be true.

An issue that looms large with regard to the nature of corresponding points involves the fixity or permanence of the relationship. If the hookup is a flexible one, over what range can it be shifted? What induces such changes? Are these apparent shifts changes in steady-state associations or transient alterations specific to novel or restricted viewing conditions? This issue and others are treated in Chapters 11 and 14.

EYE MOVEMENTS, LOCAL SIGN, AND CORRESPONDING POINTS

In addition to the considerations involving the purely sensory system using conditions in which the eyes remain fixed in position on the object of regard, eye movements must be made in response to directional judgments based on local signs and corresponding points.

For monocular horizontal saccadic movements, Henson (1976) found the actual movement to consist of two components: the main saccade and the corrective saccade. The main saccade falls short of positioning the primary line of sight on the initially peripheral target by about 10 percent of the amplitude required. For example, for an object presented at a peripheral angle of 30° the main saccade covers only about 27°. The remaining 3° is provided by the subsequent corrective saccade.

The signal that determines how much initial eye movement is required was previously identified as the local sign. Its center of projection is at the entrance pupil, whereas the mechanics of the actual movment take place, to a first approximation, around a center of rotation located some 9 mm behind it (Alpern, 1969). For objects at 40 cm, a change in fixation of 30° produces an angle through which the eye must turn of only 29.45°, a difference of about 2 percent. Since this required response is smaller than the original stimulus, some correction must be made or else the eye would overshoot and the corrective movement would always be in the opposite direction from the main one, which is not the case according to Henson.

Furthermore, consider that at a point 30° off the primary line of sight, the directional discrimination is no better than about 1.67°. Then the initial stimulus for interfixational movment can be no more accurate than 30° ± 1.67°, an uncertainty of about ± 6 percent. From this fact we would predict that the main saccade should leave the eye in a relatively overshot or undershot position randomly. Therefore, Henson's finding of consistent undershoots as large as 10 percent means that eye movements are performed in a way that cannot be accounted for entirely on the basis of fixed eye sensory local signs. Thus the initial motor response of the eye may be directed by a map that is a rescaled local sign map. If this is the case for normal subjects, then perhaps some other rescaling is involved in patients with eye movement abnormalities.

For binocular eye movements, we would expect an even more complicated relationship between the sensory side involving corresponding points and the motor side involving binocular versional or vergence movements. The most critical relationship would be expressed as changes in the vergence angle as the two eyes move. However, this issue best awaits our studies of the empirical longitudinal horopter (see Chapter 11).

SPATIAL PERCEPTION AND THE MOVING EYE

The fact that the eye is capable of fixation and movement throughout a large portion of the visual field without disrupting the stability of perceptions resulting from local signs suggests the operation of a special mechanism. This is usually considered to be a cancellation process associated with an innervational record modified by proprioceptive information from the stretch receptors, which act as a feedback loop to alter the actual muscle contraction associated with a given innervational command without participating directly in conscious perception (Ludvigh, 1952a). However, the issue is far from settled, and Matin (1975) presented evidence that questions that the process is entirely due to an outflow of commands from the cortex. Also it has been shown that the eye becomes less sensitive to light and form during rapid eye movements, a process known as *saccadic suppression* (MacKay, 1970), and this might contribute to stable spatial perceptions (see Chapter 8). At any rate, the fact that some slight motion is perceived during almost all voluntary eye movement and that this transient shift in visual direction can be measured may mean simply that the cancellation processes are less than perfect (Matin, 1975).

The system must be able to stabilize the scene during saccades and detect motion of an object in the surroundings as it is displaced across the retina of a fixed eye or tracked by a moving eye. For this latter differentiation, Robinson (1972) reported that cells in the colliculus of the monkey respond differently to image displacement and to eye movement pursuit. This mechanism could provide an electrophysiological basis for signaling perceptual centers as to the real state of affairs in the environment and the eye.

Abnormal conditions exist in which the gaze into a particular portion of the visual field is restricted. Such patients initially experience a gross apparent motion upon attempting to fixate objects in this region; if they are asked to point with their finger at the object, patients point past it. Explanation of this phenomenon involves some mismatch among the afferent retinal signs, the efferent innervational signs, and possibly the gamma efferents associated with the muscle spindles (Ludvigh, 1952b). A cumbersome form of adaptation is believed to result from eventual use of voluntary effort. Lesions of the vestibular apparatus cause a swimming motion of the environment that is correlated with the slow phase of nystagmoid movement of the eyes (Cogan, 1966). For a more thorough discussion of the role of outflow and inflow in the stabilization of visual perceptions, see Matin (1975).

Notes

1. The binocular center of projection also can be considered to be located on the Vieth-Mueller circle at the point of intersection with the perpendicular bisector of the interpupillary line (Jones, 1980).

REFERENCES

Alpern, M. (1969), "Specification of the direction of regard," *The Eye*, vol. 3, Academic, New York, 5–12.

Andersen, E. E., and Weymouth, F. W. (1923), "Visual perception and the retinal mosaic," *American Journal of Physiology*, 64, 561–591.

Andrews, D. P. (1967), "Perception of contour orientation in the central fovea; Part II, Spatial integration," *Vision Research*, 7, 999–1013.

Barlow, H. B. (1963), "Slippage of contact lenses and other artifacts in relation to fading and regeneration of supposedly stable images," *Quarterly Journal of Experimental Psychology*, 15, 36–51.

Brown, K. T. (1953), "Factors affecting differences in apparent size between opposite halves of a visual meridian," *Journal of the Optical Society of America*, 43, 464–472.

Cline, D., Hofstetter, H. W., and Griffin, J. R. (1980), *Dictionary of Visual Science*, Chilton, Philadelphia, 10.

Cogan, D. G. (1966), *Neurology of the Extraocular Muscles*, Charles C Thomas, Springfield, Ill., 184–239.

Cornsweet, T. N. (1970), *Visual Perception*, Academic, New York, 312–364.

Ditchburn, R. W. (1973), *Eye Movements and Visual Perception*, Clarendon Press, Oxford, 275–284.

Fender, D. H., and Nye, P. W. (1962), "The effects of retinal image motion in a single pattern recognition task," *Kybernetik*, 1, 192–199.

Flom, M. C., Weymouth, F.W., and Kahneman, P. (1963), "Visual resolution and contour interaction," *Journal of the Optical Society of America*, 53, 1026–1032.

Freeman, R. D. (1966), "Alignment detection and resolution as a function of retinal location," *American Journal of Optometry*, 43, 812–817.

Fry, G. H. (1961), "Eye-body co-ordination in the perception of space," *Transactions of the International Ophthalmic Optical Congress*, Crosby-Lockwood, London, 16–33.

Graham, C. H. (1965), "Visual space perception," *Vision and Visual Perception*, Wiley, New York, 504–547.

Heath, G. G. (1953), personal communciation.

Helmholtz, H. (1925), *Handbook of Physiological Optics*, vol. 3, Optical Society of America, New York, 124–127.

Henson, D. B. (1976), "Investigation into corrective saccadic eye movements," Ph.D. thesis, Indiana University, Bloomington.

Hering, E. (1942), *Spatial Sense and Movements of the Eyes*, American Academy of Optometry, Baltimore, 38–43.

Holmes, G. (1918), "Disturbances of vision by cerebral lesions," *British Journal of Ophthalmology*, 2, 353–384.

Hubel, D. H., and Wiesel, T. N. (1962), "Receptive fields, binocular interaction, and functional architecture in the cat's visual cortex," *Journal of Physiology*, 160, 106–154.

Johnson, C. A., Keltner, J. L., and Balestrery, F. (1978), "Effects of target size and eccentricity on visual detection and recognition," *Vision Research,* 18, 1217–1222.

Jones, R. (1980), personal communication.

Keesey, U. T. (1960), "Effects of involuntary eye movements on visual acuity," *Journal of the Optical Society of America,* 50, 769–774.

LeGrand, Y. (1967), *Form and Space Vision,* Indiana University, Bloomington, 139, 220–202, 232–233, 237.

Ludvigh, E. (1952a), "Possible role of proprioception in the extraocular muscles," *Archives of Ophthalmology,* 48, 436–441.

Ludvigh, E. (1952b), "Control of ocular movements and visual interpretation of the environment," *Archives of Ophthalmology,* 48, 442–448.

Ludvigh, E. (1953), "Direction sense of the eye," *American Journal of Ophthalmology,* 36, 139–143.

Luneburg, R. K. (1950), "The metric of binocular space," *Journal of the Optical Society of America,* 40, 627–642.

MacKay, D. M. (1970), "Elevation of visual threshold by displacement of retinal image," *Nature,* 225, 90–92.

Mandelbaum, J., and Sloan, L. L. (1947), "Peripheral visual acuity," *American Journal of Ophthalmology,* 30, 581–588.

Masterton, R. B., and Glendenning, K. K. (1978), "Phylogeny of the vertebrate sensory systems," *Handbook of Behavioral Neurobiology,* vol. 1, Plenum, New York, 1–38.

Matin, L. (1975), "Eye movements and perceived visual direction," *Handbook of Sensory Physiology,* vol. VII/4, Springer-Verlag, Berlin, 332–340.

Ogle, K. N. (1950), *Researches in Binocular Vision,* Saunders, Philadelphia, 10–17.

Ogle, K. N. (1962), "Spatial localization through binocular vision," *The Eye,* vol. 4, Academic, New York, 271–324.

Prichard, R. M., Heron, W., and Hebb, D. O. (1960), "Visual perception approached by method of stabilized images," *Canadian Journal of Psychology,* 14, 67–76.

Randall, H. G., Brown, D. J., and Sloan, L. L. (1966), "Peripheral visual acuity," *Archives of Ophthalmology,* 75, 500–504.

Riggs, L. A. (1965), "Visual acuity," *Vision and Visual Perception,* Wiley, New York, 321–349.

Riggs, L. A., Armington, J. C., and Ratliff, F. (1954), "Motions of the retinal image during fixation," *Journal of the Optical Society of America,* 44, 315–321.

Robinson, D. A. (1972), "Eye movements evoked by collicular stimulation in the alert monkey," *Vision Research,* 12, 1795–1808.

Sherman, H. L. (1947), *Drawing by Seeing,* Hinds, Hayden, and Eldredge, New York.

Stigmar, G. (1970), "Observations on vernier and stereo acuity with special reference to their relationship," *Acta Ophthalmologica,* 48, 979–998.

Stockley, L. A. F., and Jenkins, T. C. A. (1970), "An analysis of binocular visual acuities," *Transactions of the International Ophthalmic Optical Congress,* British Optical Association, London, 420–428.

Tschermak, A. (1952), *Introduction to Physiological Optics,* Charles C Thomas, Springfield, Ill., 135–140.

Walls, G. L. (1943), "Factors in human visual resolution," *Journal of the Optical Society of America,* 33, 487–505.

Walls, G. L. (1954), "The filling-in process," *American Journal of Optometry,* 31, 329–341.

6

VISUAL DISTANCE: EMPIRICAL CUES AND STEREOPSIS

> The attention paid to an instructor is a constant regardless of the size of the class. Thus as class size swells, the amount of attention paid per student drops in direct ratio.
>
> *Richard Herrnstein*

DISTANCE DISCRIMINATION

Stereopsis is a perceptual phenomenon that provides rather precise information about an object's distance relative to another object. Sometimes in the interest of simplifying communications, optometrists use the term *depth perception* as synonymous with *stereopsis*. However, the ease with which one-eyed people, clearly deprived of stereopsis, can perform many tasks involving judgments of depth indicates that there is much more to depth perception than is implied by the process known as stereopsis. Certainly depth can be appreciated in two-dimensional displays such as photographs, paintings, and television pictures. Animals with very little or no binocular overlap can perform some amazingly fine, spatially guided activities (Walls, 1942).

From what characteristics of the world around us does such information come? What sort of information is it? How good is it? The various bits of information are often called *cues*, like those of an actor. Cues are considered empirical because they are acquired by experience. Sometimes the information is referred to as *clues*, as in a mystery story, and described as monocular because it does not require binocular vision. These various descriptions imply a series of different stimulus relationships that somehow produce an overall impression of depth. While this impression is usually quite good, it can be fooled by a clever arrangement of objects or other novel stimulus conditions (Ogle, 1962a).

APPARENT SIZE

Apparent size refers to the fact that the size of an object, as determined by the difference in the visual directions of its extreme parts, is a function of apparent distance. In Figure 6–1, if we know how far *A* is from *B*, because it is a familiar object, we can surmise the distance from *B* to *C* because these dimensions are related geometrically by the tangent of the angle θ, the visual angle. This is not to say that failing to know of the tangent relationship precludes the use of this information. What it does imply is that if we see a person far away, the perception of that person's size will constitute a very small part of the visual field. If the person is close at hand, the apparent size will constitute a larger portion of the field even though, of course, the physical size remains constant. Through experience with this kind of situation, the observer learns to interpret changes in apparent size of familiar objects as meaning that an object of constant physical size has been moved to different distances.

For unfamiliar objects, the distance estimate can be grossly in error. Furthermore, as shown in Figure 6–2, if shape and position can be adjusted, an infinite number of object locations can be made to produce identical retinal images, and the cue can become totally unreliable (Ogle, 1962a).

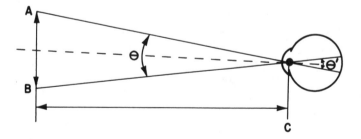

Figure 6–1.   The visual angle, θ, and the size-distance relationship.

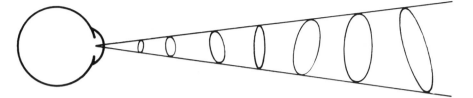

Figure 6–2.   Different shapes, slants, and distances of objects producing the
same size and shape of the retinal image.

SIZE CONSTANCY

In everyday activities, there is an additional factor in the size-distance
relationship called *size constancy*. A familiar object tends to be judged
the same size no matter at what distance it is seen. For this to happen,
the retinal image size must be supplanted in the decision-making process by a familiarity with the real size of the object. Figure 6–3 illustrates
one aspect of this relationship.

Holway and Boring (1941) conducted an experiment to study size
constancy. They arranged for the observer to see two objects, one sit-
uated at a fixed distance, which could be adjusted in size by an observer
and is called the *test object*, and the other, called the *standard object*,
presented at various distances with its size adjusted by the experimenter
so that it always subtends a constant visual angle.

If an observer sets the size of the test object on the basis of the
visual angle, then the setting will not have to be altered as the standard
object is presented at different distances. Plotting distance of the standard object as the independent variable and size of the test object as
the dependent variable will produce a straight line parallel to the abscissa. However, if an observer matches the size of the test object to
that of the standard object independent of its distance, then the settings
will fall along a line with a positive slope. After the abscissa is rescaled
in terms of the size of the standard object, the slope of this data line
should be equal to 1 when size constancy determines the results.

Figure 6–4 shows the result of such an experiment. When the view
was unrestricted, the data tended to follow the prediction for size constancy. When the field was restricted to test and standard objects, the
data approached the prediction based on visual angle. If this seems
confusing, consider another kind of experimental design in which the
standard object has a fixed size and is displayed at different distances
while the observer matches the size of a test object to it. Figure 6–5
shows the expected results. The advantage of this alternate example is

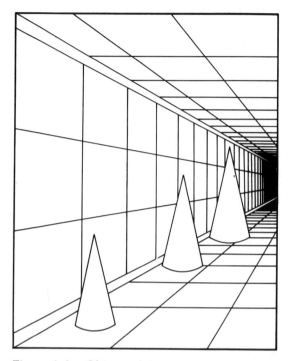

Figure 6–3.   Objects of the same physical size appear larger when set into the
context of geometric perspective cues.

that the size constancy data now plot along a line of zero slope, as does any mathematical constant.

This experiment also illustrates that under normal conditions observers tend to demonstrate size constancy; but when size is the only cue, the visual angle forms the basis for perception. Furthermore, Brunswick (1949) reported that attitude changes can greatly influence which of these two perceptual sets predominates. Introspection, or an analytic approach, such as might be used by an artist attempting to reproduce a scene, favors the visual angle mode, whereas everyday activity, which is usually more synthetic and holistic, favors the constancy mode.

To get distance information out of this relationship, we can consider that the subject compares the apparent size as determined by the visual angle with some kind of memory image of the real size of the object. Obviously this kind of operation depends on object recognition, familiarity, and experience.

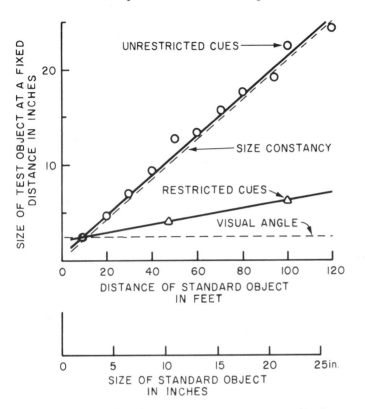

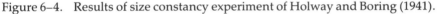

Figure 6–4. Results of size constancy experiment of Holway and Boring (1941).

SHAPE CONSTANCY

Shape constancy presents an analogous cue to that of size constancy. Thouless (1931) found that an ellipse, described by the ratio of the length of the short axis to that of the long axis, which matched a circle viewed at various olbique angles followed the predictions based on the visual angle when other cues were reduced and demonstrated constancy when they were not.

ABSOLUTE AND RELATIVE DISTANCE JUDGMENTS

Another important aspect involving all distance perceptions is the judgment of absolute distance as distinct from relative distance. Absolute distance involves estimating the distance of an object from the egocen-

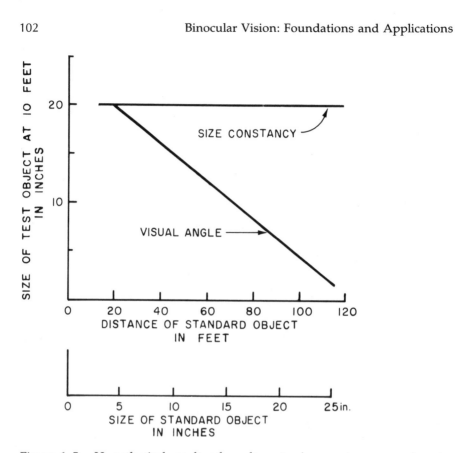

Figure 6–5.   Hypothetical results of an alternate size constancy experiment.

ter, whereas relative distance judgments refer to the relationship of distances among objects. Relative depth information would indicate, for example, which of two targets is closer to the observer without necessarily providing any hint about the absolute distance of either.

We have only to recall how easily the visual system can be fooled about the level of absolute brightness (Cornsweet, 1970) to suggest that absolute depth cues can be most inaccurate and subject to significant systematic errors as a result of a lack of experience in a particular local environment. However, as with judgments involving absolute brightness, judgments about absolute depth cues can be bettered by trial and error.

In addition, the nature of the response required of a subject to determine the veridicality of absolute distance judgments usually involves some complex visual-motor interactions. For objects in the immediate surround, some means of touching the object with a hand and arm screened from the subject's view has been used (Fry, 1961). For greater distances, either a verbal response estimating distances in feet and inches (or meters and centimeters) (Hamilton, 1964) or some other behavioral response, such as throwing darts in an alleyway screened from the visual objects, has been used (Gogel, 1962). Within the range of several meters of a subject, this perception is different depending on whether or not the eyes of the observer are allowed to fixate on the various targets (Fry, 1950).

It would seem that absolute depth can be mediated by such cues as apparent size, aerial perspective, and geometric perspective, whereas interposition, motion parallax, and light, shade, and shadow appear to contribute only relative depth information, as does stereopsis.

RELATIVE DISTANCE JUDGMENTS BASED ON APPARENT SIZE

Experimental studies of relative distance judgments using the size cue show that the smallest change in linear distance that can be detected increases with increasing test distance. This increase is such that the ratio of the incremental threshold distance to the distance of the object from the observer is roughly a constant, another example of Weber's law (Ogle, 1962a). However, at large distances, beyond about 30 m, the value of the fraction begins to increase. This fact has led investigators to suggest that visual space is bounded, which simply means that objects beyond some distant point are not seen to be significantly farther from the observer than is this limiting surface (Hering, 1942). The location of this boundary varies depending on the conditions used to determine it. For example, the boundary would be different for a subject looking up at a night sky full of stars than for a subject tested in the hallway of a small office.

Figure 6–6 presents the data of Teichner et al. (1955), which show some of the scatter produced in different surroundings. These are the results of an experiment in which the subject sees a standard target at a fixed distance and a test target that is slowly moved until the subject reports that it is a different size, which means that a detectable difference in distance exists between the two targets. Evaluation of this and other data indicate that the size cue is capable of signaling changes in distance as small as 1 percent of the total viewing distance. Under optimum conditions, a good observer can report a size change when a test target is at 101 or 99 cm and a standard target is at 100 cm. This experiment requires that the observer make these judgments while viewing the targets monocularly in order to prevent stereopsis from

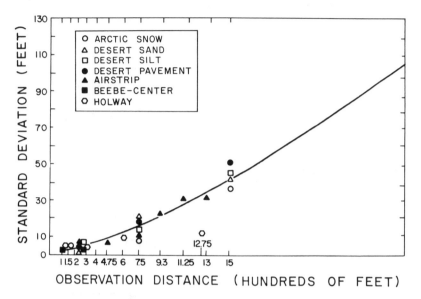

Figure 6–6.   Data gathered from a number of surroundings illustrate the sensitivity of the size-distance relationship as a function of distance (Reprinted by permission from Teichner et al., 1955).

functioning, for, as we will see, stereopsis is considerably more accurate than size, up to a certain viewing distance.

For everyday viewing, detection at the 1 percent level is too fine a judgment to expect. This can be demonstrated by monocularly viewing through a 1 percent overall magnification lens and noting how hard it is to see any change in the appearance of the surround. Perhaps a 2 or 3 percent size change is a more operational level for this cue.

INTERPOSITION (OVERLAY)

When two objects are almost lined up and viewed from a particular position, the relatively nearer object will conceal a part of the relatively farther object, as seen in Figure 6–7. This figure also shows that ambiguous discontinuities in the outlines of representations such as these can produce paradoxical perceptions of space (Graham, 1965). Couple overlay with vernier judgments and a potentially powerful space cue is created. This is so because very small offsets can be detected and usually overlay can indicate the relative depth involved.

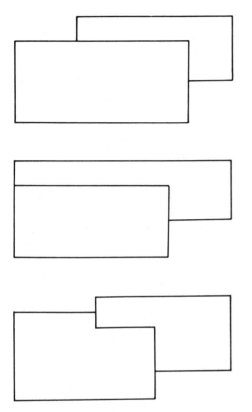

Figure 6–7.   Overlay, or interposition.

AERIAL PERSPECTIVE

Among other things, the atmosphere contains water vapor, smoke, and dust. These particles tend to scatter light, so that the longer the path-length of light through the atmosphere, the less distinct will be the contours of objects and the less saturated will be their colors. Green-horns have been known to spend hours tracking toward mountains in the Rockies that appeared to their pollution-conditioned perceptions to be a short hike away. They have been fooled because the relatively clear, less dense atmosphere of these Western mountainous regions causes judgments of absolute distance to be in error (LeGrand, 1967).

LIGHT, SHADE, AND SHADOW

The pattern of light and shade as it falls on solid objects provides an effective cue to enhance the impression of depth. The shading imparts a three-dimensional texture to objects. Light, usually coming from above, is blocked by objects creating shadows which help us to detect the relative depth of things. Furthermore, the brighter of two objects will usually appear closer (Gibson, 1950).

GEOMETRIC PERSPECTIVE

The factors comprising geometric perspective include size cue, overlay, and light, shade, and shadow. Geometric perspective deals with the geometric attributes of projecting three-dimensional space onto a two-dimensional surface. This projection takes place through a center of projection, also known as the *station point* (Ogle, 1962a), and represents physically parallel lines converging toward the horizon onto a vanishing point, as well as a decrease in detail and a crowding of picture elements, called *gradients* (Gibson, 1950).

Photographs and television pictures use all these various empirical cues to impart a sense of depth to the display. To enhance this impression of depth, view them with one eye closed, so as to suspend the stereoscopic impression of the picture plane, and adjust the viewing distance so that the entrance pupil of the eye roughly coincides with the station point of the camera lens used to create it. This viewing position minimizes distortions and is at a distance that roughly equals the diagonal dimension of the screen or picture, if the lens used was a so-called normal focal-length lens. For scenes that have been enlarged or reduced by using a telephoto or wide-angle lens, this distance is altered (Ogle, 1962a). For a more detailed discussion of some of these aspects of geometric perspective, see, for example, Pirenne (1970). Figure 6–8 depicts some of these principles.

ROLE OF MOTION PERCEPTION IN THE APPRECIATION OF DEPTH

The visual system operates on the basis of detecting changes in stimulus size, position, brightness, etc. Many of these changes can contribute to the perception of motion. It would appear that object identification or recognition is not required; rather, the system considers that successive views in time represent movement of components such as points, lines, or other local constituents, based on an affinity to identify such parts with one another and so extract the changing position as the result of a movement (Ullman, 1979).

For foveal vision, the slowest movement detectable is usually cited

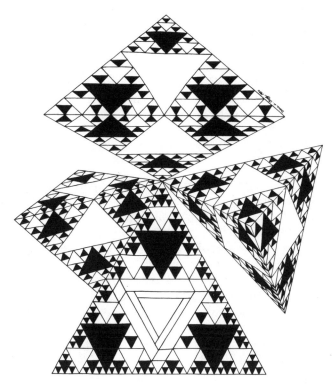

Figure 6–8. A drawing by Diane Jung, 1980, illustrates some attributes of geometric perspective cues used to create the impression of depth.

as 1 arcminute/s. In the periphery this is elevated to about 34 arcminutes/s at an eccentricity of 20° (McColgin, 1960). At optimal speeds, the minimum detectable displacement is similar to the vernier threshold at the fovea, but lower in the periphery (LeGrand, 1967). Apparently this relative enhancement of displacement detection of moving objects in the periphery acts as an early-warning device that invites voluntary saccades to bring the target onto the fovea to facilitate recognition.

With small displacements of bright objects moving slowly over the peripheral retina, both a critical distance and time exist. This conforms to Bloch's law, and such targets stimulate vision in a manner equivalent to a stationary stimulus of an equal number of quanta (Bouman and van den Brink, 1953). This sets a lower limit on motion detection in these regions.

Gibson (1950) considered that both direction and distance judgments made by an observer moving through space were facilitated by the velocity flow, which necessarily causes apparent shape changes as objects accelerate radially from a focus at the point to which the movement is directed. Regan and Cynader (1979) demonstrated that certain cells found in the visual cortex of the cat respond to changes in size. Regan and Beverley (1979) found the psychophysical function of such cells in the human cortex. Such dynamic changes in perceived size are considered quite useful in automobile driving (Allen, 1970).

MOTION PARALLAX

The relative motion of two or more points that accompanies lateral displacements is called *motion parallax*. The term is familiar to optometrists who use it to locate features in the ocular media of the eye. This same localization by relative motion operates in the everyday world. Figure 6–9A shows an eye looking at three objects that are lined up laterally on the primary line of sight. Figure 6–9B indicates how the situation changes when the eye moves a small distance to the left while maintaining fixation on the middle target. The speed and direction of the apparent movement of the near and far targets yield information as to their relative locations.

Figure 6–9C shows a composite view by using two targets with the appropriate angles labeled. This diagram represents the angular change as the eye moves through the distance s. Then, when s = distance, v = velocity, and t = time,

$$\rho = \theta - \theta' \tag{6-1}$$

and $\quad s = vt \tag{6-2}$

so $\quad \theta = \dfrac{d_1}{vt} \quad$ and $\quad \theta' = \dfrac{d_2}{vt} \tag{6-3}$

Thus $\quad \rho = \dfrac{d_1}{vt} - \dfrac{d_2}{vt} \quad$ or $\quad \rho = \dfrac{d_1}{s} - \dfrac{d_2}{s} \tag{6-4}$

If we restrict the velocity to exclude very slow and very fast movements, then a threshold angle ρ_t can be determined (Ogle, 1962a). Parallax sensitivity turns out to be quite good, and it is useful in sorting out space relationships in otherwise ambiguous surroundings (Graham, 1965). Certain animals use it to good advantage and as a substitute for stereopsis (Walls, 1942).

COMPARISON OF SOME DEPTH CUES

Some of these various cues can be expressed in terms of thresholds. In Table 6–1 we compare these. Table 6–1 shows angular thresholds and

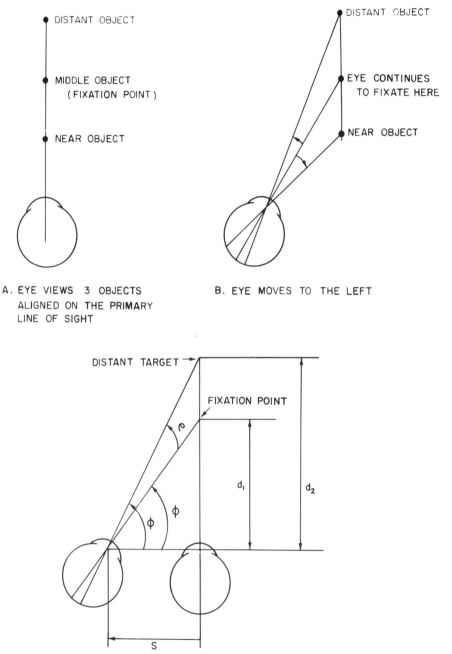

Figure 6–9.   Various aspects of motion parallax.

Table 6–1.   Comparison of Threshold Values

Cue	Typical Thresholds (arcseconds), Graham (1965) and Ogle (1962b)	Percentage Δd
Vernier	2 to 5	0.06 to 0.14
Stereopsis	6 to 10	0.17 to 0.27
Parallax	7 to 28	0.19 to 0.78
Size	—	1.0 to 3.0

equivalent Δd values for a viewing distance of 100 cm. These are typical threshold values that are cited in the literature. This does not mean that vernier thresholds are really better than stereopsis or parallax. It is safest to consider all three as about equally accurate. Size cues are extremely gross by comparison at this distance, but size plays an important part in helping us to sense distance under certain circumstances.

OTHER ATTRIBUTES SOMETIMES CONSIDERED CUES

From time to time other ocular functions are designated as cues to the perception of depth. Among these are accommodation, convergence, and proprioception (Ogle, 1962a).

The single fact that makes it unlikely that accommodation can act as a useful cue is its relative imprecision. The depth of focus, lag of accommodation, and microfluctuations (Alpern, 1969) all combine to produce a maximum sensitivity of about ±0.50. At the far end of the range, this would be equivalent to a linear range of 2 m to infinity. At 40 cm (2.5 D) a range of imprecision is produced of some 17 cm (from 50 to 33 cm), or a Δd of some 43 percent. With all the other more accurate cues to depth available, it is hard to see what a cue of this poor precision could contribute to the perception of distance (Ogle, 1962a).

Convergence presents a similar picture (Graham, 1965). Even though convergence is a binocular cue, it is a minor one at best (Gogel, 1962). Rashbass and Westheimer (1961) suggested that convergence changes are always correct as to direction and magnitude even though the subject is verbally reporting an incorrect location of target position. Furthermore, Stewart (1951) found that this is so, even when other depth cues would lead to opposite spatial judgments from those provided by binocular disparity. These results imply that the information used to control the movement of the eyes in convergence is unavailable to the perceptual system.

Other experiments have demonstrated that proprioception associated with the extraocular muscles is subconscious. The data from the muscle spindles modify the innervation to the muscle without entering directly into consciousness (Ludvigh, 1952).

STEREOPSIS

Stereopsis is the apparently innate, direct, simple sensation of the depth dimension. All the factors listed as empirical infer that a third dimension exists, but stereopsis provides a direct means of appreciating or sensing it (Ogle, 1962b). For the majority of the population, a simple demonstration of its existence suffices. For the others, no amount of effort to explain or demonstrate it seems sufficient.

Operational Formula for Calculating Binocular Disparity

The stimulus attribute that leads to the perception of stereopsis is binocular disparity. Here we refer to binocular disparity in the most general sense as that angular disparity between any two object points in the field of view. Figure 6–10A shows the two eyes viewing two objects and labels the appropriate angles used in the specification of binocular disparity. From this figure note that

$$\eta = \alpha - \alpha' \tag{6-5}$$

where η is the binocular disparity angle and α and α' are the binocular subtense angles. Since

$$\alpha = \frac{2a}{d} \quad \text{and} \quad \alpha' = \frac{2a}{d + \Delta d} \quad \text{in radians} \tag{6-6}$$

we know

$$\eta = \frac{2a}{d} - \frac{2a}{d + \Delta d} \tag{6-7}$$

which is equivalent to

$$\eta = \frac{2a\,\Delta d}{d^2 + d\,\Delta d} \tag{6-8}$$

When the binocular disparity is at the threshold level, the term $d\,\Delta d$ is small and for most purposes insignificant; it can be dropped with almost no loss of accuracy. Therefore, the binocular disparity in radian measure is

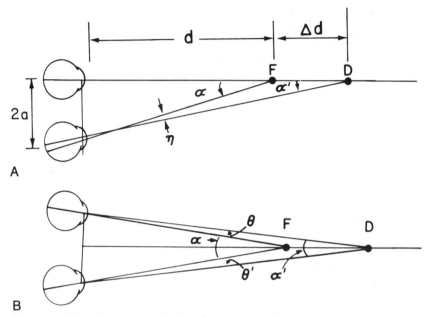

Figure 6–10.   Geometric relationships involved in binocular disparity.

$$\eta = \frac{2a \, \Delta d}{d^2} \tag{6–9}$$

To convert to arcseconds,

$$\frac{180}{\pi} = 57.296 \times 360 = 206{,}265 \text{ arcseconds/rad} \tag{6–10}$$

So the operational formula becomes

$$\eta = \frac{2a \, \Delta d}{d^2} \, 206{,}265 \text{ arcseconds} \tag{6–11}$$

Figure 6–10B shows the specification of binocular disparity for objects located along the midsagittal plane and relates binocular subtense angles to angles of eccentricity or retinal angles.

Our main interest is in η when it is at the threshold level. This sort of threshold can be determined by a number of psychophysical methods.

PSYCHOPHYSICAL METHODS OF MEASURING THE THRESHOLD OF STEREOPSIS

In discussing the basic methods of psychophysics as applied to measuring the threshold of stereopsis, we refer to the apparatus of Howard and Dolman (Howard, 1919). It consists of two rods, one movable and the other fixed, mounted behind a rectangular aperture that obscures the ends of the rods and in front of a plane background. Figure 6–11 shows the various aspects of such an apparatus.

Method of Adjustments

The method of adjustments (Gescheider, 1976) requires that the experimenter place the movable rod at some offset position and allow the observer to position it at a location judged equidistant from the fixed rod. This process is repeated, say six times, with randomly chosen amounts and directions of offset. The results produce a small scatter of the settings which can best be characterized by its mean deviation. The mean deviation, then, constitutes the Δd value in Equation (6–11) and, together with the interpupillary distance (P.D.) of the observer and the distance from the observer to the fixed rod, provides sufficient information to calculate the threshold of stereopsis. Table 6–2 shows a set of data gathered and analyzed in this way.

Method of Limits

For the method of limits (Gescheider, 1976), the observer is asked to judge when the movable rod is just noticeably different (JND) in distance from the fixed rod. The average range is used as the Δd value in Equation (6–11). Table 6–3 illustrates this.

Method of Constant Stimuli

The method of constant stimuli is considerd the most accurate of all the classical methods of psychophysics. It is the standard method with which all others are compared and upon which the various theories of thresholds for a number of different visual functions are based (Gescheider, 1976). Unfortunately, this method is too time-consuming to use in a clinical setting, although modifications of the usual procedure

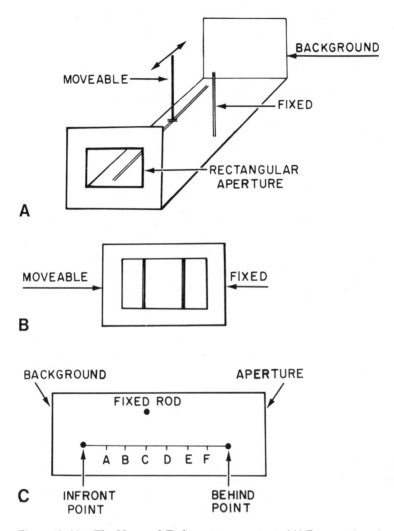

Figure 6–11. The Howard-Dolman two-peg test. *(A)* Perspective view. *(B)* View
seen by the subject. *(C)* Plan detail showing 100 percent correct
response points and division of resulting interval into six positions, to be used in determining the threshold by the method of
constant stimuli.

have been suggested for specialized clinical testing of both visual acuity
(Sloan, 1968) and stereopsis (Hofstetter and Bertsch, 1976).

For stereopsis thresholds, the usual technique consists of first finding a position of the movable rod that is always seen as closer than the

Table 6–2. Determining the Threshold of Stereopsis by the Method of Adjustment

Trial Number	Initial Offset	Movable-Rod Setting (m)	Deviation from Mean
1	Front	3.02	0.02
2	Behind	3.03	0.03
3	Front	2.98	0.02
4	Behind	2.99	0.01
5	Front	2.97	0.03
6	Behind	3.00	0.00

Mean = 3.00 Mean deviation = 0.02

$$\eta = \frac{0.064 \times 0.02 \times 206{,}265}{9} = 29.34 \text{ arcseconds}$$

Interpupillary distance P.D. (I.D.) = 64 mm; test distance = 3 m.

Table 6–3. Determining the Threshold of Stereopsis by the Method of Limits

Trial Number	JND Nearer (m)	JND Farther (m)	Range (m)
1	3.98	—	0.02
2	—	4.02	0.02
3	3.99	—	0.01
4	—	4.01	0.01
5	3.95	—	0.05
6	—	4.04	0.04
7	3.96	—	0.04
8	—	4.03	0.03
9	3.97	—	0.03
10	—	4.06	0.04

I.D. = 64 mm   d = 4.00   Average range = 2.90 mm

$$\eta = \frac{0.064 \times 0.029 \times 206{,}265}{16} = 23.93 \text{ arcseconds}$$

fixed rod and then finding a position in which it is always seen as farther than the fixed rod. This range is divided into five or six equal intervals, and the movable rod is presented to an observer in these positions a certain number of times following a random ordering of positions. Figure 6–11C and Table 6–4 present an example of the layout of the apparatus and the type of data generated by using this method. Note that each of the observer's responses is forced into one or the other of the two categories.

From the percentage of near responses for each position, a graph such as Figure 6–12 is prepared. Far responses could be used also. When the points are connected by straight lines, we can estimate the mean and standard deviation of the data, assuming that the curve generated is a reasonable approximation of a cumulative normal frequency distribution (Ogive). The estimate of the mean is the value on the abscissa that corresponds to the 50 percent response level. One standard deviation above the mean is at the 84 percent level, and one standard deviation below is at 16 percent value (Ogle, 1962b). Figure 6–12 illustrates this. In this example, the standard deviations are $+3.25$ and -5.75 cm. Theoretically these should be equal, and they would be more nearly so if a cumulative normal frequency curve had been fitted to the data. However, a part of this inequality is the result of the relatively high number of near responses that occurred when the target was in positions D, E, and F. For simplicity, we average these two estimates as our Δd value and calculate the threshold. By using these data, an interpupillary distance of 64 mm, and a test distance of 6 m, we find η_t equal to 16.5 arcseconds.

Because estimates as made above are best refined by nonlinear curve fitting, which is complicated, analysis can be facilitated by transforming percentage of responses to produce a first-order function. This can be done on probability graph paper in which percentages are spaced out according to Z scores of a normal cumulative frequency distribution

Table 6–4.   Sample Response Tally and Percentage of Near Responses for Movable-Rod Positions in Figure 6–11c in Random Order for 20 Trials at Each Position

Movable-Rod Position (cm)		Number of In-front Responses	Number of Behind Responses	Percentage of Near Responses
A	-4	18	2	90
B	-2	15	5	75
C	0	10	10	50
D	$+2$	9	11	45
E	$+4$	5	15	25
F	$+6$	3	17	15

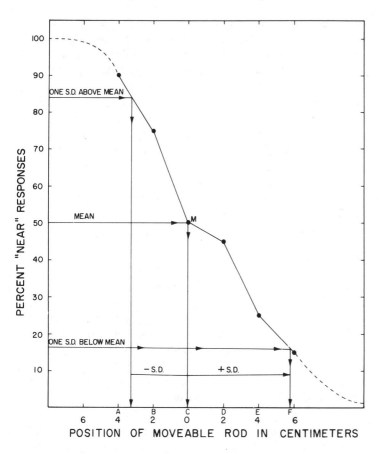

Figure 6–12.   Percentage of near responses as a function of the movable rod.

(Crow et al., 1960). Another approach is to convert percentages to probits. Probits are Z scores plus a constant (5), which renders all values as greater than zero (Finney, 1947). The advantage of these refinements is mainly in terms of maximizing the accuracy of the threshold estimates and the ease with which departures from linearity can be detected. Nonlinearity indicates that some contaminating factors are influencing the judgments. A probability plot is analyzed as described earlier. In probit analysis, the reciprocal of the slope is the estimate of the standard deviation.

In addition to its accuracy, the constant-stimuli method produces an estimate of the equidistant point. At this point the subject is most likely to see the movable rod as being at the same absolute distance as the fixed rod, and it corresponds to the 50 percent point. Displacement of this position from the physically equidistant point can reflect a response bias or an inequality in the size of the two ocular images in the horizontal meridian. The latter is known as a form of *aniseikonia* (see Chapter 13). Furthermore, this point is subject to the influence of depth cues other than binocular disparity. For example, if the fixed rod is made larger than the movable rod, then this equidistant position is shifted to a point closer to the observer than the point occupied when both rods were the same size (Hirsch et al., 1948). In this instance a monocular size cue has influenced the perception of stereopsis (see Chapters 8 and 13).

Staircase Method

A modified method of limits has been proposed by Cornsweet (1962). First the subject is presented with a large binocular disparity. If it is correctly judged, the next disparity presented has a lower value. If the initial response is incorrect, the disparity is increased. Continuing to reduce the disparity in steps, as long as the subject's responses are correct, and increasing it when he or she is wrong produce a method of tracking the threshold. Figure 6–13 illustrates such a record for threshold data reported by Stigmar (1970) which give the appearance of a staircase.

Because the subject may learn to anticipate the changes in disparity, Cornsweet suggested that the double random staircase be used. This consists of an ascending and a descending series interposed by some random process. For stereopsis, this would consist of designing a crossed-to-uncrossed step function and another for uncrossed-to-crossed values. These two intertwining series will converge on a relatively constant value and then track around the equidistant point. Thus the standard deviation of these judgments would be equal to the threshold, where the disparities used are directly specified. Staircase methods lend themselves to computer control, and automated devices designed to measure stereopsis are currently employed in several specialized clinical facilities in the United States.

SOME STIMULUS PARAMETERS

Other factors have been shown to influence the stereoscopic threshold. These include the angular size of the test objects, the luminance of the

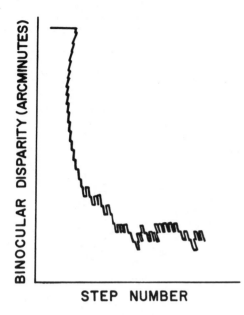

STEP NUMBER

Figure 6–13.   Staircase method applied to measuring the threshold of stereopsis (replotted from Stigmar, 1970).

background, the duration of the presentation, and the region of the retinas stimulated (Amigo, 1964).

Angular Size

Figure 6–14 presents the data of Anderson and Weymouth (1923), which show the change in threshold size that results from using objects of different angular size. Note that as the target is made longer, the threshold values decrease, up to an angular size of about 30 arcminutes. The apparatus consists of three rods; the center rod is movable, and is the one on which the subject was asked to fixate. Two fixed rods are separated laterally at an angular distance of about 26 arcminutes. For larger angular sizes, no significant change in threshold occurred. We can relate this information to retinal topography. With increasing angular size the threshold decreases until it reaches a size roughly equal to the subtense angle of each fovea. Further increases have no effect on the threshold of stereopsis.

In this figure, as with various other illustrations, the threshold is plotted on a logarithmic arcsecond scale. While this information also

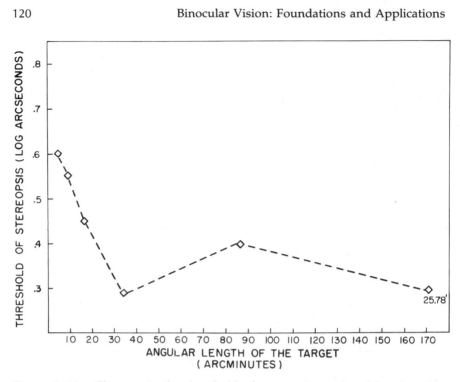

Figure 6–14. Changes in the threshold of stereopsis produced by changing
the angular length of the test objects (replotted from Andersen
and Weymouth, 1923).

can be displayed on a linear scale, the log scale magnified the differences
at the lower end. Because the thresholds involved are so small, this
scale proves the most informative and is widely used (Hofstetter, 1968).

Background Luminance

Figure 6–15 presents the data of Lit (1959) which show how the threshold of stereopsis decreases when it is tested in increasingly bright surroundings. The subject was fully adapted to each level of retinal
illuminance before thresholds were determined. This figure shows that
stereopsis at scotopic levels is a much less sensitive judgment. It also
shows a further increase in sensitivity from the cone detection threshold
up to a level of about 10 trolands.

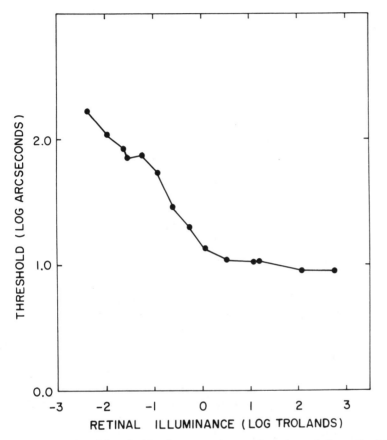

Figure 6–15. Threshold of stereopsis as a function of the retinal illuminance of the background (replotted from Lit, 1959).

Duration

Figure 6–16 presents data from a study by Ogle and Weil (1958) which show that the threshold of stereopsis changes as a function of the presentation time over a range of exposures from about 7.5 to about 1000 ms. The investigators attempted to use these data as evidence to support a dynamic theory of stereoscopic acuity, which is an extension of the mean local sign theory discussed previously. Shortess and Krauskopf (1961) repeated this experiment, using both stabilized and normal viewing conditions, and found no significant differences between thresholds measured under these two conditions. As previously pointed out, this tells us nothing about the actual role of scanning.

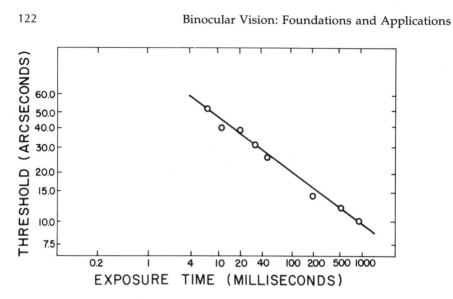

Figure 6–16.   Threshold of stereopsis as a function of exposure time of test
objects (replotted from Ogle and Weil, 1958, and reprinted by
permission from Archives of Ophthalmology 1958;59:4–17.
Copyright 1958, American Medical Association).

The fact that the threshold decreases as the exposure time increases
may be due to the effect somewhat similar to that known as Bloch's
law. The stereoscopic mechanism, like other perceptual phenomena,
requires a certain critical exposure to achieve its greatest sensitivity.
Longer exposures than this critical value produce no additional gain,
whereas shorter ones produce a less sensitive response (Riggs, 1965).
Such a mechanism is thought to be independent of the influences of
eye movements.

Eccentricity

Most stereopsis data are obtained by using a two-rod apparatus as
described earlier. The subject fixates one of the rods while judging the
relative position of the other, which is located at a variable lateral displacement. This has the effect of imaging one rod on more and more
peripheral retinal points. Figure 6–17 presents data from studies by
Hirsch and Weymouth (1948) and Ogle (1950) which indicate the expected rise in the stereoscopic threshold as the movable target is positioned in more peripheral parts of the field. The slight trend for the
thresholds to fall and then rise at small separations also was found by
Stigmar (1970) for vertically separated test objects (see Chapter 5).

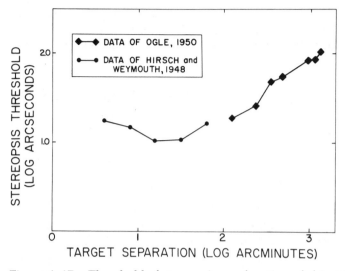

Figure 6–17.   Threshold of stereopsis as a function of object (target) separation [replotted from Hirsch and Weymouth (1948) and Ogle (1950)].

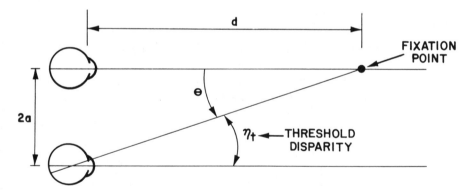

Figure 6–18.   Absolute limiting distance for stereopsis is determined by geometric relationships presented here.

Limiting Distance

Because stereopsis depends on binocular disparity, which in turn depends on the fact that the eyes are laterally separated, there exists a distance beyond which stereopsis is of no use whatsoever. In Figure 6–18, which of necessity is drawn on a greatly distorted scale, the fixation point occupies a position such that the angle formed by this point, the eye, and the parallel to the primary line of sight of the other eye is equal to the observer's threshold of stereopsis. Any object located farther than this fixation distance produces a binocular disparity which is smaller than the threshold and cannot be seen to be at a greater distance (Ogle, 1962b).

This limiting distance can be calculated from the relationships shown in the figure:

$$\eta_t = \theta \tag{6–12}$$

$$\eta_t = \frac{2a}{d} \tag{6–13}$$

$$d = \frac{2a}{\eta_t} \tag{6–14}$$

where η_t is expressed in radians. For example, if η_t is 10 arcseconds, the limiting distance is 1.32×10^3 m, or about 0.8 mi. On an open stretch of highway, oncoming traffic exceeds this distance so often as to render stereopsis useless as a basis for most decisions involved in driving (Allen, 1970).

COMPARISON WITH OTHER CUES

The fact that stereopsis operates over a limited range can form the basis for determining how the linear distance corresponding to a given angular threshold changes as a function of fixation distance. Using the ratio of Δd to d, we can compare stereopsis with other depth cues. We set $\Delta d/d$ to some percentage, assume a threshold level and an average interpupillary distance, and solve Equation (6–11) for d:

$$\frac{\Delta d}{d^2} = \frac{\eta t}{2ak} \qquad k = 206{,}265 \text{ arcseconds/rad} \tag{6–15}$$

$$\frac{\Delta d}{d} = 0.01 \tag{6–16}$$

$$d = \frac{0.02ak}{\eta t} \tag{6–17}$$

Table 6–5 presents the results of such a process for several values of $\Delta d/d$.

Such calculations are approximate because the exact formula for η has not been used. More precisely, the proximal linear interval is different from the distal linear interval:

Table 6–5.   Approximations of Distance at Which $\Delta d/d$ reaches 1, 2, and 5 Percent for Various Values of Threshold of Stereopsis

Threshold of Stereopsis (arcseconds)	d at Which $\Delta d/d = 0.01$ (m)	d at Which $\Delta d/d = 0.02$ (m)	d at Which $\Delta d/d = 0.05$ (m)
5	26.4	52.8	132.0
10	13.2	26.4	66.0
20	8.8	13.2	33.0
30	4.4	8.8	22.0
40	3.3	6.6	16.5

$$\text{Proximal } \eta_t = \frac{2a\ \Delta d}{d^2 - d\ \Delta d} \qquad \text{Distal } \eta_t = \frac{2a\ \Delta d}{d^2 + d\ \Delta d} \qquad (6\text{--}18)$$

Because of the angular nature of the threshold, the corresponding linear intervals start to diverge at about 10 m when $\eta_t = 40$ arcseconds and at about 30 m when $\eta_t = 10$ arcseconds. Schor and Flom (1969) pointed this out; their illustration is reproduced here as Figure 6–19. Considering this, we can see that other cues, such as size, overtake stereopsis at rather short distances. While a comparison of thresholds can be somewhat misleading in terms of predicting the actual behavior of observers, it does serve to emphasize that stereopsis becomes less efficient with increasing viewing distance.

Visual space appears bounded at a distance that is in excess of the limiting distance of stereopsis. Based on the size-distance relationship, this is suggested by the increase in the Weber fraction at great distances. Beyond a certain distance, the subtense angle of any object will not change further with further increases in distance, owing to the limitations of diffraction (Walsh, 1958). In this range, changes in brightness due to the inverse-square law constitute the only stimulus parameter that can be translated to a relative depth interpretation.

Placing a physical obstacle such as the walls of a room in the field of view bounds space in a different way. In this situation, the boundary makes the accurate localization of objects presented at binocular disparities such that physically equivalent objects would be located beyond the wall somewhat difficult. Such boundaries also occur when certain optical instruments such as stereoscopes and haploscopes are used. These devices are also known to produce a certain amount of proximal

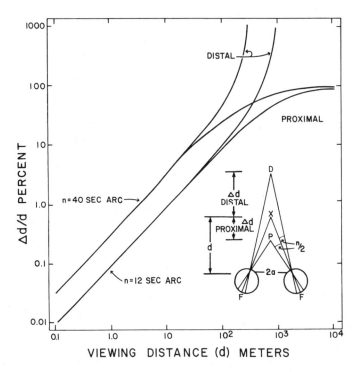

Figure 6–19.   Ratio of least detectable distance Δd to viewing distance d, as a function of the viewing distance (Reprinted by permission from Schor and Flom, 1969).

convergence, accommodation, and what has been termed an *awareness of nearness* (Hofstetter, 1951).

HYPOTHESES ABOUT DEPTH PERCEPTION

This description of the various factors involved in depth perception included some hint as to how these stimulus attributes might be used in everyday seeing. The combination of these various aspects implies some hypotheses that can form the basis for a pragmatic theory of visual perception.

Such a theory would assign top priority to physiological processes and would have as its goal the explanation of perception in physical, chemical, and anatomic terms. It would attempt to link these events with sensory observations through the hypothesis that ". . . whenever two stimuli cause physically indistinguishable signals to be sent from the sense organ to the brain, the sensations produced by these stimuli, as reported by the subject in words, symbols or actions, must be indistinguishable" (Brindley, 1970).

While such a theory might explain much about how we see, it would still fail to predict all perceptual phenomena. These failures may be a statement of our lack of understanding of the structures and functions of the visual system. However, perhaps another theory would provide us with a more fruitful framework to help understand visual perception. Psychology provides us with many such hypotheses (see, for example, LeGrand, 1967; Graham, 1965).

Information theory is a useful adjunct to the physiological theory. It concerns itself with the most general way in which information can be generated, transmitted, received, and analyzed. It involves mathematical formulations for each step and has resulted in revolutions of progress in communications. It also has allowed for the construction of devices to enhance and analyze photographic and video pictures and even made it possible to make machines that can recognize printed letters (Uhr, 1966). The application of information theory to the processes of visual perception involves estimating certain parameters and terms in a mathematical formulation and determining to what extent this process predicts what is seen. While its application to vision is only beginning, it holds great promise (see, for example, Charnwood, 1950; Ullman, 1979).

In a more practical sense, when a number of cues exist, the most accurate cue will be the most reliable, and it will determine the precision with which spatial judgments can be made (Brunswick, 1949). For example, within a certain range, stereopsis usually serves this role.

Furthermore, a subject's imprecision in performing certain visual judgments can improve with practice. Optometrists are obliged to provide some of this training by performing visual examinations. Repeated examinations on subsequent days, or even months or years later, produces more and more training and improved performance (Hofstetter, 1948).

Finally, we know that the act of perception involves more than just those areas of the brain known as the visual pathways (see Chapter 12). Visual neurology has described some of the effects on vision of nonstriate cortical lesions as follows:

- Visual agnosia: inability to understand or interpret visual stimuli.
- Metamorphopsia: change in the apparent size or shape of objects.
- Visual disorientation: inability to relate to visual stimuli occur-

ring throughout the visual field or confined to the right or left half.

- Anosognosia: failure of a patient to recognize a visual disability caused by a hemianopia or blindness (Brindley, 1970).

REFERENCES

Allen, M. J. (1970), *Vision and Highway Safety*, Chilton, Philadelphia, 22–28.

Alpern, M. (1969), "Accommodation," *The Eye*, vol. 3, Academic, New York, 217–254.

Amigo, G. (1964), "The stereoscopic threshold of the human retina," *Journal of the American Optometric Association*, 35, 3–15.

Andersen, E. E., and Weymouth, F. (1923), "Visual perception and the retinal mosaic," *American Journal of Physiology*, 64, 561–591.

Bouman, M. A., and van den Brink, G. (1953), "Aboslute thresholds for moving point sources," *Journal of the Optical Society of America*, 43, 895–898.

Brindley, G. S. (1970), *Physiology of the Retina and Visual Pathway*, E. Arnold, London, 129–138.

Brunswick, E. (1949), *Systematic and Representative Design of Psychological Experiments*, University of California, Berkeley.

Charnwood, J. R. B. (1950), *An Essay on Binocular Vision*, Hatton, London, 89–97.

Cornsweet, T. N. (1962), "The staircase-method in psychophysics," *American Journal of Psychology*, 75, 485–491.

Cornsweet, T. N. (1970), *Visual Perception*, Academic, New York, 270–310.

Crow, E. L., Davis, F. A., and Maxfield, M. W. (1960), *Statistics Manual*, Dover, New York, 152–162.

Finney, D. A. (1947), *Probit Analysis*, Cambridge University, England.

Fry, G. A. (1950), "Visual perception of space," *American Journal of Optometry*, 27, 531–553.

Fry, G. A. (1961), "Eye-body co-ordination in the perception of space," *Transactions of the International Ophthalmic Optical Congress*, Lockwood, London, 16–33.

Gescheider, G. A. (1976), *Psychophysics, Methods and Theory*, Wiley, New York, 20–38.

Gibson, J. J. (1950), *The Perception of the Visual World*, Houghton Mifflin, Boston.

Gogel, W. C. (1962), "Convergence as a determiner of absolute size," *Journal of Psychology*, 53, 91–104.

Graham, C. H. (1965), "Visual space perception," *Vision and Visual Perception*, Wiley, New York, 504–547.

Hamilton, J. E. (1964), "Effect of observer elevation on the moon illusion," M.S. thesis, Indiana University.

Hering, E. (1942), *Spatial Sense and Movements of the Eyes*, American Academy of Optometry, Baltimore, 20–28.

Hirsch, M. J., and Weymouth, F. W. (1948), "Distance discrimination, II, Effect on threshold of lateral separation of the test objects," *Archives of Ophthalmology*, 39, 224–231.

Hirsch, M. J., Horowitz, M. W., and Weymouth, F. W. (1948), "Distance discrimination, III, Effect of rod width on threshold," *Archives of Ophthalmology*, 39, 325–332.

Hofstetter, H. W. (1948), "The function of visual training in optometric practice," *The O-Eye-O*, 14, 8–11.

Hofstetter, H. W. (1951), "The relationship of proximal convergence to fusional and accomodative convergence," *American Journal of Optometry*, 28, 300–308.

Hofstetter, H. W. (1968), "Absolute threshold measurements with the diastereo test," *Archivos de la Sociedad Americana de Oftalmologia y Optometria*, 6, 327–342.

Hofstetter, H. W., and Bertsch, J.D. (1976), "Does stereopsis change with age?" *American Journal of Optometry and Physiological Optics*, 53, 664–667.

Holway, A. H., and Boring, E. G. (1941), "Determinants of apparent size with distance variant," *American Journal of Psychology*, 54, 21–37.

Howard, H. J. (1919), "A test for the judgment of distance," *American Journal of Ophthalmology*, 2, 656–675.

LeGrand, Y. (1967), *Form and Space Vision*, Indiana University, Bloomington, 117–119, 228–231.

Lit, A. (1959), "Depth-discrimination thresholds as a function of binocular differences of retinal illumination at scotopic and photopic levels," *Journal of the Optical Society of America*, 49, 746–752.

Ludvigh, E. (1952), "Possible role of proprioception in the extraocular muscles," *Archives of Ophthalmology*, 48, 436–441.

McColgin, F. H. (1960), "Movement thresholds in peripheral vision," *Journal of the Optical Society of America*, 50, 774–779.

Ogle, K. N. (1950), *Researches in Binocular Vision*, Saunders, Philadelphia, 64–68.

Ogle, K. N. (1962a), "Perception of distance and size," *The Eye*, vol. 4, Academic, New York, 247–268.

Ogle, K. N. (1962b), "Spatial localization through binocular vision," *The Eye*, vol. 4, Academic, New York, 271–320.

Ogle, K. N., and Weil, P. M. (1958), "Stereoscopic vision and the duration of the stimulus," *Archives of Ophthalmology*, 59, 4–17.

Pirenne, M. H. (1970), *Optics, Painting, and Photography*, Cambridge University, England.

Rashbass, C., and Westheimer, G. (1961), "Disjunctive eye movements," *Journal of Physiology*, 159, 326–338.

Regan, D., and Beverley, K. I. (1979), "Visually guided locomotion: Psychophysical evidence for a neural mechanism sensitive to flow patterns," *Science*, 205, 311–313.

Regan, D., and Cynader, M. (1979), "Neurons in area 18 of cat visual cortex selectively sensitive to changing size: Nonlinear interactions between responses to two edges," *Vision Research*, 19, 699–711.

Riggs, L. A. (1965), "Visual acuity," *Vision and Visual Perception*, Wiley, New York, 321–345.

Schor, C., and Flom, M. (1969), "The relative value of stereopsis as a function of viewing distance," *American Journal of Optometry*, 46, 805–809.

Shortess, G. K., and Krauskopf, J. (1961), "Role of eye movements in stereoscopic acuity," *Journal of the Optical Society of America*, 51, 555–559.

Sloan, L. L. (1968), "Clinical measurement of visual acuity," *Sympoisum on the Measurement of Visual Function*, National Academy of Science, Washington, 16–23.

Stewart, C. R. (1951), "A photographic investigation of lateral fusional movements of the eyes," Ph.D. thesis, Ohio State University, Columbus.

Stigmar, G. (1970), "Observations on vernier and stereo acuity with special reference to their relationship," *Acta Ophthalmologica*, 48, 979–998.

Teichner, W. H., Kobrick, J. L., and Dusek, E. R. (1955), "Common place viewing and depth discrimination," *Journal of the Optical Society of America*, 45, 913–920.

Thouless, R. H. (1931), "Phenomenal regression to the real object," *British Journal of Psychology*, 21, 339–359.

Uhr, L. (1966), *Pattern Recognition*, Wiley, New York.

Ullman, S. (1979), *The Interpretation of Visual Motion*, M.I.T., Cambridge.

Walls, G. L. (1942), *The Vertebrate Eye*, Cranbrook, Bloomfield Hills, MI, 247–365.

Walsh, J. W. T. (1958), *Photometry*, Constable, London, 141–142.

7

PANUM'S SPACE

Thought is only a flash between two long nights, but this flash is everything.

Henri Poincaré

MEASUREMENT OF PANUM'S SPACE

When we described the relationship known as corresponding points, we mentioned Panum's observation that haplopia (single vision) occurred for objects located over a range of space surrounding the horopter. Objects can be imaged any place within a small area on the two retinas and still be seen as single.

Figure 7–1 illustrates a schematic arrangment used for measuring the horizontal extent of Panum's space. In this example, with the subject fixating F, an object is displaced outward along the line of sight E_lH until diplopia is detected. In the figure, this occurs at D. Then the object is returned to H and displaced inward until diplopia again occurs, this time at P. From the location of H, D, P, E_l, and E_R, angles θ_p and θ_d can be calculated. The sum of these two angles constitutes the horizontal extent of Panum's space for one eccentric angle (Ogle, 1962a). Points P and D are the proximal (crossed) and distal (uncrossed) threshold points, respectively, and they can be determined by any of the psychophysical methods previously discussed. Their location with respect to H is of a statistical nature, as are all threshold points (Stevens, 1951).

Sometimes the most useful form of these data is in terms of the diplopia thresholds θ_p, the proximal threshold angle, and the distal threshold angle θ_d. These can be treated separately or combined in an arithmetic mean (Mitchell, 1966). The diplopia threshold is roughly equal to the angular size of Panum's space divided by 2.

Measurements of Panum's space can include measurements in the

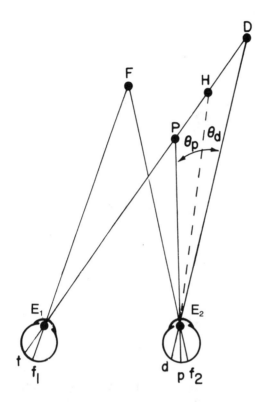

Figure 7–1.   Schematic arrangement for measuring the horizontal extent of
Panum's space.

vertical direction. This takes a circular form if eye movements are controlled and an elliptical shape with its long axis horizontal if eye movements are not controlled (Mitchell, 1966). Our main interest centers on
the horizontal dimensions since they are involved in creating horizontal
binocular disparities.

FUSIONAL INTERFERENCE

Measurements of Panum's space indicate it has a minimum angular
extent at the fixation point and increases toward the periphery of the
binocular visual field. However, measurements along the midsagittal
plane, at or near the object of regard, are difficult because a binocular
disparity is created as the target is moved off the horopter. Not only
can binocular disparity lead to the perception of stereopsis and diplopia,

but also it is the primary stimulus for fusional eye movements, which are impelling for disparities at or around the point of fixation (Ludvigh and McKinnon, 1966).

Some measurements in this region of the binocular field have been greatly influenced by fusional movements and produced results as large as 4 times the real size of the diplopia thresholds. For example, as the target is brought inward to an ever-nearer position, the subject might unwittingly respond to this change in binocular disparity by performing a convergent movement of the eyes. Diplopia would occur when the fixation stimulus and the movable object were separated by a distance that produced a disparity in excess of the angular size of Panum's spatial area, the sum of the crossed-disparity and uncrossed-disparity diplopia thresholds. A similar chain of events could occur for distal measurements, and the experimenter might conclude that Panum's space was as much as 2 times its actual angular size (Ogle, 1950).

PANUM'S SPACE AND THE RESOLUTION LIMIT

These problems of measurement at or around the primary lines of sight become important when the diplopia threshold is compared with the monocular resolution threshold (LeGrand, 1967). Figure 7–2 illustrates this comparison by presenting the data of Ogle (1950) for diplopia thresholds and the data of Clemmesen for monocular resolution (LeGrand, 1967). These two loci appear essentially the same over the range of values plotted, but for a 1° eccentricity the diplopia threshold appears to be significantly larger. By extrapolating from these data and referring to other data that directly determined the size of Panum's space at the fovea, we find a big discrepancy between these two measures. Woo (1974a) compiled the values found by various investigators; these range from 3.4 to 23 arcminutes. The 12-arcminute value found by Ogle (1950) is the most frequently cited as the foveal size of Panum's space.

Whatever the difference, it would be essentially eliminated if the binocular resolution threshold were compared with the diplopia threshold, because they are geometrically equivalent. Figure 7–3 illustrates this. To measure resolution, a target is superimposed on F and displaced laterally in the objective frontoparallel plane until a separate direction can be detected. In this diagram, this happens at P'. To determine the half-size of Panum's space (diplopia threshold) the target is moved along the line Fe_R until diplopia is detected. This occurs at point P. Notice the P and P' subtend the same angle θ at the left eye and,

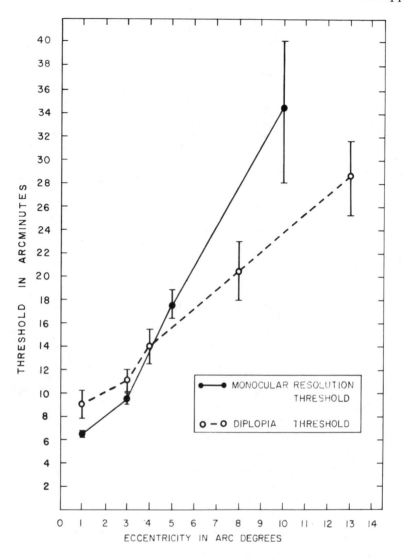

Figure 7–2.   Comparison of monocular and binocular resolution thresholds
              (replotted from LeGrand, 1967).

therefore, represent two different ways of displacing the target to produce the same angular offset (Woo, 1970).

For targets in the foveal region, Woo (1974a) compared the diplopia
threshold with the monocular separation threshold and found them
very similar. He used a small fixation target that allowed subjects to

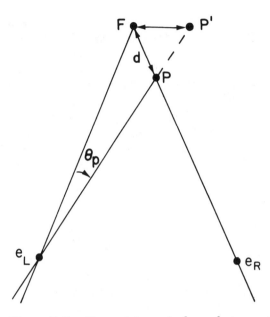

Figure 7–3.   Geometric equivalence between the angular size of the diplopia
              threshold and the binocular resolution threshold.

detect any fixational shifts greater than about 1 arcminute and presented
the test target for very short exposure times. His results suggest that
the phenomenon known as Panum's space is no more than a consequence of the resolution properties of the visual system, as first suggested by LeGrand (1967).

Richards (1971) suggested that the crossed and uncrossed limits
are mediated by separate neural mechanisms. He shows some data
suggesting that the proximal limit remains constant in angular size
while the distal limit increases with decreasing fixation distance.

DIRECTIONAL SHIFT

Ogle (1950) commented on a unique phenomenon associated with
Panum's space that he called *directional shift*. Diplopia means that two
visual directions are discernible, and haplopia implies that these two
are reduced to a single binocular visual direction. Ogle considered that
the shift from two directions to one could be accomplished if the haplopic direction were somewhere between the two previously diplopic
ones, or if it coincided with one of the two monocular visual directions
that existed in diplopia.

Woo (1970) considered that, at the threshold level, this was a simple consequence of resolution: Two targets are resolved when the appropriate lines of sight form an angle of sufficient magnitude, and only one is resolved when they do not. Nevertheless, when an object moves from a position in which it is seen double with wide separation between the two images to a position below the diplopia threshold, a unique directional shift does occur. Here, Ogle (1962b) and Sheedy and Fry (1978) found that this shift forms the basis for a valid method of determining a kind of ocular dominance (see Chapter 13). This directional shift produces a visual direction that is uniquely binocular in most subjects.

STEREOGRAMS

Figure 7–4 shows another method of arranging stimuli to produce diplopia, stereopsis, and fusional eye movements. As indicated in this figure, we can display lines on two cards and arrange to present these to the two eyes separately in a stereoscope, so that the viewer will directly sense the depth dimension. In this figure, lines of sight are drawn from the two entrance pupils e_L and e_R to three objects: a fixation point F, a distal point D, and a proximal point P. The projection of these lines onto any plane, such as dd', produces a relationship of lateral displacement among D_L, F_L, and P_L and among D_R, F_R, and P_R, shown here as vertical lines (Wheatstone, 1838).

If one of the two subsets of lines is moved laterally while the interpoint relationship is maintained as shown in the figure, then a position can be found that will allow fusion of the two subsets. Fusion is required under these circumstances in order to see depth. But once it is accomplished, we can replace the real-space points or lines with their projections and retain most of the depth information (LeConte, 1881). The stereoscopic depth is essentially the same whether we have points in real space or on cards properly positioned before the eyes in a stereoscope. Conversely, we can space any set of lines on two cards, arrange these before the eyes, and project them into space to a predictable location. This is the most important aspect in the concept of projection.

One curious thing about such targets, called *stereograms*, is that fusion of the two components is necessary before depth appears. Even when the position of the stereograms is prearranged to eliminate the need for fusional eye movements, it takes some noticeable time for a stereoscopic perception to emerge. The reason is not altogether clear, but apparently stereograms often contain extraneous information other

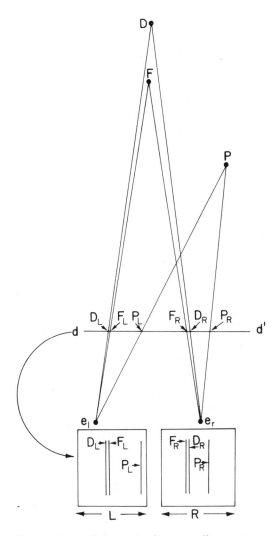

Figure 7–4. Schematic diagram illustrating construction of a stereogram.

than binocular disparity that may well interfere with the immediate perception of depth. This lag time has been noted to decrease somewhat if the stereograms have a minimum of surface-texture details. These details apparently signal that an opaque surface is being viewed, and the offset in the lines, which constitutes binocular disparity, has to be seen through this surface. Accomplishing appreciation of depth under such conflicting circumstances takes a noticeable amount of time (see Chapters 8 and 9).

Because most early workers used only stereograms and many optometrists still test stereopsis exclusively by this method, sometimes it is believed that stereopsis requires fusion and some noticeable viewing time to appreciate it (Miles, 1949).

To measure Panum's space with such an apparatus requires that a series of stereograms be prepared, each one displaying a separate binocular disparity. As an alternative, black lines on transparent sheets of plastic can serve as targets, and the relative displacement of these lines, called *decentration*, can be changed to vary the resulting binocular disparity. A more recent approach utilizes signal generators and cathode-ray tubes to produce stereograms.

STEREOPSIS OUTSIDE PANUM'S SPACE

Throughout the literature on Panum's space are reports that it is the result of a special mechanism. Ogle (1950) speaks of it as "Panum's fusional area," which implies that this is the only region of space seen binocularly, because it is here that some functional differences between binocular and monocular vision can be demonstrated. For example, some investigators claimed that stereopsis is limited to this zone even though Helmholtz (1925), Hering (1942), and others [including Wright (1951) and Ogle (1952)] have shown that stereopsis is possible with double images.

Many of these studies show that the threshold of stereopsis increases as the measuring point is moved to locations more remote from the horopter. Figure 7–5 illustrates this increase in threshold as a function of binocular disparity for three peripheral angles. The small arrows mark the position of the horopter for each of these eccentricities (Blakemore, 1970). Figure 7–6 shows the spatial limts of stereopsis surrounding the horopter.

Ogle (1953) reported that this range could be divided into two regions: a range of patent stereopsis and a range of qualitative stereopsis. The patent range includes Panum's space and the surrounding diplopic region. In this zone, observers are capable of directly sensing an increase in perceived depth accompanying an increase in binocular disparity. The area known as qualitative is outside this and so always diplopic and farther from the horopter. Here, the observer is rather uncertain about relative depth changes and sees a movable target as vaguely located behind or in front of a fixed reference target. This region is characterized by a lack of increase in perceived depth with increasing binocular disparity. Westheimer and Tanzman (1956) and Reading (1970) reported above-chance stereoscopic responses outside the ranges

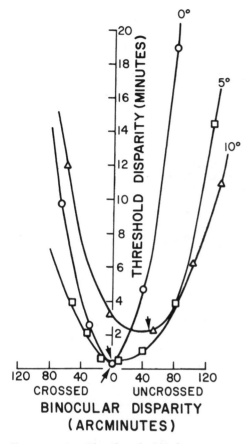

Figure 7–5.   The threshold of stereopsis increases for three peripheral angles
               when the sensitivity is measured for points at increasing distances
               from the horopter surface (Blakemore, 1970).

found by Ogle (1952). Figure 7–7 illustrates a schematic arrangement
of targets positioned to measure extrahoropteral stereopsis.

The fact that stereopsis can be sensed with diplopic images means
that Worth's grade 3 fusion (Worth, 1903) needs some modification.
For this purpose, it would be appropriate to use the term *fine stereopsis*
since it describes the small thresholds associated with Panum's space
(see Chapters 3, 9, and 10). Based on this information, it should be easy
to see how a patient with a small-angle strabismus might be able to
demonstrate a gross form of stereopsis. For example, a 3° esotrope
might be able to perceive depth if the binocular disparity of the test
objects was greater than about 60 arcseconds.

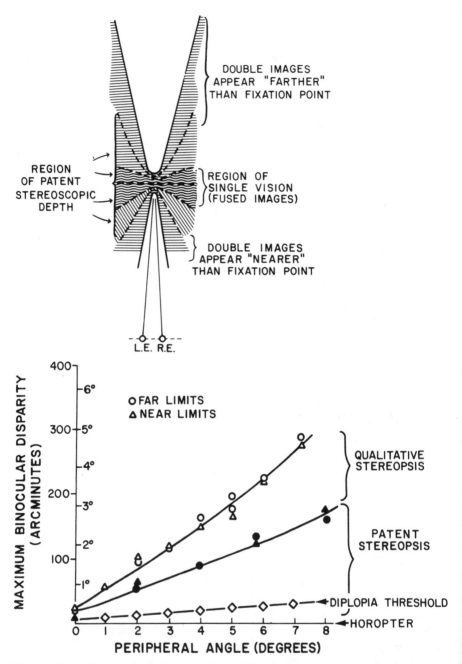

Figure 7–6.   The size of the areas in which stereopsis is possible *(bottom)* as
a function of peripheral angle and *(top)* as a schematic diagram,
relative to the fixation point (Ogle, 1952, Reprinted by permission
from Archives of Ophthalmology 1952; 48:50–60. Copyright 1952,
American Medical Association).

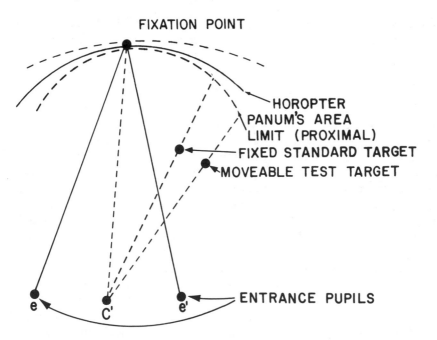

Figure 7–7. Schematic diagram illustrating objects positioned to measure the
threshold of stereopsis outside Panum's space.

PANUM'S SPACE AND FIXATION DISPARITY

There is another condition associated with Panum's space, *fixation disparity*. When requested to bifixate a given point, some subjects fail to
do so by a very small amount. This error is usually between 0.5 and
10 arcminutes. If it were larger than about 12 arcminutes, diplopia
would occur or binocular suppression would shut out one percept, and
the nomenclature would shift from fixation disparity to microstrabismus
or monofixation syndrome (Parks, 1971).

Fixation disparity causes the two diplopia thresholds to appear to
be of unequal size, although the size of Panum's area remains essentially
unaffected (Ogle, 1950). In the absence of fixation disparity, the crossed
diplopia threshold is found to be roughly the same size as the uncrossed
diplopia threshold. Any small remaining discrepancy is due to the fact
that at least some observers demonstrate a temporal-nasal difference
in directional sensitivity. Woo and Reading (1978) found statistically
significant differences in the proximal and distal limits and a concurrent
temporal-nasal monocular resolution difference with three subjects. For

these observers, the distal (uncrossed) diplopia threshold was found to be slightly larger than the proximal (crossed) diplopia threshold.

SPREAD OF PANUM'S SPACE

The size of Panum's space is variable depending on the conditions under which it is measured. Short exposures and precise fixation control reduce its size to that determined by the underlying binocular resolution mechanism. Long exposures and less precise control of fixation increase its size. Apparently, eye movements cause most of this expansion. For example, using long exposure times while measuring fixation disparity with various amounts of forced vergence, Hebbard (1960) estimated that the foveal size of Panum's area was some 23 arcminutes, while Woo (1974b) showed that its size increased from 1.0 to 4.0 arcminutes when the exposure time was increased from 5 to 100 ms.

Bagolini and Campobianco (1965) reported that patients with small-angle strabismus have greatly enlarged areas over which they perceive single vision. For one patient this was as large as 70 arcminutes when it was measured along the midsagittal plane. Such an abnormal expansion might be the result of some eye movement abnormality or innervational shift in such observers.

FIXATION DISPARITY VERSUS BINOCULAR DISPARITY

Sometimes it is easy to confuse fixation disparity and binocular disparity. Binocular disparity is the stimulus for such sensory experiences as stereopsis, which requires no motor activity whatsoever. Fixation disparity is the difference between the binocular subtense angle of the point to be fixated and the actual angle formed by the intersection of the two primary lines of sight; it results from a mismatch between the stimulus to fusion and the fusional response. Some of this confusion could be avoided by referring to this phenomenon as *retinal slip*, as proposed by Ames and Gliddon (1928), or *vergence error*, or *discrepancy*, as suggested by Hebbard (1960).

Fixation disparity is purely motor in the sense that subjects are unaware that their eyes are not quite pointed where they should be. Only because such a condition is believed to lead to discomfort (Mallett, 1969) is there any kind of sensory consequence. Undoubtedly, such symptom-causing processes are not mediated directly by the visual sensory system.

FIXATION DISPARITY, PANUM'S SPACE, AND
CORRESPONDING POINTS

Fixation disparity provides us with a way to look at the tightness of correspondence across the two retinas. For example, suppose we choose to present a single fusion stimulus at a peripheral angle of 4°, degrees. Then, referring to Figure 7–2, we would expect the precision of the alignment of the primary lines of sight to be governed by the resolution capabilities of this peripheral region. According to these data, we would expect fixation disparities to assume values in a range of ±14 arcminutes. These would be the largest values of fixation disparity to be found in a group of otherwise normal subjects. Moving the fusion lines out to 8° would yield a tolerance of about ±24 arcminutes. At 12° this would be about ±32 arcminutes. In other words, within the limits of variability among subjects, the precision of alignment of the primary lines of sight, as measured by fixation disparity, should be dictated by the resolution limits of the regions of the two retinas to which the binocular fusion targets are presented (LeGrand, 1967).

This hypothesis is supported by the clinical observation that the central fusion-lock targets produce the smallest range of fixation disparity measurements in a group of patients, whereas the peripheral fusion-lock targets produce a larger range in the same patients. Ogle et al. (1949) report that fixation disparity values do increase on some subjects as a central blank area in a binocular display of acuity letters is increased in angular size. However, if a simple square frame or circle is used as the only binocular fusion stimulus, the fixation disparity is reported to not change with increasing angles of eccentricity (Sheppard, 1951; Ogle et al., 1967). However, several details about these latter studies remain unclear, and a more systematic investigation is needed.

Alder (1957) measured peripheral disparity changes during viewing of a cental point, a form of nonius horopter determination. The increase in disparity at three eccentric points in three subjects is very similar to the increase in fixation disparity with peripheral fusion stimuli reported by Ogle et al. (1949) for one of their subjects. Alder also found no simple increase in fixation disparity with peripheral fusion targets, consisting of circles. However, considering this relationship with forced vergences, he reported that the expected trend was demonstrated.

Perhaps a part of these different findings can be accounted for by the demonstrable reduction in fixation disparity as a function of exposure time (Schor, 1979). Suppose we could objectively measure eye position to an accuracy of a few arcminutes. Then by monitoring eye position during fixation disparity measurements and correcting the data to reflect the real position of the eyes relative to the targets, perhaps some of these conflicting reports might be resolved.

Another approach might be to use binocular stabilized images, as Fender and Julesz (1967) did. Unfortunately, their results must be questioned because it is known that stabilized images are not really fixed on the retina. This plus the use of random dot targets (see Chapter 8) caused a general expansion in the size of Panum's space. This reported enlargement may be no more than an inadvertent measurement of the patent range of stereopsis (Woo, 1970).

UNCOMPENSATED PORTION OF HETEROPHORIA

Ames and Gliddon (1928) proposed that heterophorias were made up of a compensated and an uncompensated component. They suggested that the amount of prism or lenses necessary to neutralize a vergence slip is a measure of the uncompensated part. This amount causes the eyestrain symptoms that must be dealt with clinically, and Mallett (1969) suggested that prescriptions based on this principle produce great satisfaction among patients with binocular problems.

According to Hebbard (1960), any dissimilarity between the images in the two eyes, such as differences in size, shape, or clarity, will cause an increase in fixation disparity, as will foveal suppression.

Carter (1960) suggested that it is usual for both eyes to share equally in the deviation. Only those patients with a history of abnormal suppression associated with vergence stress or previously manifest oculomotor deviations exhibit large monocular components. Mallett (1969) considered that these cases should be corrected by locating the neutralizing prism in front of the eye manifesting the deviation.

It is prudent to include fixation disparity measurements in a clinical routine in addition to heterophoria measurments by both objective (cover test) and subjective (Von Graffe's method) means. This has been illustrated by Saladin and Sheedy (1978), who found that measurements based on heterophorias best discriminated between normal and abnormal subjects.

Figure 7–8 shows four different response patterns of changing fixation disparity with forced prism vergence (Carter, 1964). Ogle et al. (1967) considered type 2 the most likely to be symptom-free. Often type 1 can be converted to type 2 with vergence training. However, because measurements of these functions require special instrumentation, Mallett (1969) suggested that the objective of such a procedure has been met when the patient can maintain a given amount of fixation disparity

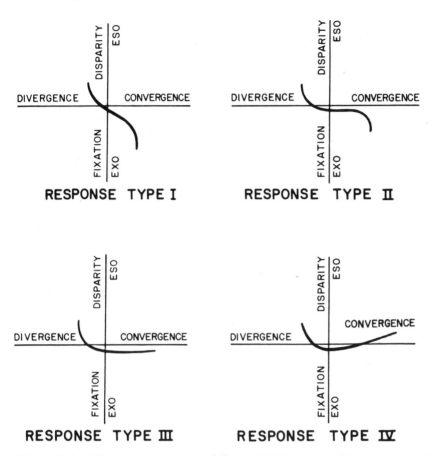

Figure 7–8.   The response types of Carter (1964, reprinted by permission).

while viewing through four prism diopters, base in for esodeviations and base out for exodeviations. Types 3 and 4 are associated with sensory anomalies including abnormal suppression (Carter, 1964). For these, neutralization of the deviation in a prescription is useless without first eliminating the abnormal suppression.

Carter (1960), among others, emphasized the effect of instrumentation on fixation disparity, and Mallett designed a distance and near test that seems to produce a very good simulation of word-reading tasks. Payne et al. (1974) found that prescriptions based on Mallett's technique were more successful in a group of exodeviation patients than those based on adjustments of the fusional reserves (Alpern, 1969).

Charnwood (1951) suggested that fixation disparity measurements with a test that also presents a binocular disparity reduces their magnitude. However, Palmer (1961) reported that such displays caused a shift in fixation disparity to a greater exodeviation when an uncrossed binocular disparity was used.

Figure 7–9 shows fixation disparity measurements with forced vergences using varying-size fusion-free areas. Charnwood (1951) pointed out that, given the shift of the central flat portion of these curves, as the fusion stimuli are moved peripherally, a different motor response to forced vergence is revealed. As we will see, this can be considered as a slip between the sensory corresponding-point relationship and that for the motor system. Such an innervational translation is known as *anomalous correspondence* (see Chapter 14).

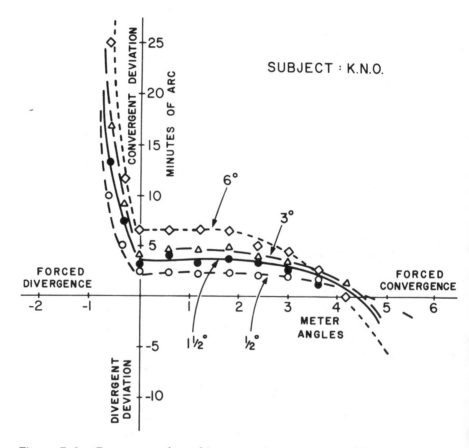

Figure 7–9.   Responses of a subject to various amounts of forced vergence with different peripheral fusion stimuli (Ogle, 1950).

OVERVIEW

The physiological basis of Panum's space appears to be identical with that subserving binocular resolution, as originally suggested by Le-Grand. What is special about this spatial area is that it represents the region in which objects are seen singly at unique binocular visual directions. It is also the region in which binocular interactions are at their very best. Clearly, binocular function is not limited to Panum's space since stereopsis is possible with diplopic percepts.

The role of eye movements as they relate to Panum's space needs further elaboration. While clearly the goal of fusional activity is to bring objects of interest into this region, fixation disparity and related issues seem to require further study.

From a clinical point of view, achieving binocular vision means overcoming diplopia and obtaining fine stereoscopic perceptions. Since clinical measurements usually require prolonged viewing, which allows the eyes considerable freedom of movement, the foveal size should be considered to be about 12 arcminutes.

Because gross binocularity is possible outside this area, the clinician should not be surprised at unqualified reports of binocularity in a wide range of conditions considered to exclude binocular function. Such reports require a more precise specification of the level of function and the status of binocular vision, not only during a range of specificable tests but also throughout the daily activities of the patient.

Corrections of fixation disparity form an effective basis of solving some problems experienced by patients with binocular vision. However, these corrections are best utilized in a context that measures the quality of sensory fusion as well as various other oculomotor relationships.

REFERENCES

Alder, A. V. (1957), "The binocular induced phi movement as a method of measuring binocular fixation disparity," M.S. thesis, Indiana University, Bloomington.

Alpern, M. (1969), "Types of eye movements," *The Eye*, vol. 3, Academic, New York, 65–174.

Ames, A., and Gliddon, G. H. (1928), "Ocular measurements," *Transactions of the Section on Ophthalmology*, 102–175.

Bagolini, B., and Capobianco, N. M. (1965), "Subjective space in comitant squint," *American Journal of Ophthalmology*, 59, 430–442.

Blakemore, C. (1970), "The range and scope of binocular depth discrimination in man," *Journal of Physiology*, 211, 599–622.

Carter, D. B. (1960), "Studies in fixation disparity, III, The apparent uniocular components of fixation disparity," *American Journal of Optometry*, 37, 408–419.

Carter, D. B. (1964), "Fixation disparity with and without foveal contours," *American Journal of Optometry*, 41, 729–736.

Charnwood, J. R. B. (1951), "Retinal slip," *Transactions of the International Optical Congress*, British Optical Association, London, 165–172.

Fender, D., and Julesz, B. (1967), "Extension of Panum's fusional area in binocular stabilized vision," *Journal of the Optical Society of America*, 57, 819–830.

Gescheider, G. A. (1976), *Psychophysics, Methods and Theory*, Wiley, New York, 20–38.

Hebbard, F. W. (1960), "Foveal fixation disparity measurements and their use in determining the relationship between accommodative convergence and accommodation," *American Journal of Optometry*, 37, 3–26.

Helmholtz, H. (1925), *Handbook of Physiological Optics*, vol. 3, Optical Society of America, New York, 403–426.

Hering, E. (1942), *Spatial Sense and Movements of the Eyes*, American Academy of Optometry, Baltimore, 29–32.

LeConte, J. (1881), *Sight, on Exposition of the Principles of Monocular and Binocular Vision*, Appleton, New York.

LeGrand, Y. (1967), *Form and Space Vision*, Indiana University, Bloomington, 200–211, 303–313.

Ludvigh, E., and McKinnon, P. (1966), "Relative effectivity of foveal and parafoveal stimuli in eliciting fusional movements of small amplitude," *Archives of Ophthalmology*, 76, 443–449.

Mallett, R. F. J. (1969), "Fixation disparity in clinical practice," *Australian Journal of Optometry*, 52, 97–109.

Miles, P. W. (1949), "Limits of stereopsis due to physiological diplopia," *American Journal of Ophthalmology*, 32, 1567–1573.

Mitchell, D. E. (1966), "Retinal disparity and diplopia," *Vision Research*, 6, 441–451.

Ogle, K. N. (1950), *Researches in Binocular Vision*, Saunders, Philadelphia, 64–93.

Ogle, K. N. (1952), "Disparity limits of stereopsis," *Archives of Ophthalmology*, 48, 50–60.

Ogle, K. N. (1953), "Precision and validity of stereoscopic depth perception with double images," *Journal of the Optical Society of America*, 43, 906–913.

Ogle, K. N. (1962a), "Spatial localization through binocular vision," *The Eye*, vol. 4, Academic, New York, 271–324.

Ogle, K. N. (1962b), "Ocular dominance and binocular retinal rivalry," *The Eye*, vol. 4, Academic, New York, 409–417.

Ogle, K. N., Martens, T. G., and Dyer, J. A. (1967), *Oculomotor Imbalance in Binocular Vision and Fixation Disparity*, Lea & Febiger, Philadelphia, 57–64.

Ogle, K. N., Mussey, F., and Prang, A. DeH. (1949), "Fixation disparity and the fusional processes in binocular single vision," *American Journal of Ophthalmology*, 32, 1069–1087.

Palmer, D. A. (1961), "Measurement of the horizontal extent of Panum's area by a method of constant stimuli," *Optical Acta*, 8, 151–159.

Parks, M. M. (1971), "The monofixation syndrome," *Symposium on Strabismus*, Mosby, St. Louis, 121–153.

Payne, C. R., Grisman, J. D., and Thomas, K O. (1974), "A clinical evaluation of fixation disparity," *American Journal of Optometry*, 51, 88–90.

Reading, R. W. (1970), "The threshold of distance discrimination for objects located outside of Panum's area," *American Journal of Optometry*, 47, 99–105.

Richards, W. (1971), "Independence of Panum's near and far limits," *American Journal of Optometry*, 48, 103–109.

Saladin, J. J., and Sheedy, J. E. (1978), "Population study of fixation disparity, heterophoria, and vergence," *American Journal of Optometry*, 55, 744–750.

Schor, C. M. (1979), "The influence of rapid prism adaptation upon fixation disparity," *Vision Research*, 19, 201–211.

Schor, C. M., and Tyler, C. W. (1981), "Spatio-temporal properties of Panum's fusional area," *Vision Research,* 21, 683–692.

Sheedy, J. E., and Fry, G. A. (1978), "The perceived direction of the binocular image," *Vision Research,* 19, 201–211.

Shephard, J. S. (1951), "A study of the relationship between fixation disparity and target size," *American Journal of Optometry,* 28, 391–404.

Stevens, S. S. (1951), "Mathematics, measurement, and psychophysics," *Handbook of Experimental Psychology,* Wiley, New York, 1–49.

Westheimer, G., and Tanzman, I. J. (1956), "Qualitative depth localization with diplopic images," *Journal of the Optical Society of America,* 46, 116–117.

Wheatstone, C. (1838), "On some remarkable and hitherto unobserved, phenomena of binocular vision," *Philosophical Transactions,* London, 8, 371–394.

Woo, G. C. S. (1970), "The basis for Panum's area," Ph.D. thesis, Indiana University, Bloomington.

Woo, G. C. S. (1974a), "Temporal tolerance of the foveal size of Panum's area," *Vision Research,* 14, 633–635.

Woo, G. C. S. (1974b), "The effect of exposure time of the foveal size of Panum's area," *Vision Research,* 14, 473–480.

Woo, G. C. S., and Reading, R. W. (1978), "Panum's area explained in terms of known acuity mechanisms, *British Journal of Physiological Optics,* 32, 30–37.

Worth, C. (1903), *Squint: Its Causes, Pathology, and Treatment,* Blakiston, Philadelphia.

Wright, W. D. (1951), "The role of convergence in stereoscopic vision," *Proceedings of the Physical Society,* London, 46, 289–297.

8
SPECIAL ASPECTS INVOLVING STEREOPSIS

Round numbers are always false.

Samuel Johnson

PULFRICH STEREOPHENOMENON

An interesting phenomenon involving stereopsis was reported first by Pulfrich (1922). He surmised that the binocular view of the path of a swinging pendulum should appear distorted if one eye viewed it through a filter that created an asymmetry of retinal illuminances between the two eyes. This was no small accomplishment because he was monocular and never saw the effect that bears his name (Christianson and Hofstetter, 1972).

When a neutral density filter is placed over one eye, it reduces the retinal illuminance to this eye. Furthermore, if the filter is sufficiently dense, it initiates the process of dark adaptation. Both changes cause an increased time gap between the onset of a stimulus and of its perception (Dodwell et al., 1968). For binocular viewing of a stationary object, these changes produce a tilting of frontally placed objects, so that they appear closer on the side with the filter (Cibis and Haber, 1951). If the target moves, it causes a different match-up of messages arriving at the cortex at any one time and creates a kind of temporal disparity. The same perception can be produced by taking a stereo movie, cutting the film down the middle, and reattaching it with the right half slipped down one or more frames. Projecting the result produces the Pulfrich phenomenon (Julesz and White, 1969). See Figure 8–1.

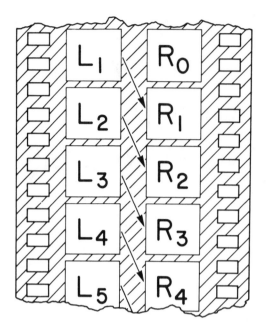

Figure 8–1.   Schematic diagram of a piece of movie film, used for three-dimensional projection, illustrates how a change of one frame (or more) can be used to produce the Pulfrich stereophenomenon (Julesz and White, 1969).

Figure 8–2 illustrates the resulting disparity created by a black line P moving from left to right at velocity v. At one particular instant, this produces visual direction impressions R and L, which will combine to form the binocular projection to S. The difference in depth of this point Δd is related to the difference in latency Δt between the two monocular percepts by the geometry of similar triangles (Lit, 1949):

$$\frac{v(\Delta t)}{2a} = \frac{-\Delta d}{\Delta d - d} \tag{8–1}$$

$$\Delta t = \frac{-2a(\Delta d)}{v(\Delta d - d)} \tag{8–2}$$

The direction of the displacement reverses if the filter is placed over the other eye. This provides a way to derive a vicarious form of stereoscopic perception while viewing a moving two-dimensional display such as a video picture. When a TV screen is viewed binocularly with one eye looking through a filter, such as a sunglass lens, any motion will cause the images to appear displaced in depth. Switching

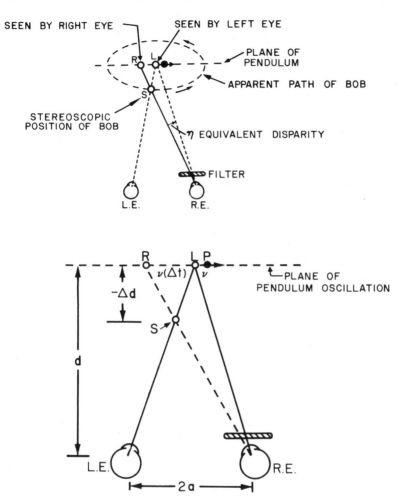

Figure 8–2.   Geometry of the Pulfrich stereophenomenon (Ogle, 1962).

the filter to the other side turns this displacement around. While this is an enjoyable observation, no claim is made that it is a complete substitute for viewing real three-dimensional projections or holographs (Enright, 1970).

The phenomenon can be observed under any circumstances in which there is a significant difference in retinal illuminance between the two eyes. Such conditions are encountered in patients with anisocoria or unilateral opacities of the ocular media. Any moderate mismatch in optical density of sunglass lenses can bring this about also. This phenomenon causes problems because it produces a false distance perception of any and all objects in motion.

From time to time, observations are reported which seem to call into question the latency-difference basis of this effect. For example, Katz and Schwartz (1955) reported that the ellipsoidal displacement was seen by 12 patients viewing a display in which the moving object was seen in different parts of the field by each eye in succession, and Harker (1967) has offered an explanation based on saccadic suppression. Nevertheless, the latency hypothesis is generally accepted as the reason for this effect.

Because the reaction time, which is mainly based on latency, changes rather systematically as a function of retinal location (Rains, 1963), theoretically some distortion of frontal movement should occur naturally since the latency-eccentricity function is asymmetric with respect to the fovea. This seems to be the case if the diplopic images are viewed in motion. Diplopia tends to accentuate latency differences between retinal points. However, familiarity with the phenomenon produces a strong expectancy in most observers.

CONTRAST AND STEREOPSIS

Ogle and Weil (1958) failed to find any decrease in stereo sensitivity over a range of binocular contrasts from 0.15 to almost 0.015. Apparently, as long as a contour is detectable, it can serve as the basis for binocular disparity information (see Chapter 12). Furthermore, Charnwood (1950), Ogle and Groch (1956), and Gillott (1957) failed to find any increase in the threshold of stereopsis when the image to one eye was dimmed. However, Lit (1959) and Reading and Woo (1972) reported that measurable changes did occur.

DELAY BETWEEN PRESENTATION OF TWO IMAGES

Binocular vision is at its best when it occurs with simultaneous stimulation of retinal points. Delaying the delivery of one of the pair of disparate images causes an increase in the threshold of stereopsis. For a given exposure time and level of retinal illuminance, there exists a critical delay time at which the threshold rises exponentially (Ogle, 1963). Depending on the exposure time, the critical delay time occurs between about 60 and 200 ms. Regardless of the exposure time, only relatively small changes in the threshold occur over the first 40 or 50 ms of delay (Wist and Gogel, 1966).

If the effect of introducing a delay between the presentations of a stereo pair is equivalent to the latency change that accounts for the Pulfrich phenomenon, then dimming the component presented first should tend to restore stereo sensitivity. However, Reading and Woo (1972) found that either delay or dimming reduced sensitivity, regardless of which image was changed. This suggests that binocular disparity information is encoded at the retinal level by a means involving both latency and intensity.

Stereopsis is possible with afterimages (Ogle and Reihner, 1962). There is one amazing report that eidetic images produced stereopsis when a time delay of 24 h occurred between presentations of the first and second components of a stereogrammetric pair to a particular subject (Stromeyer and Psotka, 1970).

COLOR AND STEREOPSIS

The binocular observation of a red light and a blue light, located at the same physical distance, often will cause the red one to appear closer than the blue. This phenomenon, called *chromostereopsis*, is thought to be due to the decentration of the primary lines of sight nasally from the optical axes of the two eyes. This offset causes a chromatic dispersion of the light, which displaces the blue part of the spectrum more nasalward than the red. Such a displacement means that the blue will have a relatively less crossed disparity (or more uncrossed disparity) and so will be seen at a greater distance than is the red. This explanation has been supplemented by Vos (1960). He suggested that an asymmetric Stiles-Crawford effect (Stiles and Crawford, 1933) frequently may be an antagonistic factor. He confirmed that approximately 50 percent of the observers see the red as closer and the blue was closer for the other 50 percent.

Pennington (1970) confirmed that the threshold of stereopsis is higher for blue wavelengths than for the red and green. He rejected the effects of chromatic aberration as a basis for this fact and suggested that it may be due to larger summative areas for the blue mechanism, as reported by Brindley (1954). He also found that some subjects showed the greatest stereo sensitivity for red lights whereas others showed it for green. Jonkers and Kylstra (1963) reported that minimizing brightness contrast, so that the differences between targets and backgrounds were mainly due to differences in chromaticity, also reduced stereoscopic sensitivity.

TELESTEREOSCOPE AND PERCEIVED DEPTH

Helmholtz (1925) invented a binocular instrument that he called the *telestereoscope*. Figure 8–3 illustrates the optical principle involved. It is a modified Wheatstone stereoscope that extends the baseline of the observer. By expanding the interpupillary distance, the range of distances over which stereopsis can be appreciated is greatly extended, and each separation in depth between objects in the field of view produces an enlarged binocular disparity.

This principle is used to construct stereoscopic rangefinders, and even prism binoculars, such as are used to view sporting events, include a modest optical expansion of the interpupillary distance (Jacobs, 1943). However, this latter instrument produces a much greater angular magnification than the magnification of binocular disparities caused by a small extension of the baselines, and the resulting view is decidedly flat (Wallach and Zuckerman, 1963). Ideally, a set of 7X binoculars should expand the interpupillary distance by this same factor. Unfortunately, such a match would produce an instrument with about a 45-cm separation between its optical centers, hardly a handy device to use while viewing a football game.

Actually, this flatness demonstrates that the perceived depth re-

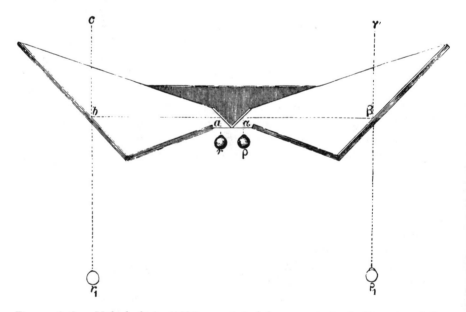

Figure 8–3.   Helmholtz's (1925, reprinted by permission) diagram of the telestereoscope.

sulting from a given binocular disparity is a function of perceived distance. Ordinary binoculars produce a perception of a reduction in apparent distance rather than an increase in apparent size, demonstrating size constancy, as previously discussed. Because of the relationship between perceived depth and perceived absolute distance, the depth appears relatively reduced. While viewing conditions can be arranged so that the perceived depth resulting from a given amount of binocular disparity is independent of absolute distance judgments (Foley, 1967), usually it is related inversely to the square of the perceived distance (Kaufman, 1974).

PSEUDOSCOPE AND PERCEPTUAL CONFLICT

Wheatstone (1838) arranged two right-angle prisms as illustrated in Figure 8–4*A* and called the resulting instrument a *pseudoscope*. As indicated, this reverses the images seen by each eye and so reverses the direction of all binocular disparities. Viewing geometric forms through

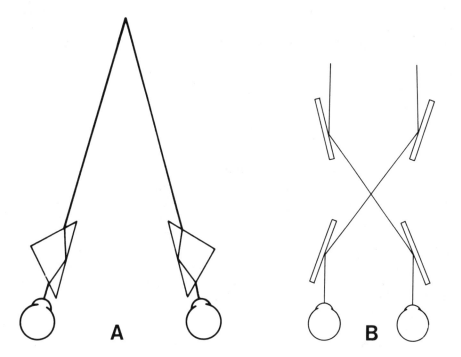

Figure 8–4.   (A) Wheatstone's (1839) diagram of the pseudoscope. (B) Le-Grand's (1967) modification using mirrors.

a pseudoscope produces a reversal of the resulting perceptions of depth, provided that shadows or overlay cues do not intervene. It does not cause landscapes or human faces to appear reversed. Apparently, familiar objects with strong memory images prevent the reversed disparities from producing their predicted results (Helmholtz, 1925). Mirrors also have been used to construct pseudoscopes, as shown in Figure 8–4B (LeGrand, 1967).

Gogel (1954) measured stereoscopic distance matches to the figure like that illustrated in Figure 8–5. The geometric perspective of this figure is such that the left end appears to be more distant then the right; binocular disparity cues are just the opposite. When the subject matches a binocular disk to the same apparent distance as the left end of this figure, she or he tends to set it at a point physically behind this edge. Such behavior indicates that perspective cues have a pronounced influence on depth matching.

Not only are the averages of matching settings displaced in a direction that indicates an influence of the perspective cue, but also the variability is increased over that obtained by depth matching at the middle of the figure. Hirsch et al. (1948) found a similar displacement and increase in variability of equidistant settings, using a two-rod stereo apparatus with one rod twice as wide as the other. Later, when describing perceptions involved with aniseikonia, we will see that sometimes the stereoscopic perception of depth can be virtually shut out of consciousness when its information is at odds with that from other cues (see Chaper 13).

MOTION AND STEREOPSIS

Studies of dynamic visual acuity have shown that the correlation between visual acuity with fixed test objects and that performed with moving objects is only fair (Burg, 1967). Luria and Weissman (1968) measured stereopsis and found a low correlation between static and dynamic stereoscopic thresholds. Figure 8–6 shows how the threshold increases as the speed of rotation increases. This figure also shows the data of Cutler and Ley (1963) which illustrate the decrement in binocular resolution as a function of the angular speed of the target. In monocular viewing, the increase in threshold of resolution is even greater.

Such kinetic performances are due to the inability of the oculomotor system to accurately track a target moving at high speed, to optical smearing, and to a process known as *saccadic suppression* (Alpern, 1969). Saccadic suppression may be due to pressure exerted by the vitreous on the retina (Richards, 1969) or to a decrease in sensitivity of

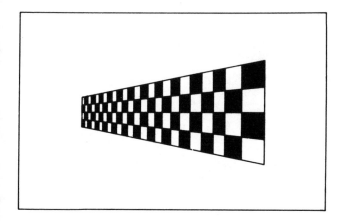

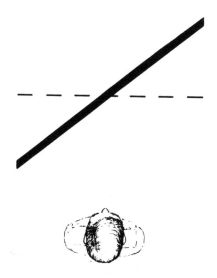

Figure 8–5.   An experimental arrangement designed to create conflict between binocular disparity and perspective cues (Gogel, 1954).

the cells in the lateral geniculate body (Brindley, 1970), cortex (Armington and Bloom, 1974), or brainstem (Zuber and Stark, 1966). Apparently, saccadic suppression reduces the sensitivity of the system during eye movements so that perceptions will be stabilized.

A comparison of the data presented in Figure 8–6 indicates that their effect is a differential one. Perhaps this indicated difference is a result of the fact that two different mechanisms are involved or that

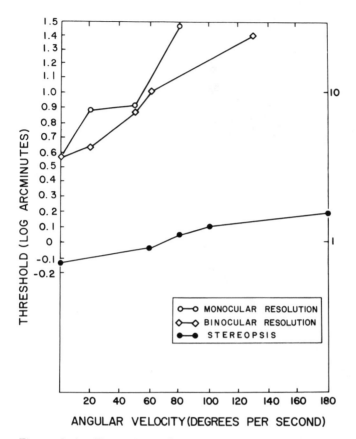

Figure 8–6.   Dynamic performances (Luria and Weissman, 1968; Cutler and
              Ley, 1963).

saccadic suppression acts differentially. If so, stereoscopic information
would appear to have a higher priority or suffer less reduction in sensitivity than does resolution.

However, when the target oscillates in and out of the plane of
fixation, according to Tyler (1971), the system is less able to detect
motion than it is monocularly. This reduction in sensitivity to stereoscopic depth movement was reported also by Ludvigh (1942) and Julesz
and Payne (1968).

FIELD SIZE AND STEREOPSIS

Luria (1969) reported that over a certain range of angular values the
threshold of stereopsis increases with decreasing field size. The effect

appears to be separate from those produced by altering the angular size or the angular separation of the stimuli, as discussed earlier. Luria and Kinney (1971) attribute the effect to instrument myopia, an increase in accommodation with decreasing field size, as reported by Hennessy and Leibowitz (1971). However, some other explanation may be required since defocusing may or may not alter stereoscopic sensitivity (see Chapter 10).

EYE MOVEMENTS AND STEREOPSIS

Wright (1951) measured the threshold of stereopsis with subjects steadily fixating one target and compared these data with thresholds measured when subjects moved their eyes to successively fixate each of two targets. He concluded that convergence enhanced stereo sensitivity. However, Rady and Ishak (1955) and Ogle (1956) consider that the effect of eye movements is very small. The lack of increased sensitivity derived from eye movement processes demonstrates again the separateness of these activities from those involved in depth discrimination (Mitchell, 1970).

PANUM'S LIMITING CASE AND RANDOM-DOT STEREOPSIS

Figure 8–7 illustrates stereograms that produce a stereoscopic perception know as *Panum's limiting case* (Panum, 1858) and the real-space equivalence. The limit illustrated is that two objects seen by one eye combine with one object seen by the other eye to form a stereoscopic impression of depth (Ronne, 1956). According to Hering (Ogle, 1962), the one point in the left eye serves a double function. When the left-eye point combines with both right-eye points, it participates in two different distance perceptions: one yielding the projection C' to A and the other C' to B. This is limiting because the elimination of one more line or point suspends stereopsis. As has been suggested, no relative depth is possible unless two or more points, or their stereogrammetric representations, are contained in the binocular visual field and are close enough to the horopter to allow the stereoscopic mechanism to work.

Ogle (1962) stated that the depth is perceived no matter which of the two lines is fused with the single line. Nevertheless, changes in fusion reverse the directions of the resulting binocular disparities. This alters the perception of the unfixated point from being closer to being farther than the fixation point. Furthermore, he reported that the stereo-

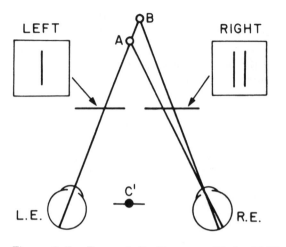

Figure 8–7.   Panum's limiting case (Ogle, 1962).

scopic perception washes out with only momentary exposures of the unfixated point. Apparently, this form of stereopsis requires longer exposure times than the more usual one. Perhaps this difference represents the additional time needed for some further neural process to accomplish the double coupling required in this situation.

The first random-dot stereogram was produced by Aschenbrenner in 1954 (Shipley, 1971). Julesz (1960) generated these by having a computer go through a large matrix of dots, randomly choosing to blacken each cell or leave it white. With duplicate dot patterns as backgrounds, he then arranged to produce crossed binocular disparity by shifting small center zones from one to eight rows laterally toward one another. Since this shift left blank spaces, he had the plotter fill them up, using the original randomizing process. Figure 8–8 illustrates this process for a much smaller matrix (Julesz, 1960) and presents one of his large matrix stereograms (Julesz, 1965).

Monocularly the stereograms reveal no particular pattern, and the two halves do not appear in any way different despite the small offsets in their centers. However, when it is viewed in a stereoscope, a contour emerges that demarcates the offset areas from the surround, and this region is seen as being in a different-depth plane (Julesz, 1960). As Julesz points out, these targets allow for the demonstration of stereopsis by using patterns that do not contain monocularly recognizable forms.

The refilled blank spaces are uncorrelated between the members of the stereogrammetric pair. Nevertheless, these appear in the same-

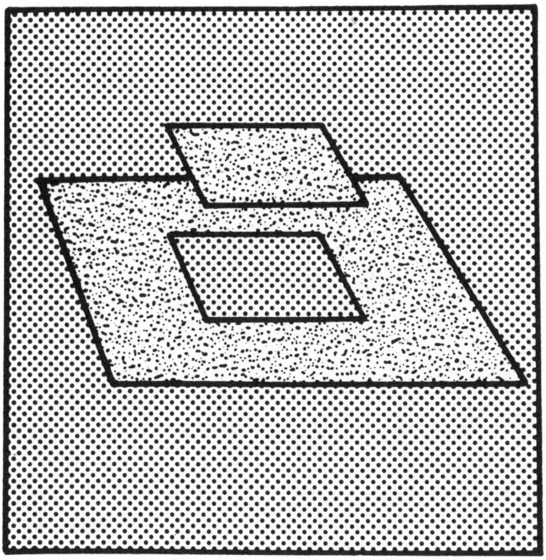

A

a	b	a	c	d	f
g	e	h	d	c	b
e	f	A	G	a	g
e	a	D	B	e	c
f	c	d	e	f	e
d	g	c	h	b	a

a	b	a	c	d	f
g	e	h	d	c	b
e	A	G	c	a	g
e	D	B	d	e	c
f	c	d	e	f	e
d	g	c	h	b	a

B

Figure 8–8.   (A) A schematic representation of the resulting perception (Julesz, 1965). (B) A small dot matric of random brightnesses (Julesz, 1960. Copyright 1960, American Telephone and Telegraph Company. Reprinted by permission).

depth plane as the offset centers. Julesz (1964) considered this phenomenon an example of Panum's limiting case.

Julesz and Spivack (1967) described two processes involved in random-dot stereopsis, *local stereopsis* and *global stereopsis*. They felt that upon taking up the view of these stereograms, the brain is required to establish the required match-ups of the two images of the dots or clusters of dots. This pattern matching is done dot by dot and cluster by cluster and is designated local stereopsis. Global stereopsis involves a similar kind of pattern matching over rather larger areas, to find elements with the same disparity value. For example, the process might be described as follows. Upon presentation of a random-dot stereogram, a local pattern-matching process or coupling occurs, and localized clusters of dots appear in depth. Once this is complete, the depth form emerges in the central area because of a rather more global process that identifies this area as being at a different depth.

Fender and Julesz (1967) considered that fusion was a prerequisite for the perception of stereopsis with random-dot patterns. We have already seen that this is true, regardless of the character and amount of contour information, for all stereogrammetric displays (see Chapter 7). Furthermore, Julesz (1963) demonstrated a stereoscopic perception that survives a 20 percent magnification of one image. This latter effect also has been achieved by using conventional contours (Reading and Tanlamai, 1980). Nevertheless, random-dot patterns are unique and produce some effects that would seem difficult to explain in terms of a simplified understanding of corresponding points. Chang (1976) did a study with these patterns in which he found no difference between the threshold of stereopsis measured with random-dot patterns and line targets. He suggested that these patterns are special because they provide a sufficiently dense packing of dots to mask such effects as binocular rivalry. The targets also allow fusion a free reign, so that the point of intersection of the primary lines of sight can float over a rather large range of angular disparities and still permit the perception of stereopsis (Woo, 1970).

Harwerth and Rawlings (1977) have shown decrements in random-dot stereo sensitivity with decreasing exposure time. In one subject, responses were reduced to the chance level when the duration was 0.5 s, whereas the other reached this level at 0.25 s. However, Julesz (1964) reported perceptions of rather large random-dot disparities at exposure times of 0.08 s. A comparison with similar studies involving conventional line targets (see Chapter 6) indicates that this aspect of random-dot stereopsis may be no more than an elaborate instance involving Panum's limiting case.

STABLE BINOCULAR DEPTH PERCEPTION WITH MOVING EYES

Perhaps these concepts can be used to explain how eye movements during steady fixation can produce changes in binocular disparity as large as 7 or 8 arcmintues (Fender and Julesz, 1967) while stereoscopic perceptions remain unaffected. One solution would be that, once fixation and fusion have occurred, a coupling process occurs between corresponding points and certain noncorresponding points that receive roughly similar patterns. This process fixes the depth relationships of objects in the field of view, and the association endures throughout the fixational pause. According to this schema, the only binocular disparities that can be consciously appreciated would be those that existed at the onset of the initial act of fixation and those that occur subsequently as a result of sufficient movement of objects in the field of view, movement of the head, or movement of the eyes. This cental insensitive zone, or disparity dead zone, could be either the result of a cancellation process associated with eye movements at an unconscious level or simply the chance combination of monocular insensitive zones. Similar hypotheses have been suggested, or implied, by Fender and Julesz (1967) and Ditchburn (1973).

Random-dot patterns are useful clinical devices, as we discuss in Chapter 9, and say something about the sequence of processing of visual information in the visual cortex, as presented in Chapter 12.

STEREOANOMALY: STEREOBLINDNESS

Richards (1971) chose to measure some subjects' stereoscopic perceptions of diplopic images by using a three-category forced-choice technique. In this study, the subject had to respond to each binocular disparity presented by classifying its relative location with regard to a fixation plane as "front, on plane, or behind." He hypothesized that binocular disparity was processed by separate groups of neurons depending on whether it was crossed, uncrossed, or zero. If this were so, he reasoned that application of the usual two-category technique would not uncover anomalies.

For example, if the crossed-disparity system were lacking, an anomalous subject operating in the usual two-category way would sense uncrossed disparities and respond directly. For crossed disparities, there is no depth effect, but the anomalous subject can see that this class of stimuli does not appear the same as the normally processed uncrossed ones. Therefore, the subject can learn to say "front" to these and thus tend to mask the anomaly. Plotting percentage of correct responses as a function of binocular disparity produces a pattern like that identified with subject MW in Figure 8-9. Richards also found the opposite response pattern, like subject AE. Subject AE is considered to be lacking in the uncrossed binocular disparity detectors.

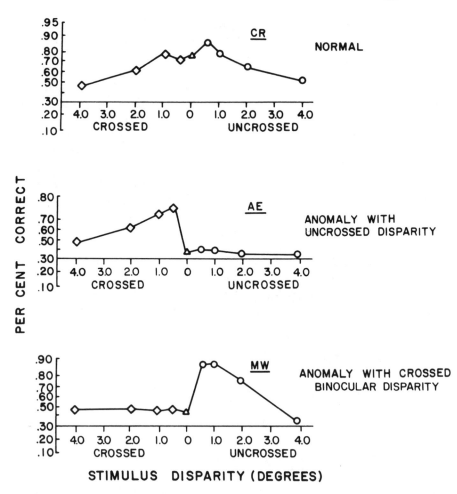

Figure 8–9.   Percentage of correct responses to various large amounts of binocular disparities (Reprinted by permission from Richards, 1971).

Figure 8–9 also presents a third response pattern (CR) which is considered normal. Notice that for CR the correct response rate for zero disparity is not the highest value recorded. However, this is slightly misleading since what is plotted at zero is the response rate to a monocularly presented stimulus. Furthermore, if we consider the test distance used and assume an average interpupillary distance for the observers, the projection of 2° and 4° of uncrossed disparities produces an intersection behind the subject's head; yet the correct response rate for this subject is no different than for a ±1° of binocular disparity.

Exactly what a correct response should be under such circumstances is not altogether clear.

Four other subjects performed depth-matching settings. The data for three are presented in Figure 8–10. The ordinate is the binocular disparity at which the subject sets an object to match it to the depth of another object, which is set at the values indicated on the abscissa. Note that for depth matches of binocular disparities that are smaller than the diplopia threshold, all three subjects' settings appear normal.

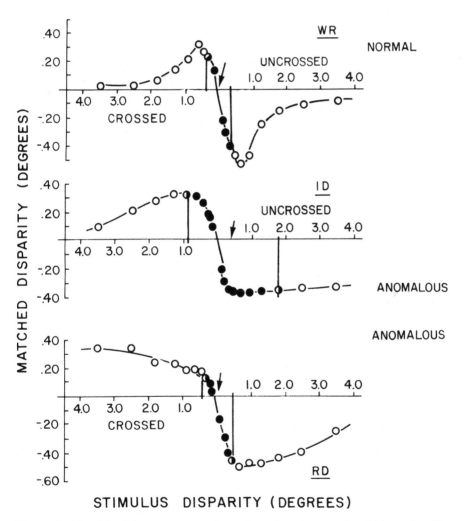

Figure 8–10.   Matching responses to various large amounts of binocular disparities (Reprinted by permission from Richards, 1971).

The condition presented for subject ID and RD is best described as an anomaly of stereo perception for objects located outside Panum's area.

In this report, Richards did not attempt to systematically correlate stereoanomalies with oculomotor anomalies. However, he performed another study of some 150 subjects drawn from a college community and found that 2.7 percent of these were stereoblind to large disparities. He suggested that this percentage was very close to the incidence of strabismus (Richards, 1970). In Figure 8–10 the filled circles represent reports of haplopia, and the half-filled ones reports of diplopia. From this we can get some rough idea of the size of Panum's area and, by approximation, find a disparity at which the two primary lines of sight most likely intersected. Two of these subjects appear to have normal-size areas and no deviation. Subject ID seems to have had about 24 arcminutes of exodeviation and a very large Panum's space. Based on this information, this subject might have had a microheterotropia or some other form of binocular sensory anomaly. Stereoanomalies may be the result or the cause of some of these anomalies. Only future study may show which causes the other.

REFERENCES

Alpern, M. (1969), "Types of movements," *The Eye*, vol. 3, Academic, New York, 65–174.

Armington, J. C., and Bloom, B. (1974), "Relations between the amplitudes of spontaneous saccades and visual responses," *Journal of the Optical Society of America*, 64, 1263–1271.

Brindley, G. S. (1954), "The summation areas of human color-receptive mechanisms at increment threshold," *Journal of Physiology*, 124, 400–408.

Brindley, G. S. (1970), *Physiology of the Retina and Visual Pathway*, Williams and Wilkins, Baltimore, 103.

Burg, A. (1966), "Visual acuity as measured by dynamic and static tests: A comparative evaluation," *Journal of Applied Psychology*, 50, 460–466.

Chang, F. W. L. (1976), "Determination of the minimum threshold of stereopsis with random dot patterns," Ph.D. thesis, Indiana University.

Charnwood, J. R. B. (1950), *An Essay on Binocular Vision*, Hatton, London, 599–622.

Christianson, S., and Hofstetter, H. W. (1972), "Some historical notes on Carl Pulfrich," *American Journal of Optometry*, 49, 944–947.

Cibis, P. A., and Haber, H. (1951), "Anisopia and preception of depth," *Journal of the Optical Society of America*, 41, 676–683.

Cutler, G. H., and Ley, A. H. (1963), "Kinetic visual acuity," *British Journal of Physiological Optics*, 20, 119–127.

Ditchburn, R. W. (1973), *Eye Movements and Visual Perception*, Clarendon Press, Oxford, 375–376.

Dodwell, P. C., Harker, G. S., and Behar, I. (1968), "Pulfrich effect with minimal differential adaptation of the eyes," *Vision Research*, 8, 1431–1443.

Enright, J. T. (1970), "Stereopsis, visual latency, and three-dimensional moving pictures," *Amercian Scientist*, 58, 536–545.

Fender, D., and Julesz, B. (1967), "Extension of Panum's fusional area in binocular stabilized vision," *Journal of the Optical Society of America*, 57, 819–830.

Foley, J. M. (1967), "Binocular disparity and perceived relative distance: An examination of two hypotheses," *Vision Research*, 7, 655–670.

Gillott, H. F. (1957), *The Effect on Binocular Vision of Variations in the Realtive Size and Levels of Illumination of the Ocular Images*, British Optical Assoc., London, 56–69.

Gogel, W. C. (1954), "Perception of the relative distance position of objects as a function of other objects in the field," *Journal of Experimental Psychology*, 47, 335–342.

Harker, G. S. (1967), "A saccadic suppression explanation of the Pulfrich phenomenon," *Perception and Psychophysics*, 2, 423–426.

Harwerth, R. S., and Rawlings, S. C. (1977), "Viewing time and stereoscopic threshold with random-dot stereograms," *American Journal of Optometry and Physiological Optics*, 54, 452–457.

Helmholtz, H. (1925), *Handbook of Physiological Optics*, vol, 3, The Optical Society of America, New York, 307–312.

Hennessey, R. T., and Leibowitz, H. W. (1971), "The effect of a peripheral stimulus on accommodation," *Perception and Psychophysics*, 10, 129–132.

Hirsch, M. J., Horowitz, M. W., and Weymouth, F. W. (1948), "Distance discrimination, III, Effect of rod width on threshold," *Archives of Ophthalmology*, 39, 325–332.

Jacobs, D. H. (1943), *Fundamentals of Optical Engineering*, McGraw-Hill, New York, 253–258.

Jonkers, G. H., and Kylstra, P. H. (1963), "Brightness contrast and color contrast in stereoscopic vision acuity," *Ophthalmologica*, 145, 139–143.

Julesz, B. (1960), "Binocular depth perception of computer-generated patterns," *Bell System Technical Journal*, 39, 1125–1162.

Julesz, B. (1963), "Stereopsis and binocular rivalry," *Journal of the Optical Society of America*, 53, 994–999.

Julesz, B. (1964), "Binocular depth perception without familiarity cues," *Science*, 145, 356–362.

Julesz, B. (1965), "Texture and visual perception," *Scientific American*, 212, 38–48.

Julesz, B., and Payne, R. A. (1968), "Differences between monocular and binocular stroboscopic movement perception," *Vision Research*, 8, 433–444.

Julesz, B., and Spivack, G. J. (1967), "Stereopsis based on vernier cues alone," *Science*, 157, 563–565.

Julesz, B., and White, B. (1969), "Short term visual memory and the Pulfrich phenomenon," *Nature*, 222, 639–641.

Katz, M.S., and Schwartz, I. (1955), "New observation of the Pulfrich effect," *Journal of the Optical Society of America*, 45, 523–524.

Kaufman, L. (1974), *Sight and Mind*, Oxford, New York, 275–278, 321–322.

LeGrand, Y. (1967), *Form and Space Vision*, Indiana University, Bloomington, 304–305.

Lit, A. (1949), "The magnitude of the Pulfrich stereophenomenon as a function of binocular differences of intensity at various levels of illumination," *American Journal of Psychology*, 62, 159–181.

Lit, A. (1959), "Depth-discrimination thresholds as a function of binocular differences of retinal illumination at scotopic and photopic levels," *Journal of the Optical Society of America*, 49, 746–752.

Lit, A. (1960), "Effect of target velocity in a frontal plane on binocular spatial localization at photopic retinal illumination levels," *Journal of the Optical Society of America*, 50, 970–973.

Ludvigh, E. (1942), "Relative effectiveness of make-and-break and continuous tracking in range at various rates of change on angular disparateness," *Office of Scientific Research and Development*, Report 55794, U.S. Navy, Washington.

Luria, S. M. (1969), "Stereoscopic and resolution acuity with various fields of view," *Science*, 164, 452–453.

Luria, S. M., and Kinney, J. A. S. (1971), "Peripheral stimuli and stereoacuity for navy divers working under water," *Naval Submarine Medical Center*, Report 654.

Luria, S. M., and Weissman, S. (1968), "Relationship between static and dynamic stereo acuity," *Journal of Experimental Psychology*, 76, 51–56.

Mitchell, D. E. (1970), "Properties of stimuli eliciting vergence eye movements and stereopsis," *Vision Research*, 10, 145–162.

Ogle, K. N. (1956), "Stereoscopic acuity and the role of convergence," *Journal of the Optical Society of America*, 46, 269–273.

Ogle, K. N. (1962), "Special topics in binocular spatial localization," *The Eye*, vol. 4, Academic, New York, 349–407.

Ogle, K. N. (1963), "Stereoscopic depth perception and exposure delay between images to the two eyes," *Journal of the Optical Society of America*, 53, 1296–1304.

Ogle, K. N., and Groch, J. (1956), "Stereopsis and unequal luminosities of the images to the two eyes," *Archives of Ophthalmology*, 56, 878–895.

Ogle, K. N., and Reihner, L. (1962), "Stereoscopic depth perception from afterimages," *Vision Research*, 2, 439–447.

Ogle, K. N., and Weil, M.A. (1958), "Stereoscopic vision and the duration of the stimulus," *Archives of Ophthalmology*, 59, 4–17.

Panum, P. L. (1858), *Physiologische Untersuchungen uber das Sehen mit zwei Augen*, Schwerssche, Kiel, 76.

Pennington, J. (1970), "The effect of wavelength on stereoacuity," *American Journal of Optometry*, 47, 288–294.

Pulfrich, C. (1922), "Die stereoskopie im Dienste der isochromen und heterochromen Photometrie," *Naturwissenschaften*, 25, 553–564, 569–601, 714–722, 735–743.

Rady, A. A., and Ishak, I. G. H. (1955), "Relative contributions of disparity and convergence to stereoscopic acuity," *Journal of the Optical Society of America*, 45, 530–534.

Rains, J. D. (1963), "Signal luminance and position effects in human reaction time," *Vision Research*, 3, 239–251.

Reading, R. W., and Tanlamai, T. (1980), "The threshold of stereopsis in the presence of differences in magnification of the ocular images," *Journal of the American Optometric Association*, 51, 593–595.

Reading, R. W., and Woo, G. C. S. (1972), "Some of the time factors associated with stereopsis," *American Journal of Optometry*, 49, 20–28.

Richards, W. (1969), "Saccadic suppression," *Journal of the Optical Society of America*, 59, 617–623.

Richards, W. (1970), "Stereopsis and stereoblindness," *Experimental Brain Research*, 10, 380–388.

Richards, W. (1971), "Anomalous stereoscopic depth perception," *Journal of the Optical Society of America*, 61, 410–414.

Ronne, G. (1956), "The physiological basis of sensory fusion," *Acta Ophthalmologica*, 34, 1–26.

Shipley, T. (1971), "The first random-dot texture stereogram," *Vision Research*, 11, 1491–1492.

Stiles, W. S., and Crawford, B. H. (1933), "The luminous efficiency of rays entering the eye pupil at different points," *Procedures of the Royal Society*, London, B–133, 428–450.

Stromeyer, C. F., and Psotka, J. (1970), "The detailed texture of eidetic images," *Nature*, 225, 346–349.

Tyler, C. W. (1971), "Stereoscopic depth movement: Two eyes less sensitive than one," *Science*, 174, 958–961.

Vos, J. J. (1960), "Some new aspects of color stereoscopy," *Journal of the Optical Society of America*, 50, 785–790.

Wallach, H., and Zuckerman, C. (1963), "The constancy of stereoscopic depth," *American Journal of Psychology*, 76, 404–412.

Wheatstone, C. (1838), "On some remarkable, and hitherto unobserved, phenomena of binocular vision," *Philosophical Transactions*, London, 8, 371–394.

Wist, E. R., and Gogel, W. C. (1966), "The effect of inter-ocular delay and repetition interval on depth perception," *Vision Research*, 6, 325–334.

Woo, G. C. S. (1970), "The basis of Panum's area." Ph.D. thesis, Indiana University.

Wright, W. D. (1951), "The role of convergence in stereoscopic vision," *Proceedings of the Physical Society*, London, 64, 289–297.

Zuber, B. L., and Stark, L. (1966), "Saccadic suppression: Elevation of visual threshold associated with saccadic eye movements," *Experimental Neurology*, 16, 65–79.

9

CLINICAL ASPECTS OF STEREOPSIS

> Never go to a doctor whose office plants
> have died.
>
> *Erma Bombeck*

RATIONALE FOR CLINICAL PROCEDURES

The procedures used in testing stereopsis in a clinical setting usually
are quite different from those employed in a laboratory setting. While
most clinical tests are based on psychophysical methods, they are sufficiently informal in their administration that the clinician frequently
uses them without even realizing it. Furthermore, in accordance with
the clinical axiom of "a minimum number of measurements for maximum accuracy," a series of simplified tests of visual functions exist that
are intended to screen the normals from the abnormals without necessarily assigning a specific classification or numerical value to the results. For stereopsis, a screening test can be performed by presenting
a test object of a disparity of 40 arcseconds or less to see whether the
patient can correctly perceive the depth configuration. Such a test does
not specify the patient's threshold angle; it simply indicates that the
patient has passed or failed.

Any clinical routine of examination procedures has to be efficient
because of the time and energy expended. Nevertheless, there is ample
leeway in the usual examination routine for some special testing of such
things as glare sensitivity, color vision, and stereopsis as well as special
investigations, in certain cases, into issues involving disease, strabismus, aniseikonia, and so on.

We can consider clinical practice to include a core of activities that a clinician does routinely and almost without regard to the patient's signs and symptoms. In fact, these things would not be done for a patient only if it would waste time in getting the proper and immediate care, as in an ocular emergency, or the problem were obvious, simple, and restricted, as in adjusting a frame. One reason for this core is that it develops a profile of information that screens out the relatively high-incident problems, provides facts about the features of the patient's visual mechanism that form the basis for deciding on the best course of solving her or his problems, and establishes a certain data baseline by which to assess change at subsequent points. Stereopsis tests belong in this core or routine of clinical examination techniques.

CLINICAL TESTS FOR STEREOPSIS

We describe several clinical tests for stereopsis. They are divided into real-depth and projected-depth tests. Some tests are administered at the near point while others are for distance testing. For still others, distance is used as the independent variable. In the clinical situation, it is easiest to consider as the threshold value the binocular disparity angle for which the patient is correct 100 percent of the time.

Real-Depth Tests

In real-depth tests, a test object is physically moved out of the plane of one or more other test objects. These tests are easily administered to patients with very little experience in judging depth. Care must be taken to align the patient in the proper position so as to prevent geometric perspective cues from being created by an oblique view of the test objects. The patient must keep the head steady and free from movement to avoid responses based on motion parallax.

Two-Rod Stereo Test.   The apparatus for the two-rod stereo test, used mainly in laboratory settings, is shown in Figure 6–11 (Howard, 1919). In the clinic, the method of adjustments is utilized most frequently (see Chapter 6), and a table of threshold values for different mean deviations of the settings and interpupillary distances is prepared to simplify the analysis of the findings. For example, Table 9–1 presents mean deviations and corresponding threshold values in arcseconds for an interpupillary distance of 64 mm and a test distance of 6 m. The method of adjustment is discussed in Chapter 6. Although the test is not suitable

Table 9–1. Mean Deviations and Corresponding Thresholds for 6-m
Test Distance, Given Interpupillary Distance of 64 mm

Mean Deviation (cm)	Binocular Disparity (arcseconds)
1	3.67
2	7.33
3	11.00
4	14.67
5	18.33
6	22.00
7	25.67
8	29.34
9	33.00
10	36.67

for routine use, it serves as a standard with which all others can be compared because of its great accuracy in determining the threshold of stereopsis (Weymouth and Hirsch, 1945).

Stereoptor. Figure 9–1 shows a sketch of the view of this instrument as seen by the patient. It consists of four separate test configurations. These slide into place before an illuminated aperature and are composed of three variable-width strips, of which one is moved out of the plane of the other two by about 2.5 mm. The width of each strip is arranged so that usually one of the wider strips is placed behind the plane of the others while the thinnest is usually moved in front of this plane. This arrangement places the size cues in direct conflict with the binocular disparity cues. The design was intended to help the practitioner decide whether the patient was properly responding to the binocular disparity cue. However, size cues that directly contradict binocular disparity may confound stereoscopic perceptions and produce an artificially elevated threshold (Sloan and Altman, 1954).

The test was designed to be administered by first demonstrating it at a near distance, say 40 cm, and then retreating to 2 m and exposing, in turn, all eight target positions while the patient keeps the head perfectly still. The additional four positions come about by turning the instrument upside down and reexposing the original four. The process is repeated at ever-closer distances until the patient calls all eight positions correctly. Targets should be covered with the hand while they are being changed. This test uses distance as the independent variable and is designed to be employed between 2 and 3 m.

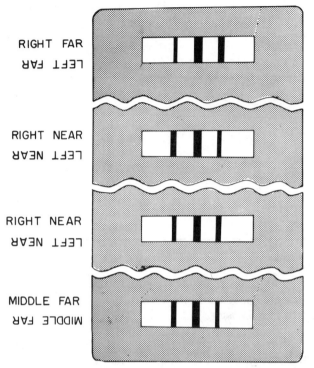

RIGHT FAR
LEFT FAR

RIGHT NEAR
LEFT NEAR

RIGHT NEAR
LEFT NEAR

MIDDLE FAR
MIDDLE FAR

Figure 9–1. Views seen by the subject of the stereopter. The instrument is turned upside down to obtain eight separate depth configurations.

For analysis of the results, Verhoeff proposed the use of a stereopsis scale that was reminiscent of the decimal visual acuity scale. The distance in centimeters at which the patient calls all eight positions correctly is divided by 100. Then this can be expressed as a decimal stereoscopic acuity or, as Verhoeff (1942) proposed, converted to a Snellen-like fraction. Table 9–2 summarizes this kind of notation and allows conversions from Verhoeff's scale to threshold angles in arcseconds. At least one other scale has been commonly used (Fry, 1942); it was empirically determined by Shephard and is expressed in terms of percentages. For example, 100 percent stereopsis corresponds to a threshold value of 16 arcseconds. Other values can be approximated by

$$\log \eta = 2.85 - 0.0176(\text{percent stereo}) \tag{9–1}$$

Nevertheless, the threshold angle notation and log threshold are the best ones (Hofstetter, 1968).

Table 9–2. Analysis of Stereoptor Test Data

Distance (m)	Binocular Stereoscopic Decimal Acuity of Verhoeff	Binocular Disparity When I.D. = 64 mm (arcseconds)
2	2.0	8.25
1.5	1.5	14.67
1.0	1.0	33.00
0.9	0.9	40.74
0.8	0.8	51.57
0.7	0.7	67.35
0.6	0.6	91.67

The test distance at which a patient correctly detects the displacement of all eight targets on the stereopter can be converted to binocular stereoscopic decimal acuity and threshold angle. Binocular disparity is based on Δd = 2.5 mm and I.D. = 64 mm.

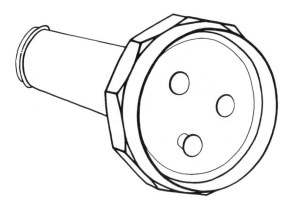

Figure 9–2.   A perspective view of the diastereo test.

Diastereo.   Hofstetter has directed the development of a simple, inexpensive test for stereopsis (Pardon, 1962). His group used a flashlight and mounted a diffusing lens over the front of it. On its face, three dots were attached. The front surface of one dot was moved forward about 9.1 mm. Figure 9–2 illustrates a view seen by the patient (Reisman, 1965).

This test is administered by positioning the Diastereo on the midsagittal plane of the subject with the face of the instrument parallel to the face plane at a distance of 6 m. With the examiner's hand over the instrument, it is rotated to one of eight different positions and exposed for a second or so. The patient is asked to refrain from moving the head and to respond by identifying the position of the protruding dot: up, down, left, right, up and left, up and right, down and left, or down and right. This process is repeated at decreasing distances until the patient calls all eight positions correctly. By scaling off an examination room floor or wall and preparing a table like Table 9–3, this test can be used most quickly and efficiently by the practitioner (Koetting and Mueller, 1962). It is as sensitive as any of the more elaborate and expensive stereo tests available, and it is highly reliable (Hofstetter and Bertsch, 1976).

For all real-depth testing devices, large target offsets or short viewing distances with fixed offsets can produce accurate distance judgments based on apparent size. Tables 9–1, 9–2, and 9–3 include those conditions in which apparent size changes are less than 1 percent (see Chapter 6). When values outside these ranges are used, binocular test results should be directly compared with monocular results to determine whether binocular performance is superior.

Projected-Depth Tests

Most of these tests are presented easily and quickly. However, the patient should be allowed sufficient viewing time for the stereopsis impression to "develop." A small number of patients find that the appreciation of a stereo effect with these tests is very difficult, whereas they respond readily to real-depth tests. This could be due to a reluctance to believe that objects can be seen in some plane other than that of the face of the instrument (see also Chapters 7 and 8).

Table 9–3.　Threshold Angle of Stereopsis for Corresponding Test Distances of the Diastereo

Distance (m)	Binocular Disparity (arcseconds)	Distance (m)	Binocular Disparity (arcseconds)
6.00	3.34	3.50	9.81
5.75	3.63	3.25	11.37
5.50	3.97	3.00	13.35
5.25	4.36	2.75	15.88
5.00	4.81	2.50	19.22
4.75	5.32	2.25	23.73
4.50	5.93	2.00	30.03
4.25	6.65	1.75	39.23
4.00	7.51	1.50	53.39
3.75	8.54	1.25	76.88

Δd = 9.1 mm and I.D. = 64 mm.

Stereograms. Figure 9–3 shows how binocular disparity is created with a Brewster stereoscope (see also Chapter 7). Also called *binocular parallax*, the binocular disparity is the difference between the angles labeled θ_L and θ_R. These are the subtense angles at the eyes for a pair of common points on two stereograms A and A' and B and B'. When the stereograms are located in the focal plane of the stereoscope's lenses, angle $\theta_R = \theta'_R$ and $\theta_L = \theta'_L$. It is easy to show that

$$\eta = \frac{\overline{AA'} - \overline{BB'}}{f'}\ 206{,}265\ \text{arcseconds/rad} \tag{9-2}$$

The expression $\overline{AA'} - \overline{BB'}$ is called *decentration.*It is used because of the ease with which it can be measured on a stereogram by a millimeter ruler. For example, if $\overline{BB} > \overline{AA'}$, then B will be seen farther away from the patient than A. This helps the clinician in appraising a patient's responses. The following equation is extremely handy for calculating target positions on a stereogram that will produce a given binocular disparity (Fry, 1942):

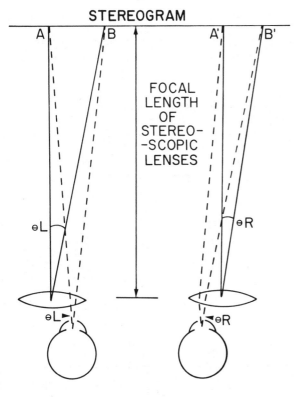

Figure 9–3. Optical principles of the Brewster stereoscope as they apply to generating binocular disparity (Fry, 1942).

$$\eta = \frac{decentration}{f'} \ 206{,}265 \ \text{arcseconds/rad}$$

The Keystone Telebinocular contains a pair of $+5 = D$ lenses and is used to administer the Visual Skills series of tests. The stereopsis card of this series (DB–6D) has 12 rows of symbols with one symbol on each row appearing in a closer plane than the others. Table 9–4 shows the row number, symbol, decentration, and binocular disparity for this test (Fry, 1942). The test presents disparity values only as low as about 83 arcseconds, and as we explain later, creates certain questions about what is actually being measured. Other Keystone tests are available that have disparities as small as about 8 arcseconds, but the Visual Skills version is just not sensitive enough.

Vectographic Tests.   Vectography uses polarizing material on the test objects only. Therefore, the background is much brighter and the contrast greater than in conventional polarizing display techniques (Valyus, 1962). For vectographic display, the stereograms overlap and so require no stereoscope to produce fusion. Since zero-disparity points have no offset, they can be left unpolarized.

Grolman Slide.   As indicated in Table 9–5 this projection slide has five rows of five circles, of which one stands out in crossed disparity

Table 9–4.   Information on Keystone Visual Skills DB-6D Stereopsis Stereogram

Row	Crossed-Disparity Symbol	Decentration (mm)	Binocular Disparity (arcseconds)
1	Cross	1.07	1103.52
2	Circle	0.70	721.93
3	Star	0.64	660.05
4	Circle	0.54	556.92
5	Square	0.44	453.78
6	Square	0.38	391.90
7	Heart	0.25	257.83
8	Cross	0.22	226.89
9	Star	0.19	195.95
10	Cross	0.10	103.13
11	Heart	0.09	92.82
12	Circle	0.08	82.51

Source: Fry (1942).

Table 9–5. Approximate Binocular Disparities for Grolman Vectographic Slide

Row	Binocular Disparity (arcseconds)
1	250
2	180
3	125
4	60
5	40

Source: Amos (1970).

Table 9–6. Binocular Disparities for Titmus Stereo Test

Row	Binocular Disparity (arcseconds)
1	800
2	400
3	200
4	150
5	100
6	80
7	60
8	50
9	40

Source: Amos (1970).

in each row. The binocular disparity of the bottom row is about 40 arcseconds, just good enough for clinical testing. The test is popular because it is conveniently contained with other slides that provide test objects for a fairly complete binocular refraction routine. Naturally, the test assesses stereopsis for distance fixation (American Optical, 1973). The standard Project-o-chart slide has only four rows of five circles each, and the smallest disparity available is 60 arcseconds (Grolman, 1966), which is not sensitive enough for most clinical purposes.

Titmus Stereo Test. This test is also produced by the vectographic process and requires the use of polarizing filters before the patient's eyes. Table 9–6 presents the binocular disparity steps available for the Titmus stereo test. It is based on a design by Wirt (1942) and intended to be used at 40 cm.

Randot Stereo Test. This vectographic test utilizes the principles of random-dot patterns (see Chapter 8) and is calibrated in arcseconds to present patterns at 600, 400, 200, 100, 70, 50, 40, 30, and 20 arcseconds in a crossed binocular disparity at 40 cm. By inverting the test plates, these become uncrossed binocular disparities (Titmus Optical Co., 1978).

Because the perception of a sufficiently large amount of binocular disparity is accompanied by the perception of a depth contour, this test removes many potential ambiguities. If a patient reports no figure outlined by the binocular contour, then he or she is not perceiving stereoscopically. One part of the test uses a configuration of circles. Here, one of the four stand out in crossed disparity while the other three are presented in uncrossed disparity. Table 9–7 shows the position of the crossed-disparity circle, and Figure 9–4 schematically shows an example of the target configuration.

Random-Dot E Test. Reinecke and Simons (1974) reported a random-dot test in which the emerging pattern was a Snellen-like letter E. By varying the test distance, as with the Stereoptor and Diastereo tests, the distance at which the outline of the E is correctly reported can be determined. However, the test was designed as a screening device since at a little over 4 m, the binocular disparity is still 63 arcseconds.

Anaglyphs. Another method of presenting stereograms is by anaglyph (LeGrand, 1967). This process prints one of the pair with red ink and

Table 9–7. Key for Randot Circle Test

Row	Crossed-Disparity Position	Binocular Disparity at 40 cm (arcseconds)
1	Top	400
2	Bottom	200
3	Right	100
4	Top	70
5	Left	50
6	Right	40
7	Bottom	30
8	Top	20

Source: Titmus Optical Co. (1978).

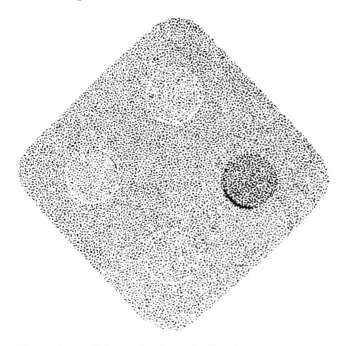

Figure 9–4. Schematic view of a Randot target.

the other with green. The patient views the resultant through a red filter before one eye, which causes the green ink to appear black on a red background, and a green filter before the other eye, which causes the red ink to appear black on a green background.

Institute for Perception Random-Dot Stereogram. Walraven (1975) described an anaglyphic random-dot stereogram developed at the Institue for Perception, Soesterberg, the Netherlands. The test consists of three screening plates of 33 arcminutes of disparity and three test plates, ranging from 480 to 15 arcseconds. Several of the plates contain a monocularly visible form and identical objects that are seen only when the observer possesses global stereopsis (see Chapter 8). This test has proved useful for detecting stereopsis in young children as well as adults. Table 9–8 reports the disparities used, and Figure 9–5 shows an example of the target form.

EXTENDING THE DISPARITY RANGE OF PROJECTED-DEPTH STEREO TESTS

Table 9–9 presents binocular disparities obtainable by using the Titmus test at 50 and 60 cm. By extending the test distance, lower binocular

Table 9–8. Binocular Disparities for Institute for Perception Stereo Test

Plate Number	Form of Binocular Contour	Binocular Disparity (arcseconds)
1	Butterfly	1980
2	Disks	1980
3	Disks, triangle, and diamonds	1980
4	Suppression test	—
	Orientation of missing sector of disk targets	
5	Down and left	480
	Up and down	240
6	Up and left	120
	Right and right	60
7	Down and right	30
	Up and left	15

disparity values can be obtained with all vectographic and anaglyphic tests. Binocular disparity is changed by the ratio of the distances involved. For example, using a test calibrated for 40 cm at a test distance of 50 cm reduces the indicated disparities by a factor of 0.80.

ESTIMATING THE AVERAGE THRESHOLD FOR A NORMAL POPULATION

One objective of testing for stereopsis is to classify patients with regard to the general population. From available data (Hofstetter, 1968; Hofstetter and Bertsch, 1976), we can estimate that the adult population mean threshold angle is about 1.16 log arcseconds with a standard deviation of about 0.21 log arcsecond given the 100 percent correct-response criterion. This information suggests that if a patient possesses a threshold of 2 arcseconds, then she or he has an exceptionally fine discrimination of stereopsis since this value is more than 2 standard deviations below the mean. In the same way, a threshold of 38 arcseconds would be an extremely poor performance because this value exceeds the estimated value of the mean by more than 2 standard deviations. On the basis of this sort of reasoning, we can expect that almost 97.5 percent of the population will have thresholds between about 2 and 38 arcseconds. If we wished to be on the lookout for trouble, we would concentrate on those values that fall above the mean by 2 standard deviations, or about 38 arcseconds. If we agree that all thresh-

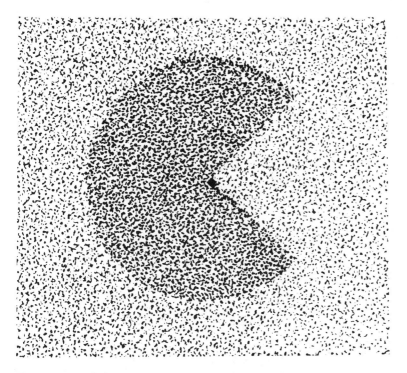

Figure 9–5. Schematic view of a target in the Institute for Perception test.

Table 9–9. Equivalent Binocular Disparities Created by Using the Titmus Stereo Test at 50 and 60 cm

Row	Binocular Disparity at 50 cm (arcseconds)	Binocular Disparity at 60 cm (arcseconds)
1	640	533
2	320	267
3	160	133
4	120	100
5	80	67
6	64	53
7	48	40
8	40	33
9	32	27

olds smaller than 38 arcseconds will be considered normal, and all above 38 arcseconds abnormal, then we will need to test at binocular disparities smaller than 36 arcseconds. The more values tested below this level, the better the test.

Using the 100 percent correct-response level facilitates the comparison of results on different clinical tests. For example, since stereogrammetric tests present targets at fixed binocular disparities, correctly perceiving the depth configuration constitutes is equivalent to the 100 percent correct-response level on such tests as the Diastereo. However, when we compare thresholds using this criterion with those determined by more formal psychophysical techniques, we must allow for this difference in method. Hofstetter and Bertsch (1976) chose the 66.67 percent correct-response level, which is equivalent to the more usual 50 percent correct-response level with a correction for guessing. They determined that the average threshold for 242 subjects was 5.5 arcseconds, a value similar to that found by Berry (1948) and others by the method of constant stimulus in laboratory settings.

COMPARISON OF TESTS

Weymouth and Hirsch (1945) suggested that the Keystone Telebinocular stereopsis test may be invalid since a distribution of thresholds determined by this test showed a marked bimodality not present in the distribution of thresholds measured on the same group of subjects by the Howard-Dolman test. Apparently, some patients respond to the visual skills stereo test on the basis of some cue other than binocular disparity. This is very undesirable in any clinical test. Cooper and Warshowsky (1977) found that the lateral displacement of one object in a stereo pair necessary to produce binocular disparity on the Titmus stereo test could be correctly judged by some subjects in terms of its resulting depth displacement even when stereo viewing conditions were suspended. All stereogrammetic tests using conventional contours may suffer from this potential problem, particularly if the subject is permitted to view the stereograms for extended periods. Random-dot tests are not subject to this same problem because of the high dot density.

Woo and Sillanpaa (1979) presented data to show that the threshold of stereopsis is smaller for crossed disparities, such as are used in most clinical tests. They suggested that both forms of disparity sensitivity should be examined. The Randot test presents both crossed and uncrossed disparities. However, uncrossed disparities also can be obtained with the Grolman slide by switching the polarizers before the two eyes, and with the Titmus by turning the test upside down. Table 9–10 shows this.

Some random-dot tests, such as that of the Institute of Perception, require recognition of the orientation of a form in depth. This kind of stereoscopic perception necessitates larger amounts of binocular disparity than those needed to perceive individual clusters of dots in stereoscopic relief (Over and Long, 1973). Thresholds determined by using this perceptual criterion are elevated (Reading and Tanlamai, 1982).

Furthermore, thresholds determined by any and all stereogrammetric tests show a lack of significant correlation with those determined by real-depth tests. The reason is that the threshold increases as the size of the errors in the apparent equidistant point increases (see Chapter 6). These errors in absolute depth judgment typically are larger for stereogrammetric test objects (Reading and Tanlamai, 1982).

USE OF TEST RESULTS

In assessing stereopsis in strabismic subjects Pardon (1962) suggested 40 arcseconds as the dividing point between normal and abnormal subjects. The result of a good stereopsis test is indispensible information in the diagnosis of microtropia, a recently identified clinical entity (Helveston and von Noorden, 1967).

This information is also useful in the evaluation of visual performance. For example, improvement in stereo sensitivity accompanying the correction of ametropia is a useful before-and-after measurement of improvement. Levy and Glick (1974) presented data on the threshold of stereopsis as measured with the Titmus stereo test through various amounts of fogging lens power. Figure 9–6 is derived from their data. It indicates mean thresholds and estimated standard deviation sizes. Such a test, with fixed increments or levels of binocular disparity, reveals a clear trend of increasing threshold with increasing plus lens

Table 9–10.   Some Clinical Tests of Stereopsis and Methods of Obtaining Uncrossed Disparities

Test	Method of Obtaining Uncrossed Disparity
Grolman	Reverse polarizers
Randot	Turn plate upside down
Institute of Perception test	Reverse red and green lenses

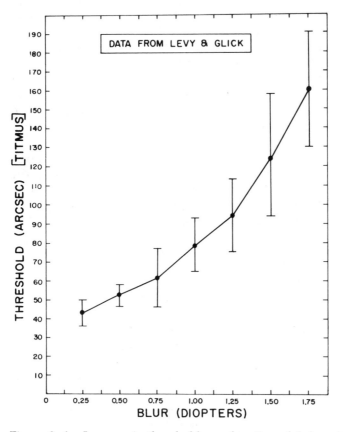

Figure 9–6.   Increase in threshold as a function of defocusing (modified from
Levy and Glick, 1974).

power. Peters (1969) obtained similar results for induced anisometropia measured by decrements in the sensitivity of space eikonometer settings.

Were these studies to be repeated with the Diastereo test, we might reasonably expect that the mean differences between 0.5-D increments in plus blur or anisometropia would produce significantly different threshold values. If this is so, then evaluating the threshold of stereopsis by a test with finely graded binocular disparities could be useful for verifying such findings as the subjective refraction and the binocular balance. In short, it would consitute a sensitive visual performance indicator. However, since stereopsis sensitivity is virtually unaffected by decreasing contrasts (see Chapter 8), and since defocusing can be considered to affect mainly retinal contrast, perhaps measurements of stereopsis are relatively insensitive to small changes in lens power.

Reading and Tanlamai (1980) found a nearly linear increase in the log threshold as a function of increasing magnification differences between the two ocular images over a range from 0 to 33 percent. This explains reports of stereopsis in monocular aphakia corrected with either contact lenses (Rosenbloom, 1953) or spectacles (Lubkin et al., 1966). As with microstrabismus, the fact that image-size differences degrade stereopsis further emphasizes the value of threshold measurement and specification as a means of differentiating fine and gross binocular function (see Chapter 13).

Nevertheless, testing patient responses to large binocular disparities establishes the operation of some form of simultaneous binocular vision. Furthermore, such tests have proved useful for the detection of amblyopia in children between about 2 and 4 years of age (Simons and Reinecke, 1974; Walraven, 1975; and Cooper and Feldman, 1978).

Ideally, stereopsis should be assessed both far and near. Such measurements are useful for detection and evaluation of binocular sensory anomalies that are accentuated at one or the other of these two locations. For example, the Diastereo can be used as a test for stereopsis with distance viewing, since the average patient should reach the 100 percent correct-response level at about 3 m. For near-point testing, a test based on random-dot design can be utilized.

OVERVIEW

Clinical stereopsis tests can be divided into two categories: real-depth and projected-depth tests. Real-depth tests have the advantage of providing nearly instantaneous perception of stereopsis and producing reliable responses from patients who have very little prior experience with depth judgments. These tests have the potential disadvantage of yielding misleading results owing to movements of the patient's head (motion parallax) or misalignment of the instrument (geometric perspective). Projected-depth tests, particularly those using vectography, can be employed conveniently and can assess stereopsis rapidly. Some small percentage of patients resist responding to these tests, apparently because they are reluctant to believe that images can be seen out of the plane of the test plate. Some small amount of time may be required for all patients to perceive stereopsis while using these devices. Furthermore, in general, projected-depth thresholds usually are slightly higher and virtually without correlation to real-depth test results.

By the 100 percent correct-response criterion, the normal binocular patient should have a threshold equal to, or less than, about 38 arc-seconds. An abnormality of binocular vision is indicated when the threshold is greater than about 40 arcseconds. Application of this information means that all patients with strabismus, abnormal suppression, moderate to large amounts of amblyopia, eccentric fixation, aniseikonia, and anomalous correspondence should fail this test.

Stereopsis threshold measurements may be useful also for comparative measurements of improvement following application of corrections of ametropia, for verification of the correctness of the binocular balance findings, and for relative measurements of progress during the course of treatment of some binocular anomalies.

REFERENCES

American Optical Co. (1973), "A new remote control A.O. custom Project-o-chart," sales literature, Southbridge, OB 8, 7.

Amos, J. (1970), "Clinical stereopsis," unpublished manuscript.

Berry, R. N. (1948), "Quantitative relations among vernier, real depth, and stereoscopic depth acuities," *Journal of Experimental Psychology*, 38, 708–721.

Chang, F. W. L. (1976), "Determination of the minimum threshold of stereopsis with random dot patterns," Ph.D. thesis, Indiana University, Bloomington.

Cooper, J., and Feldman, J. (1978), "Random-dot-stereogram performance by strabismic, amblyopic, and ocular-pathology patients in an operant-discrimination task," *American Journal of Optometry and Physiological Optics*, 55, 599–609.

Cooper, J. and Warshowsky J. (1977), "Lateral displacement as a response cue in the Titmus stereo test," *American Journal of Optometry and Physiological •Optics*, 54, 537–541.

Fry, G. A. (1942), "Measurement of the threshold of stereopsis," *Optometric Weekly*, 23, 1029–1032.

Grolman, B. (1966), "Binocular refraction, A new system" *New England Journal of Optometry*, 17, 118–130.

Helveston, E. M., and von Noorden, G. K. (1967), "Microtropia—A newly defined entity," *Archives of Ophthalmology*, 78, 272–281.

Hofstetter, H. W. (1968), "Absolute threshold measurements with the Diastereo test," *Archivos de la Sociedad Americana de Oftalmologia y Optometria*, 6, 327–342.

Hofstetter, H. W., and Bertsch, J. D. (1976), "Does stereopsis change with age?" *American Journal of Optometry and Physiological Optics*, 53, 664–667.

Howard, H. J. (1919), "A test for the judgment of distance," *American Journal of Ophthalmology*, 2, 656–675.

Julesz, B. (1971), *Foundations of Cyclopian Perception*, Chicago Univ. Press.

Koetting, R. A., and Mueller, R. C. (1962), "Evaluation of a rapid stereopsis test," *American Journal of Optometry*, 39, 299–304.

LeGrand, Y. (1967), *Form and Space Vision*, Indiana University, Bloomington, 305–306.

Levy, N. S., and Glick, E. B. (1974), "Stereoscopic perception and Snellen visual acuity," *American Journal of Ophthalmology*, 78, 722–724.

Lubkin, V., Stollerman, H., and Linksz, A. (1966), "Stereopsis in monocular aphakia with spectacle correction," *American Journal of Ophthalmology*, 61, 273–276.

Ogle, K. N. (1938), "Induced size effect," *Archives of Ophthalmology*, 20, 604–623.

Over, R., and Long, N. (1973), "Depth is visible before figure in stereoscopic perception of random-dot patterns," *Vision Research*, 13, 1207–1299.

Pardon, H. R. (1962), "A new device for stereopsis," *Journal of the American Optometric Association*, 33, 510–512.

Peters, H. B. (1969), "The influence of anisometropia on stereosensitivity," *American Journal of Optometry*, 46, 120–123.

Reading, R. W., and Tanlamai, T. (1980), "The threshold of stereopsis in the presence of differences in magnification of the ocular images," *Journal of the American Optometric Association*, 51, 593–595.

Reading, R. W., and Tanlamai, T. (1982), "Finely graded binocular disparities from random-dot patterns," *Opthalmic and Physiological Optics*, 2, 47–56.

Reinecke, R. D., and Simons, K. (1974), "A new stereoscopic test for amblyopia screening," *American Journal of Ophthalmology*, 78, 714–721.

Reisman, M. (1965), "Evaluation of a modified stereopsis test," *Indiana Journal of Optometry*, 35, 9–14.

Rosenbloom, A. A. (1953), "The correction of unilateral aphakia with corneal contact lenses," *American Journal of Optometry*, 30, 536–542.

Simons, K., and Reinecke, R. D. (1974), "A reconsideration of amblyopia screening and stereopsis," *American Journal of Ophthalmology*, 78, 707–713.

Sloan, L. L., and Altman, A. (1954), "Factors involved in several tests of binocular depth perception," *Archives of Ophthalmology*, 52, 524–544.

Titmus Optical Co. (1978), "Randot-stereotest," Instruction Manual, Petersburg, VA, 2–4.

Valyus, N. A. (1962), *Stereoscopy*, Focal, London, 114–116.

Verhoeff, F. H. (1942), "Simple quantitative test for acuity and reliability of binocular stereopsis," *Archives of Ophthalmology*, 28, 1000–1019.

Walraven, J. (1975), "Amblyopia screening with random-dot stereograms," *American Journal of Ophthalmology*, 80, 893–900.

Weymouth, F. W., and Hirsch, M. J. (1945), "The reliability of certain tests for determining distance discrimination," *American Journal of Psychology*, 58, 379–390.

Wirt, S. E. (1942), "A new near-point stereopsis test," *Optometric Weekly*, 38, 647–649.

Woo, C. G., and Sillanpaa, V. (1979), "Absolute stereoscopic thresholds as measured by crossed and uncrossed disparities," *American Journal of Optometry and Physiological Optics*, 56, 350–355.

10

DEVELOPMENT OF BINOCULAR VISION

> Anyone can do any amount of work pro-
> vided it isn't the work he is supposed to be
> doing at that moment.
>
> *Robert Benchley*

VISION: INNATE OR LEARNED?

The way in which the visual system grows to maturity is a fascinating study of some considerable practical importance that bears on broader issues involving the influences of genetics and the environment.

Practically, visual structure and visual performance, as well as visually guided behavior, help relate the system to the capacities of the person to adapt to the environment, including some of those activities collectively known as learning. If some problem develops, its early removal or remedy lifts the impediment and allows maturation to proceed.

One important theoretical issue has to do with the very nature of the development of the visual process. Basically, the early authorities in physiological optics drew up into two camps, one claiming that vision was innate (Hering, 1977) and the other that vision was learned (Helmholtz, 1925). This philosophic difference is not unlike various forms of the nature-nurture question that continues to be a relevant problem in certain issues involving biology and behavioral sciences.

Until fairly recently, the majority of information about the development of the human visual system was based on some few anatomic studies (Mann, 1928) and a wealth of observations of infants' reactions to their surroundings (Gesell et al., 1949). Recently this information has been supplemented by more extensive studies and observations taken with such modern measuring techniques as electron microscopy, electrooculography, and visually evoked responses. In addition, studies of animals have proved useful.

While a complete description of all aspects of the development of the visual system is beyond the scope of this discussion, some comments on the development of binocular vision and related visual structures and functions is desirable.

DEVELOPMENT OF THE FOVEA

Fine spatial judgments are at their best at the fovea. Development of this retinal structure precedes the onset of good visual acuity, fine stereopsis, and excellent color discrimination (Amigo, 1972b). Foveal development has been studied most extensively in the macaque (Hendrickson and Kupfer, 1976) for it parallels human development (Hollenberg and Spira, 1972). Shortly after birth, the foveal pit is well formed. Cones are progressively displaced toward the fovea, producing an increasing density at this location until about the third month. Cones elongate, decreasing in intersegment diameter by a factor of 2 which allows the receptors to be more tightly packed. However, outer segments change very little in size after birth (Hendrickson and Kupfer, 1976). At term, the lamellar biomembraneous folds are present in the outer segment, but contain large vesicles (Ordy et al., 1965). These membranes are fully formed, presumably with adult concentrations of photopigments, and any further alterations in outer-segment orientation are completed by the third month (Samorajski et al., 1965).

Hendrickson and Kupfer (1976) estimated that the dimensions and density of foveal cones in the newborn *Macaca mullata*, as determined by electron microscopy, could support an angle of resolution of about 2 arcminutes. Behavioral study of the acuity in newborn monkeys shows an average resolution angle of about 15 arcminutes at 1 week of age (Teller et al., 1978). This suggests that maturation of the central nervous system lags foveal structural development. Judging from studies of the lateral geniculate nucleus (Hickey, 1977) and visual cortex (Conel, 1939, 1959) in humans, anatomic development continues in these structures through the first 2 years (see Chapter 2).

DEVELOPMENT OF VISUAL ACUITY

It has been reported that human newborns respond to a moving light with a pursuit eye movement. Such movements are mainly conjugate, with occasional spurious horizontal vergence changes at birth (Worth, 1903) and are well developed and coordinated in all infants studied by age 6 months (Dayton et al., 1964). Compensatory eye movements also are present at 1 week and fully effective at the end of the first month (Gesell et al., 1949).

Upon display of a horizontally moving pattern of vertical stripes which can be resolved, eye movements occur that consist of slow pursuit movements as the stimulus moves across the field and a fast saccade to take up fixation again (Alpern, 1969). Infant acuity has been assessed by this means, called *optokinetic nystagmus (OKN)*, as has the acuity of a variety of subhuman species (see, for example, Pirenne, 1948). Usually the newborn is placed in the center of a large cylinder upon which equally spaced black and white vertical stripes are located. The cylinder is rotated slowly while eye movements are recorded by electrooculography (Dayton et al., 1964). Assessment of acuity involves decreasing the angular size of the stripes until no eye movements can be detected. Correlations with more conventional acuity measures in adults show close agreement (Reinecke and Cogan, 1958).

In newborns, applications of OKN by Dayton et al. (1964) indicate an average angle of resolution of about 25 arcminutes and as good as 17 arcminutes in a few neonates. This average steadily improves with age, and an extrapolation of the data from several studies (Dobson and Teller, 1978) for infants from 1 to 5.5 months of age indicates that OKN acuity should reach the adult level between 6 and 7 months.

Preferential looking (PL) involves observing the infants' eyes and head to detect any tendencies to fixate differentially various stimuli in the child's field of view (Dobson and Teller, 1978). Correlations with adult performance are less readily available for this method. Nevertheless, there is good agreement between results obtained by the PL and the optokinetic methods on infants. According to Dobson and Teller (1978), newborn acuity is better than about 20 arcminutes and improves steadily. An extrapolation based on this and other data (Dobson and Teller, 1978) indicates adultlike acuities by 6.5 to 7.4 months of age.

By summing cortical responses to temporal changes in the simulus, such as changes in the luminance, visual acuity can be measured also. To record the visually evoked response (VER), electrodes are placed on the scalp over the occipital pole, and the resulting potentials are amplified and averaged to improve the signal-to-noise ratio (Regan, 1972). Two forms of the VER exist: transient and steady-state. Transient VERs are a complex waveform of fluctuations in electric potential over a period of time following the sudden onset or offset of a flash of light. Steady-state VERs are regular cyclic responses to periodic variations in stimulus luminance, position, or size. Both forms have been utilized on infants from 1 to 6 months of age, and they indicate a steady development of acuity which reaches an adult state at 5 to 6 months of age (Marg et al., 1976; Harter et al., 1977).

Dobson and Teller (1978) pointed out that VER acuities usually are higher at any age in this development range. While a part of this superiority may be due to the intrinsic differences between criteria and methodology, they also may depend on neural signals that are demodulated or lost prior to expression at the behavioral level. Nevertheless, Woodruff (1972) reached the conclusion that infant acuity attains its adult level by 6 months of age by using simple clinical observation. Whatever the case, it should be possible to develop fine depth perception after 7 months of age.

DEVELOPMENT OF ACCOMMODATION AND VERGENCE EYE MOVEMENTS

A part of the lack of fine acuity in the early months of life may be due to an inability of the infant to accommodate. However, Ruskell (1967) cites two studies in which examiners found an average difference of 7 to 8 D between cycloplegic and manifest refractions in newborns. Using dynamic retinoscopy, Haynes et al., (1965) found some evidence of accommodative responses no earlier than 2 months of age and full development by 4 months of age. Brookman (1980) was able to demonstrate active accommodative responses as early as 2 weeks of age. According to Barber (1955), the ciliary muscle increases in size as the eye grows after birth, and it reaches full development by the seventh year.

Worth's (1903) observations showed that infants demonstrate binocular fixation and convergence during the first few months, and by age 5 to 6 months they respond to the disruption of binocular fixation. This is accomplished by a 5° to 8° prism base-out placed before one eye, and a corrective fusional eye movement is produced, indicating virtually full development of binocular fusion at this time. Aslin (1977), using corneal reflex photography, was able to detect relative convergence and divergence movements as early as 1 month of age and full development by ages 2 to 3 months. However, judgments of eye position based on the corneal reflexes are sufficiently imprecise so that the question of the accuracy of infant bifixation is left largely unanswered.

Development of accommodative convergence has not been studied directly, although strong theoretical arguments and data on adults would indicate its probably innate and invariant nature. The interested reader should see Alpern (1969) for a review of this topic.

DEVELOPMENT OF DEPTH PERCEPTION

Behavioral studies of developing depth perception depend on observing responses of infants to certain visual displays. Besides using eye movements as discussed earlier, the majority of these studies rely on some form of body movements which excludes the study of infants during the first few months. Responses of infants 6 to 14 months of age indicate body-coordinated behavior based on the ability to appreciate the depth relationships of a visual cliff (Walk and Gibson, 1961). However, such studies contain a variety of cues (Aslin and Dumais, 1979) and do not completely address the issue of empirical versus innate function. The visual cliff consists of a center board on which the subject is placed. To one side is a heavy glass plate in contact with a patterned surface. To the other side, another patterned surface is positioned a variable distance below the glass plate. The basic methodology of placing a subject on the center board and observing which way it moves has been applied to studies of depth perception in both humans and animals. Binocular and monocular performances measured by this apparatus leave some doubt as to the relevant depth cues (Greenspan, 1971).

Bower (1964), using conditioning techniques, demonstrated the operation of size constancy and motion parallax in infants 6 to 8 weeks old. This confirms the general trend that visual performance emerges much earlier than formerly believed (Duke-Elder, 1949).

Recently, Fox et al. (1980) demonstrated stereoscopic vision in infants 3.5 to 6 months old. Responses in this study consisted of observing infant head movements as a stereoscopic contour in a random-dot stereogram moved across the field of view. Above-chance responses were obtained to 45 and 134 arcminutes of binocular disparity beyond 3.5 months of age. Reinecke and Simons (1974) used the random-dot E test to study stereopsis in 111 children 2.6 to 6.8 years old. Their data indicated that the average threshold was about 103 arcseconds. Walraven (1975), using the Institute for Perception test, suggested that 240 arcseconds is a good level of binocular disparity to use as a screening criterion for children 2 to 7 years old. Amigo (1972a), using the Titmus stereo test, found an average threshold of 153 arcseconds for a group of 17 children from 3 to 3.9 years of age and 70 arcseconds for 56 children from 4 to 4.9 years of age. Hofstetter (1965), using the Diastereo, found that the average threshold was 20 arcseconds (75 percent correct) for a group of 19 subjects 6 to 10 years of age. Jani (1966) reported that only 8.9 percent of 159 children aged one to 9 years failed to pass a Diastereo screening test at 5 ft (a binocular disparity of 52 arcseconds). Beyond 8 years of age, Hofstetter and Bertsch (1976) demonstrated that there is no further change in the threshold as a function of age. Animal studies also show a development of disparity detection (see Chapter 12).

From these reports, we can conclude that normal binocular vision is in operation from 3 to 6 months of age. That is, the child can respond to large binocular disparities. At age 2½ years, failure of a young patient to perceive random-dot depth patterns of about 300 arcseconds should indicate some developmental anomaly of binocular vision. By age 5 to 8 years, stereopsis should be approaching the adult level, and the threshold should be no more than about 40 arcseconds, as discussed in Chapter 9.

Throughout these infant studies, reports exist of considerable variability in threshold values. Furthermore, infants are difficult to work with and frequently are in a state of somnolence (Gesell et al., 1949). Others become fussy and distracted and simply ignore the examiner and the attempts at testing. Clinicians frequently are forced to arrange informal tests to appeal to the young as a sort of game (Woodruff, 1972). For many functions, some of the so-called objective measurements (retinoscopy, optokinetic nystagmus, loose prism test, and cover test) are available. Where necessary, visually evoked responses can be helpful, and perhaps the development of a stereopsis test utilzing this approach would prove useful (see, for example, Regan, 1977).

Table 10–1 summarizes much of this developmental information. It includes some extrapolations and approximations based on the reports cited.

INFANT SACCADIC EYE MOVEMENTS AND LOCAL SIGN

Aslin and Salapatek (1975) reported that saccadic eye movements in 1- and 2-month-old children show that in response to an initially peripheral stimulus, the eye movement pattern consists of a series of small, steplike saccades. For example, an infant's response to a 30° peripheral target might consist of three separate saccades, each of about 10°. This could suggest that local signs have yet to develop, but the authors reported that the step size was related to the size of the peripheral angle. This latter relationship implies that the response mechanism involving eye movements is the immature one. Certainly, considerable proof exists of the innate nature of local signs (Walls, 1951). The gradual process of myelination is not complete at term (Altman, 1967), and the lack of this feature of development may well form the basis for explaining this early eye movement behavior.

Table 10–1.   Summary of Development of Some Aspects of Binocular Vision

Visual Acuity Method	Level at Birth (arcminutes)	Age When Adult Level Is Reached (months)
Calculations/anatomic development (monkey)	2	3
Optokinetic nystagmus	25	6.5 to 7.5
Preferential looking	20	6.5 to 7.5
Visually evoked potentials	20 (at 1 month of age)	5 to 6
Clinical observation	—	6

Motor Activity Method	Age at First Appearance (months)	Age When Adult Level Is Reached (months)
Follow fixation (electro-oculography)	At birth	6
Compensatory eye movements (observation)	0.25	1
Voluntary fixation (observation)	0.25 to 0.75	3
Convergence (corneal reflex)	1	2 to 3
Accommodation (dynamic retinoscopy)	0.25	4
Bifoveal fixation (clinical observation)	2	5 to 6

Stereopsis (Response Mode)	Age at First Appearance	Level (arcseconds)
Gross (head movements)	3.5 to 6 months	3000
Fine (verbal or motor response)	2.0 to 2.9 years	240
	3.0 to 3.9 years	153
	4.0 to 4.9 years	70
	5.0 to 8.0 years	≤40

All data, excepting estimates of acuity based on foveal structural development, are from studies of human infants.

VISUAL DEPRIVATION

Recordings from individual neurons in the lateral geniculate nucleus and the visual cortex produced some substantial contributions to an understanding of at least some binocular processes. Among the principal attributes of these cells which have been studied are those concerned with receptive field characteristics and ocular dominance (Hubel, 1979).

A *receptive field* of any cell in the visual system is defined as that portion of the visual field over which the introduction of a small spot of light produces, or otherwise influences, electrical responses in the neuron itself. For cells in the ganglion cell layer of the retina, and all six layers of the lateral geniculate nucleus, these fields are circular and have excitatory subcenters and inhibitory surroundings, or the converse. The interested reader should consult Brindley (1970) for a detailed discussion of these receptive field characteristics.

In the visual cortex of the monkey, receptive field organization follows a hierarchy, proceeding from cells with symmetrically circular receptive fields, which receive the axons from the geniculate and are located in layer IVc, through simple and complex cells, which are located progressively farther outward and inward from this intermediate layer (Hubel and Wiesel, 1968). These two categories of cortical cells have rectangular receptive fields (Bishop, 1973). Furthermore, these cells show a strong preference for moving line-shaped stimuli that are oriented rather precisely in a given meridian (Hubel and Wiesel, 1962). Figure 10–1 illustrates this orientation preference.

In the monkey, the species that provides the best model for studies of vision in humans, the complex cells respond binocularly: some 50 percent of the complex cells can be activated by shining a light in either eye. Among these binocular cells, a difference also exists in the weighting given to stimulation of one eye or the other. This characteristic is called *ocular dominance* (Hubel and Wiesel, 1968). As a matter of convenience, Hubel and Wiesel (1962, 1968) classified cortical cells of the cat (simple cells) and the monkey (complex cells) into seven categories of dominance. Table 10–2 shows their system of classification. In this system, categories 2 through 6 are considered binocular. Figure 10–2 illustrates the dominance distribution found in both adult and newborn monkeys.

The fact that dominance patterns are established at birth, prior to any visual experience, indicates that a genetic, innate mechanism is involved. These cells also exhibit other characteristics that are analogous

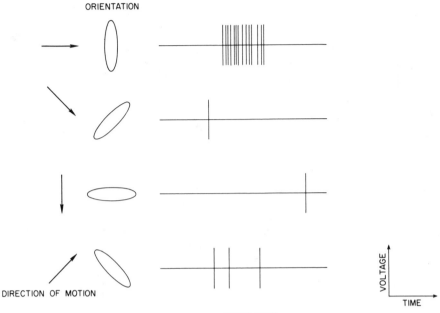

Figure 10–1.   Orientation preferences of cortical cells. *Left*, a schematic of the orientation of a slit of light; *right*, neural responses (Hubel and Wiesel, 1962).

Table 10–2.   Description of Dominance in Terms of Effect of a Stimulus Delivered to the Two Eyes

Category	Ipsilateral	Contralateral
1	No response	Exclusively
2	Much less effective	Much more effective
3	Slightly less effective	Slightly more effective
4	No difference	No difference
5	Slightly more effective	Slightly less effective
6	Much more effective	Much less effective
7	Exclusively	No response

Modified after Hubel and Wiesel (1962).

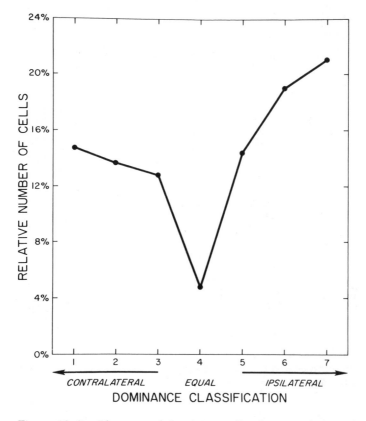

Figure 10–2.   The normal dominance distribution of cortical cells in the adult
monkey (Hubel and Wiesel, 1968).

to some of the important psychophysical phenomena associated with binocular vision, discussed in Chapter 12.

The histology of the lateral geniculate nucleus indicates that it consists of six isolated laminae. Layers 2, 3, and 5 receive inputs from the ipsilateral eye whereas layers 1, 4, and 6 receive ganglion cell axons from the contralateral eye. While lateral geniculate cells from a common location of the binocular visual field are lined up topographically in these layers, no detectable interlamellar fibers have been found by light microscopy (Brindley, 1970).

Injecting a radioactive marker into one eye leads to uptake by the ganglion cells. By the process of axonal transport, these materials are deposited in the appropriate laminae of the geniculate, and autoradiography of the visual cortex shows that measurable amounts reach this structure (Grafstein and Laureno, 1973). The pattern of irradiation in the visual cortex of monkeys is columnar. It produces a stripped pattern, often regular, but with some branchings (Hubel and Wiesel, 1969; Wiesel et al., 1974). Electrophysiological studies of cortical cells show that these stripes contain cells of similar dominance. This organizational pattern is not detectable by conventional histological techniques (Chow, 1973). Figure 10–3 illustrates the resulting pattern.

Another columnar organization is revealed only by electrophysiological recordings from single cells of the visual cortex of monkeys. This has to do with orientation preference, and penetrations of the cortex at various angles indicate that these are smaller in diameter but otherwise quite similar to the dominance columns (Hubel and Wiesel, 1974).

Starting at birth, closing one eye by lid suturing in young monkeys for 16 months produces virtually no change in the responses of geniculate cells receiving this eye's inputs. At the cortex, there is a profound shift in dominance toward the cells responding to inputs from the eye remaining open. Figure 10–4 illustrates the resulting dominance distribution (Hubel et al., 1977).

Histological evaluation of the lateral geniculate nucleus of monocularly deprived monkeys reveals a large number of undersized cells (von Noorden, 1973). Hubel (1979) felt that these neurons failed to grow

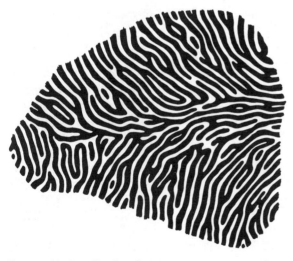

Figure 10–3.   Ocular dominance pattern in the right visual cortex following injection of a radiographic substance in the left eye (Reprinted by permission from Hubel, 1979).

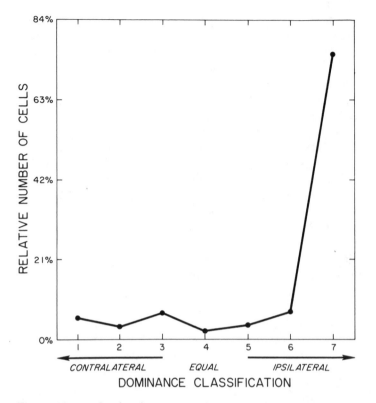

Figure 10–4. Ocular dominance distribution following monocular deprivation
of an infant monkey (Hubel, 1979).

to normal size because of the defect in the cortex brought about by imbalancing the ocular inputs during the animal's developmental period. The lateral geniculate nucleus of monocularly deprived kittens shows a similar failure of the large cells to reach normal size, although Chow (1973) reported that enzymatic activity continued. Sherman et al. (1972) reported that these abnormally small cells were irresponsive to light stimulation and were all in one category, known as *transient*, or *Y, cells*. Transient cells are thought to mediate temporal discriminations, such as flicker perception, and to be involved in reflex fixational eye movements (Ikeda and Wright, 1974). We discuss these cells in greater detail in Chapter 12.

In the cortex, routine histological techniques show no deprivation effects, but autoradiography reveals cortical columns receiving inputs from the deprived eye become smaller and there is a concurrent expansion of the columns receiving inputs from the unaffected eye (Hubel,

1979). Furthermore, using Nissl, Golgi-Cox, and Rapid Golgi stains reveals that the neurons have decreased dendritic lengths, fewer branchings of stellate cells, and smaller and less developed dendritic arborizations of the Meynert cells in the deprived visual cortex of the cat. In addition, certain neurochemical changes have been found, such as an increase in noradrenalin and dopamine (Chow, 1973).

Closing both eyes in newborn kittens produces a larger number of cortical cells that lose their orientation preference and others that become irresponsive to any form of light stimulation. However, about half of the cells maintain their usual response characteristics, receptive field organization, and dominance distribution (Hubel and Wiesel, 1965). See Figure 10–5.

Inducing an artificial strabismus by sectioning the medial rectus in one eye shortly after birth and recording when the kitten matures produces a dominance pattern in which almost all the cells are monocular. In addition, no irresponsive cells are found (Hubel and Wiesel, 1965). Figure 10–6 illustrates that almost all resulting dominances of cortical cells are ipsilateral or contralateral.

If normal monkeys 1 to 3 weeks old are injected with a radioactive amino acid, layer IVc of the visual cortex shows that the tagging material is distributed throughout, rather than forming periodic bands as it does in the adult. Segregation into columns starts before birth but is not complete until the third to sixth postnatal week. Therefore, the apparent expansion of columns seen following monocular deprivation may be no more than a persistence of terminals from the eye that remained open (Wiesel and Hubel, 1974).

Following monocular deprivation, simply reopening the eye produces very little recovery. In fact, closing the formerly unaffected eye, so as to alternately deprive the two eyes in turn, results in some recovery of the monocular cells responding to the originally deprived eye only if it is done during a certain susceptible period (Blakemore and Van Sluyters, 1974).

The suturing of eyelids, used in most deprivation studies, produces an almost total deprivation of pattern and motion as well as a substantial reduction in retinal illuminance. However, only the lack of stimulation from forms and their movements produces the effects described (Hubel, 1979). Prolonged periods in the dark can cause retinal degeneration (Walls, 1951). Lid suturing for shorter periods does not affect the retina (Chow, 1973).

Binocular deprivation appears to prevent normal maturation and cause some breakdown of the normal orientation preferences. However, it does not substantially alter the innate dominance distribution (Hubel and Wiesel, 1963). Binocular deprivation does prevent cells of

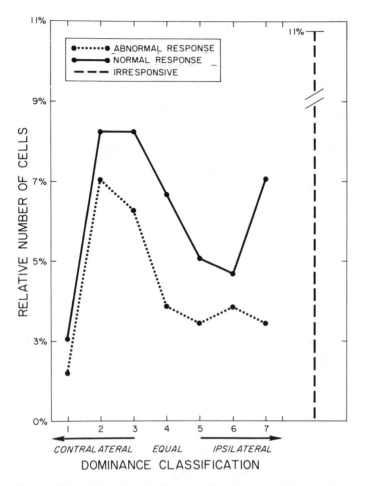

Figure 10–5. Ocular dominance distribution following binocular deprivation
             of a kitten. (Hubel and Wiesel, 1965).

similar dominance from collecting to form columns, which apparently
precedes the full development of simple and complex cells. However,
monocular deprivation seems to produce an imbalance in the ability of
the two monocular inputs to compete for synaptic space and thus dis-
rupts binocular activation of cortical neurons (Cunningham and Murphy, 1978), as do alternate occlusion and artificial strabismus (Blakemore
and Van Sluyters, 1974).

There is also a distribution of orientation preferences in monkeys
(Mansfield, 1974). For cortical neurons receiving their input from the
central 2° of the temporal retina, there are more neurons with vertical

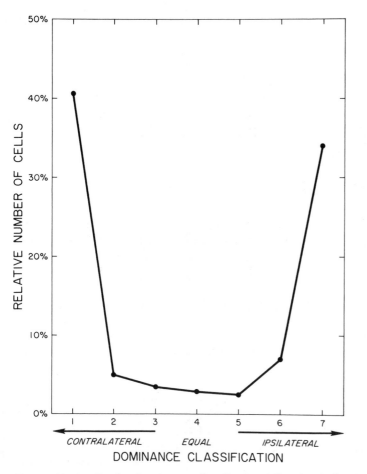

Figure 10–6.   Ocular dominance distribution following induction of an artificial
strabismus in a young kitten (Hubel and Wiesel, 1965).

and horizontal optimal orientations than at any oblique meridian. Evidence exists that these preferences can be influenced by early visual
experience in kittens (Freeman and Pettigrew, 1973) and that early-
onset astigmatism in humans causes a differential acuity which is not
of optical origin (Mitchell et al., 1973). Apparently, such effects constitute a shift in some cells' preference, since Leehey et al. (1975) demonstrated that this anisotropy is present in normal human infants 6
weeks old.
     It seems that some critical aspects of binocular vision exist which
cannot be totally prespecified and for which visual experience is nec-

essary. Because of developmental changes in eye size and separation, precise interocular interactions may depend on experience to fine-tune the cortical organization. Such developments could facilitate the processes of motor fusion and stereopsis (Cunningham and Murphy, 1978), as we discuss in Chapters 12 and 15.

Several reports have challenged some of these characteristics (Bishop, 1973, 1975; Chow, 1973). Nevertheless, the preponderance of evidence supports the general picture presented here.

SENSITIVE PERIOD

As mentioned earlier, disruption of binocular vision in young animals produces severe changes in the binocular visual system only if it occurs during a certain early period. The duration of this sensitive period can be estimated by studying the developmental anatomy of the normal system (Bishop, 1975). That is, structures that do not appear mature at any given age still may be susceptible to disruption. However, the limitation of these methods is that subtle differences in structures might not be detected. What can be determined is the earliest age at which a structure appears mature. This would set an early limit on estimates of the sensitive period.

In kittens, closing off one eye for various periods at different ages and determining the resulting dominance distributions indicate that the sensitive perod for this animal starts around the fourth week and continues at a high level through the eighth week. After this, the animal is less and less susceptible to disruption by monocular occlusion and is virtually unaffected after 4 months (Hubel and Wiesel, 1970). Reversing the occlusion after a variable period of monocular deprivation and determining the degree of recovery reveal that the sensitive period is all but over by 14 weeks of age (Blakemore and Van Sluyters, 1974). However, lateral geniculate cells continue to grow through the first 4 months of life (Garey et al., 1973).

Amblyopia has been demonstrated behaviorally in monocularly deprived monkeys. This deprivation produced no effect on the visual acuity in animals over 3 months old (von Noorden and Dowling, 1970), which corresponds rather precisely with the point at which the foveal structure reaches maturity (Hendrickson and Kupfer, 1976). Strabismus amblyopia occurred only if monkeys were made strabismic during the first week of life. Even so, recovery continued over the entire period of acuity testing, which lasted some 30 months (von Noorden and Dowling, 1970).

Clinical Implications

In humans, clinical wisdom says that a corneal scar, occurring as late as 6 years of age, causes a permanent amblyopia (von Noorden and Maumenee, 1968), and that occlusion therapy is quite effective up to age 4 years and less so from 4 to 9 years of age (Parks, 1971). The informaton tabulated in Table 10–1 indicates that normal binocular vision develops completely by around 8 years of age. Based on this, the critical period in humans is at least 8 years long.

Restricting consideration to congenital esotropes subsequently corrected cosmetically by surgery, Banks et al. (1975) correlated the degree to which adaptation to a tilting grating presented to one eye influenced the subsequent apparent tilt of a physically vertical grating, as viewed by the other eye. This phenomenon is called the *transfer of the tilt aftereffect*. Banks et al. employed an index of this transfer as an index of the restoration of binocularity, assuming that a higher index meant a better binocular function. They concluded that the sensitive period did not start until several months after birth, peaked between 1 and 3 years, and was mainly over by age 7 years.

This method of assessing binocular functon is founded on the assumption that the interocular transfer effect used and other attributes of binocular vision are mediated by identical neural processes. While this may be so, as some apparent correlation of the degree of transfer and the threshold of stereopsis in a few normal subjects shows (Mitchell and Ware, 1974), such a relationship may not be true for all strabismics (Hess, 1978). Furthermore, Taylor (1973) reported on a study of 50 congenital esotropes, diagnosed by direct observation or from infant photographs to have occurred at or before 6 months of age. Of these children 30 were considered to have received adequate surgery, which was performed between 3.5 and 23 months of age. Only three of this latter group could perceive at the 40 arcsecond level (Titmus stereo test) when they were tested 5 to 16 years later. Some 27 others had binocular functional scotomas from 24 to 190 arcminutes in diameter and centered on the object of regard. Scotoma size was rather closely correlated with measurements of the threshold of stereopsis. Perhaps the presence of such a scotoma in one eye, when viewing is binocular, could reduce the interocular tilt aftereffect, as reported by Banks et al. (1975). Perhaps congenital strabismus represents either a genetic defect or one usually associated with early irreparable damage or unrecoverable loss in the nervous system. While the nonvisual advantages of corrective surgery are important, sensitive periods based on patients who lack normal function seem inappropriate. Of course, it could turn out that abnormal and normal binocular vision develop at the same time.

Another clinical wisdom runs that the earlier the onset and the longer the duration of an untreated strabismus, the less likely that the patient will achieve a functional cure. Flom (1963, p. 198) defined a *functional cure* as follows:

1. Maintenance of bifoveal fixation in the ordinary situations of life.
2. Loss of bifixation should not occur more often than one percent of the time.
3. Vision should be clear and generally comfortable.
4. The range of bifixation should include all fields of gaze and extend from very great viewing distances to only a few centimeters.
5. Corrective lenses and reasonable amounts of prism may be worn if necessary.

To this might be added

6. The function of both foveae in binocular viewing must be explicitly demonstrable as, for example, attaining a threshold of stereopsis of 40 arcseconds or less.

Studies of some other surgical corrections, reanalyzed by Flom

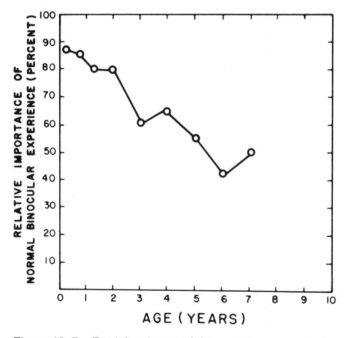

Figure 10–7.   Partial estimate of the sensitive period in humans, based on the data presented by Flom (1963).

(1963), indicated that functional cures of congenital strabismus have been recorded when the surgery took place as late as 10 years of age. Flom's reevaluation of strabismus treated by visual training indicated that the percentage of functional cures increased with age at onset from 10 percent for congenital defects to 50 percent for those occurring at or after age 7 years. Furthermore, reports continue to appear of measurable improvement after surgery and/or visual training for patients aged 7 years and older (Fletcher and Silverman, 1966; Birnbaum et al., 1977).

Direct estimates of the duration of the critical period in humans, both based on interocular transfer, range from 2.5 years (Hohmann and Creutzfeldt, 1975) to around 7 years (Aslin and Dumais, 1979). However, it seems that more thorough and systematic study will be required to precisely delineate this period. Certainly any index of binocularity should be solidly based on the functional terms such as suggested by Flom. Based on his analysis, Figure 10–6 probably represents the best available approximation of a sensitive epoch in human development. Incomplete as it might be, it is founded on standards as rigorous as those that have been applied to the development of binocular vision in the normal infant. Perhaps the critical period for humans does not end until about age 13 years or later.

BINOCULAR VISION IN CHILDREN BORN AT LOW BODY WEIGHT

Prematurity has been associated with a higher incidence of infant mortality, cerebral palsy, cataracts, and strabismus. Also it has been reported that the risk of cerebral damage increases in severity with decreasing body weight at birth. The result is a minimal cerebral damage syndrome which includes some of the various learning and behavioral disorders (Fledelius, 1976).

Fledelius (1976) studied a wide range of ocular attributes in children whose body weight at birth was 2.5 kg or less. This weight-at-birth criterion is a better, more reliable definition of prematurity than the estimation of the duration of the term. Fledelius investigated a group of these children who had reached 10 years of age.

For a comparison of binocular Snellen visual acuity, Fledelius found a significant difference between premature children and full-term children at age 10 years. His findings for stereopsis, by using the Titmus test, are seen in Table 10–3. The results in the two groups are compared with the incidence of the various categories of oculomotor deviations found in the same two groups (see Table 10–4), and they show strikingly similar percentages.

Table 10–3. Percentages of Children Attaining Various Ranges of
Binocular Disparity Detection

Binocular Disparity Correctly Detected	Percentage Premature (n = 300)	Percentage Mature (n = 237)
None	16.7	3.8
800–200	10.0	4.6
150–60	13.0	7.6
50–40	60.3	84.0

Source: Fledelius (1976).

Table 10–4. Percentages of Children with Three Categories of
Oculomotor Imbalance as Measured by the Cover Test
and Maddox Rod Test

Muscle Balance	Percentage Premature (n = 300)	Percentage Mature (n = 237)
Heterotropia	22.5	5.9
High heterophoria	11.9	11.0
Low heterophoria and orthophoria	65.6	83.1

Source: Fledelius (1976).

Unfortunately, this study contains very little information on the
development of premature eyes and vision. Furthermore, the nature
of such a study produces some preselection. Certainly, a study of the
development of visual functions in such infants would be most
informative.

REFORMULATION OF THE NATIVISTIC-EMPIRICAL ARGUMENT

Aslin and Dumais (1979, p. 50) suggested that rather than choose between an innate and acquired basis for vision, the issue should be
reformulated so that answers to the following questions could be
sought:

  1. How severely do genetic factors constrain the plasticity of binocular
      function?

2.   What environmental manipulations influence binocular functions?
3.   When during development does the environment exert its greatest influence on binocular functions?

To these might be added

4.   How do environmental manipulations influence binocular functions?

Based on the information presented in this chapter, binocular development is facilitated by normal early visual experience. That is, given a normal early binocular experience and the proper genetically determined components (Francois, 1961), development proceeds to completion. The lack of either produces a failure to develop. The interested reader should see Aslin and Dumais (1979) for more detailed discussion of the various theories of visual development.

VISUAL TRAINING IN OLDER CHILDREN

No matter what the duration of the critical period, early detection and, where possible, early correction of these visual anomalies seem essential. For older patients the issue of treatment should be resolved on a case-by-case basis. Following attention to improving the quality of sensory fusion by scrupulously thorough correcton of refractive anomalies and oculomotor imbalances, visual training should be considered. The decision to use this method to help a patient can be guided by the prognostic indices provided by Flom (1963). After a relatively short term of this kind of treatment, progress (or its absence) should be assessed realistically and future treatments determined accordingly. For those patients who show some improvement, further training is justified and desirable. When progress halts, so should the training.

OCCLUSION THERAPY

Studies of the development of binocular vision in animals reveal that the clinical practice of occluding the normal eye, to facilitate the reduction of amblyopia in the abnormal eye, may succeed in the limited context of tending to equalize the visual acuities between the two eyes. Nevertheless, such a therapeutic strategy may well prevent the development of normal binocular vision, as would alternate occlusion.

REFERENCES

Alpern, M. (1969), "Types of eye movements," *The Eye*, vol. 3, Academic, New York, 65–174.

Altman, J. (1967), "Postnatal growth of the mammalian brain," *The Neurosciences*, Rockefeller University, New York, 723–743.

Amigo, G. (1972a), "Pre-school vision study," *British Journal of Ophthalmology*, 57, 125–132.

Amigo, G. (1972b), "Visuo-sensory development of the child," *American Journal of Optometry*, 49, 991–1002.

Aslin, R. N. (1977), "Development of binocular fixation in human infants," *Journal of Experimental Child Psychology*, 23, 133–150.

Aslin, R. N., and Dumais, S. T. (1979), "Binocular vision in infants: A review and a theoretical framework," *National Science Foundation*, 77–04580, Washington.

Aslin, R. N., and Salapatek, P. (1975), "Saccadic localization of visual targets by the very young human infant," *Perception and Psychophysics*, 17, 293–302.

Banks, M. S., Aslin, R. N., and Letson, R. D. (1975), "Sensitive period for the development of human binocular vision," *Science*, 190, 675–677.

Barber, A. N. (1955), *Embryology of the Human Eye*, Mosby, St. Louis, 212–214.

Birnbaum, M. H., Koslowe, R., and Sanet, R. (1977), "Success in amblyopia therapy as a function of age: A literature survey," *American Journal of Optometry and Physiological Optics*, 54, 269–275.

Bishop, P. O. (1973), "Neurophysiology of binocular single vision and stereopsis," *Handbook of Sensory Physiology*, vol. III/3, Springer-Verlag, Berlin, 256–305.

Bishop, P. O. (1975), "Binocular vision," *Adler's Physiology of the Eye*, Mosby, St. Louis, 558–613.

Blakemore, C., and Van Sluyters, R. C. (1974), "Reversal of physiological effects of monocular deprivation in kittens: Further evidence for a sensitive period," *Journal of Physiology*, 237, 195–216.

Bower, T. G. R. (1964), "The visual world of infants," *Scientific American*, 215, 80–92.

Brindley, G. S. (1970), *Physiology of the Retina and Visual Pathway*, Williams & Wilkins, Baltimore, 95–105.

Brookman, K. E. (1980), "Ocular accommodation in human infants," Ph.D. thesis, Indiana University, Bloomington.

Chow, K. D. (1973), "Neuronal changes in the visual system following visual deprivation," *Handbook of Sensory Physiology*, vol. VII/3, Springer-Verlag, Berlin, 599–627.

Conel, J. (1939), *The Postnatal Development of the Human Cerebral Cortex*, vol. 1, Harvard University, Cambridge.

Conel, J. (1959), *The Postnatal Development of the Human Cerebral Cortex*, vol. 6, Harvard University, Cambridge.

Cunningham, T. J., and Murphy, E. H. (1978), "Ontogeny of sensory systems," *Handbook of Behavioral Neurobiology*, vol. 1, Plenum, New York, 39–71.

Dayton, G. O., Jones, M. H., Aiu, P., Rawson, R. A., Steele, B., and Rose, M. (1964), "Developmental study of coordinated eye movements in the human infant." *Archives of Ophthalmology*, 71, 865–870.

Dobson, V., and Teller, D. Y. (1978), "Visual acuity in human infants: A review and comparison of behavioral and electrophysiological studies," *Vision Research*, 18, 1469–1483.

Duke-Elder, W. S. (1949), *Text-Book of Opthalmology*, vol. 4, Kimpton, London, 3816–3822.

Fledelius, H. (1976), "Prematurity and the eye," *Acta Ophthalmologica*, Supp. 128, Scriptor, Copenhagen, 113–158.

Fletcher, M. C., and Silverman, S. J. (1966), "Stabismus: A summary of 110 consecutive cases, part 1," *American Journal of Ophthalmology*, 61, 86–94.

Flom, M. C. (1963), "Treatment of binocular anomalies of vision," *Vision of Children*, Chilton, Philadelphia, 197–228.

Fox, R., Aslin, R. N., Shea, S. L., and Dumais, S. T. (1980), "Stereopsis in human infants," *Science*, 207, 323–324.

Francois, J. (1961), *Heredity in Ophthalmology*, Mosby, St. Louis, 255–269.

Freeman, R. D., and Pettigrew, J. D. (1973), "Alteration of visual cortex from environmental asymmetries," *Nature*, 246, 259–360.

Garey, L. J., Fisken, R. A., and Powell, T. P. S. (1973), "Observations on the growth of cells in the lateral geniculate nucleus of the cat," *Brian Research*, 52, 359–362.

Gesell, A., Ilg, F. L., and Bullis, G. E. (1949), *Vision: Its Development in Infant and Child*, Hoelper-Harper, New York.

Grafstein, B., and Laureno, R. (1973), "Transport of radioactivity from eye to visual cortex in the mouse," *Experimental Neurology*, 39, 44–57.

Greenspan, S. B. (1971), "Behavioral and developmental studies of depth perception," *American Journal of Optometry*, 48, 677–688.

Harter, M. R., Deaton, K. F., and Odom, J. V. (1977), "Pattern of visual evoked potentials in infants," *Visually Evoked Potentials in Man: New Developments*, Clarendon Press, Oxford, 332–352.

Haynes, H., White B. L., and Held, R. (1965) "Visual accommodation in human infants," *Science*, 148, 528–530.

Helmholtz, H. (1925), *Handbook of Physiological Optics*, vol. 3, Optical Society of America, New York, 531–625.

Hendrickson, A., and Kupfer, C. (1976), "Histogenesis of fovea in macaque monkey," *Investigative Ophthalmology*, 15, 745–755.

Hering, E. (1977), *The Theory of Binocular Vision*, Plenum, New York, 1–8.

Hess, R. (1978), "Interocular transfer in individuals with strabismic amblyopia: A cautionary note, *Perception*, 7, 201–205.

Hickey, T. L. (1977), "Postnatal development of the human lateral geniculate nucleus: Relationship to a critical period for the visual system," *Science*, 198, 836–838.

Hofstetter, H. W. (1965), "Absolute threshold measurements with the Diastereo test," *Dublin International Optical Congress*, Dublin, 5–10.

Hofstetter, H. W., and Bertsch, J. D. (1976), "Does stereopsis change with age?" *American Journal of Optometry and Physiological Optics*, 53, 664–667.

Hohmann, A., and Creutzfeldt, O. D. (1975), "Squint and the development of binocularity in humans," *Nature*, 254, 613–614.

Hollenberg, M. J., and Spira, A. W. (1972), "Early development of the human retina," *Canadian Journal of Ophthalmology*, 7, 472–491.

Hubel, D. M. (1979), "The visual cortex of normal and deprived monkeys," *American Scientist*, 67, 532–543.

Hubel, D. H., and Wiesel, T. N. (1962), "Receptive fields, binocular interaction, and functional architecture in the cat's visual cortex," *Journal of Physiology*, 160, 106–154.

Hubel, D. H., and Wiesel, T. N. (1963), "Single-cell responses in striate cortex of kittens deprived of vision in one eye," *Journal of Neurophysiology*, 26, 1003–1007.

Hubel, D. H., and Wiesel, T. N. (1965), "Binocular interaction in striate cortex of kittens reared with artificial squint," *Journal of Neurophysiology*, 28, 1041–1059.

Hubel, D. H., and Wiesel, T. N. (1968), "Receptive fields and functional architecture of monkey striate cortex," *Journal of Physiology*, 195, 215–243.

Hubel, D. H., and Wiesel, T. N. (1969), "Anatomical demonstration of columns in the monkey striate cortex," *Nature*, 221, 747–750.

Hubel, D. H., and Wiesel, T. N. (1970), "The period of susceptibility to the physiological effects of unilateral eye closure in kittens," *Journal of Physiology*, 206, 419–436.

Hubel, D. H., and Wiesel, T. N. (1974), "Sequence regularity and geometry of orientation columns in monkey striate cortex," *Journal of Comparative Neurology*, 158, 267–294.

Hubel, D. H., Weisel, T. N., and LeVay, S. (1977), "Plasticity of ocular dominance columns in monkey striate cortex," *Philosophical Transactions, Royal Society B*, London, 278, 377–409.

Ikeda, H., and Wright, M. J. (1974), "Is amblyopia due to inappropriate stimulation of the 'sustained' pathway during development?" *British Journal of Ophthalmology*, 58, 165–173.

Jani, S. N. (1966), "The age factor in stereopsis screening," *American Journal of Optometry*, 43, 653–657.

Leehey, S. C., Moskowitz-Cook, A., Brill, S., and Held, R. (1975), "Orientational anisotropy in infant vision," *Science*, 190, 900–901.

Mann, I. (1928), *The Development of the Human Eye*, Cambridge University, London.

Mansfield, R. J. W. (1974) "Neural basis of orientation perception in primate vision," *Science*, 186, 1133–1135.

Marg, E., Freeman, R. D., Peltzman, P., and Goldstein, P. J. (1976), "Visual acuity development in human infants: Evoked potential measurements," *Investigative Ophthalmology*, 15, 150–153.

Mitchell, D. E., Freeman, R. D., Millodot, M., and Haegerstrom, G. (1973), "Meridional amblyopia: Evidence for modification of the human visual system by early visual experience," *Vision Research*, 13, 535–558.

Mitchell, D. E., and Ware, C. (1974), "Interocular transfer of visual after-effect in normal and stereoblind humans," *Journal of Physiology*, 236, 707–721.

Ordy, I. M., Samorajski, T., Collins, R. L., and Nagy, A. R. (1965), "Postnatal development of vision in a subhuman primate *(Macaca mulatta)*," *Archives of Ophthalmology*, 73, 674–686.

Parks, M. M. (1971), "Management of eccentric fixation and ARC in esotropia," *Symposium on Horizontal Ocular Deviations*, Mosby, St. Louis, 81–87.

Pirenne, M. H. (1948), *Vision and the Eye*, Chapman & Hall, London, 96–110.

Regan, D. (1972), *Evoked Potentials in Psychology, Sensory Physiology, and Clinical Medicine*, Chapman & Hall, London.

Regan, D. (1977), "Evoked potential indications of the processing of pattern, colour, and depth information," *Visual Evoked Potentials in Man: New Developments*, Clarendon Press, Oxford, 234–249.

Reinecke, R. D., and Cogan, D. G. (1958), "Standardization of objective visual acuity measurements: Optokinetic nystagmus vs. Snellen acuity," *Archives of Ophthalmology*, 60, 418–421.

Reinecke, R. D., and Simons, K. (1974), "A new stereoscopic test for amblyopia screening," *American Journal of Ophthalmology*, 78, 714–721.

Ruskell, G. L. (1967), "Some aspects of vision in infants," *British Orthoptics Journal*, 24, 25–32.

Samorajski, T., Keefe, J. R., and Ordy, J. M. (1965), "Morphogenesis of Photoreceptor and retinal ultrastructure in a sub-human primate," *Vision Research*, 5, 639–648.

Sherman, S. M., Hoffmann, K. P., and Stone, J. (1972), "Loss of specific cell type from dorsal lateral geniculate nucleus in visually deprived cats," *Journal of Neurophysiology*, 35, 532–541.

Taylor, D. M. (1973), *Congenital Esotropia: Management and Prognosis*, Stratton, New York.

Teller, D. Y., Regal, D. M., Videen, T. O., and Pulos, E. (1978), "Development of visual acuity in infant monkeys *(Macaca nemestrina)* during the early postnatal weeks," *Vision Research*, 18, 561–566.

von Noorden, G. K. (1973), "Histological studies of the visual system in monkeys with experimental amblyopia," *Investigative Ophthalmology*, 12, 727–738.

von Noorden, G. K., and Dowling, J. E. (1970), "II, Behavioral studies in strabismus amblyopia," *Archives of Ophthalmology*, 84, 215–226.

von Noorden, G. K., and Maumenee, A. E. (1968), "Clinical observations on stimulus-deprivation amblyopia (amblyopia ex anopsia)," *American Journal of Ophthalmology*, 65, 220–224.

Walk, R. D., and Gibson, E. J. (1961), "A comparative and analytical study of visual depth perception," *Psychological Monographs*, 75, 1–44.

Walls, G. L. (1951), "The problem of visual direction," *American Journal of Optometry*, 28, 55–83, 115–146, 173–212.

Walraven, J. (1975), "Amblyopia screening with random-dot stereograms," *American Journal of Ophthalmology*, 80, 893–900.

Wiesel, T. N., and Hubel, D. H. (1974), "Ordered arrangement of orientation columns in monkeys lacking visual experience," *Journal of Comparative Neurology*, 158, 307–318.

Wiesel, T. N., Hubel, D. H., and Lam, D. M. I. (1974), "Autoradiographic demonstration of ocular-dominance columns in the monkey striate cortex by means of transneuronal transport," *Brain Research*, 79, 273–279.

Woodruff, M. E. (1972), "Observations on the visual acuity of children during the first five years of life," *American Journal of Optometry*, 49, 205–215.

Worth, C. (1903), *Squint: Its Causes, Pathology, and Treatment*, Blakiston, Philadelphia, 20–23.

11

THE LONGITUDINAL HOROPTER

> The fact is the sweetest dream that labor knows.
>
> *Robert Frost*

LONGITUDINAL HOROPTER

The key concept to gaining a through understanding of binocular vision is the *horopter*. The term was introduced by a Jesuit priest, Franciscus Aguilonius in 1613, some 200 years before the onset of systematic inquiries into the nature of seeing (Shipley and Rawlings, 1970). It is perhaps the least understood concept in all visual science, one that brings sleep to the eyes of many optometrists. Nevertheless, the horopter offers a means of studying corresponding points throughout an important portion of the binocular visual field. In most clinical situations, it can be assumed that the horopter is a surface passing through the point to be fixated or close to it if fixation disparity is present. For many purposes, knowing about the horopter and its association with the fixation point is sufficient. To an investigation into the fundamental nature of binocular vision, the study of the horopter is indispensible. It holds great promise of indicating some basic facts about both normal and abnormal subjects. Unfortunately, only one study has attempted to objectively measure eye position during horopter measurements (Boucher, 1967).

In Chapter 5 the horopter is defined, and the geometric form it would assume if corresponding points were mapped out at even intervals is presented. According to Ogle (1950), a more complete definition is: for a given fixation point, the horopter is the locus of points in object space that give rise to a common primary visual direction (e.g. stimulate corresponding points). *Primary* was used by Ogle to mean that fusional eye movements were not permitted.

Although in its most general form the horopter locus might be considered to be a surface with both vercial and horizontal extents, such a simple form may not exist because of the complications of differences in vertical disparities for all object points off the plane of regard (Ogle, 1962). For practical purposes, the longitudinal horopter can be measured. Thus the horizontal or lateral positions that will stimulate corresponding points are measured. These points are corresponding in the sense that they give rise to common visual directions in the lateral dimension. To avoid the complications of vertical disparities, usually long rods are used so that the relative vertical image positions become virtually unimportant. Furthermore, such objects help position the eyes in a way that tends to eliminate cyclorotations, which can cause the ends of long rods to appear tilted in depth. Therefore, corresponding meridians are really measured with such objects (Ogle, 1962).

PHYSIOLOGICAL SIGNIFICANCE

Direct measurement of the longitudinal horopter allows comparison with the geometric horopter (the Veith-Mueller circle). If the data plotted on a locus that corresponds to a circle constructed through the point of fixation and the two centers of the entrance pupils, then we know that corresponding points are mapped out at constant intervals, symmetrically around the fixation point. Therefore, on the retinas, each pair of points lies symmetrically around the centers of each fovea at equally spaced distance increments across the temporal retina in one eye and the nasal retina in the other eye. However, if the empirical horopter locus has a shape different from the Vieth-Mueller circle, we can conclude that this orderly spaced arrangement does not exist. If this is so, perhaps we can account for the shape of the horopter in terms of the number of crossed versus uncrossed optic nerve fibers, the differences in resolution or vernier acuity across the temporal and nasal fields, or the results of monocular partition experiments, as discussed in Chapter 5.

FUNCTIONAL SIGNIFICANCE AND HOROPTER CRITERIA

While the issue of determining the exact nature of the distribution of corresponding points is basic to an exposition of binocular vision, the horopter is important from another aspect. Remember, it is the boundary between crossed and uncrossed binocular disparity. If we started at a point on the horopter and then move slightly off, the most sensitive way to detect that the point was no longer exactly on the horopter locus would be by the perception of stereopsis or a vernier kind of misalignment. Continuing to move farther from the horopter surface would allow detection of diplopia. This suggests at least three different ways to measure the longitudinal horopter: the first based on a stereoscopic perception, the second based on a special two-eyed vernier perception, and the third based on detection of diplopia. Tschermak (1942) was the first to enumerate these and other ways, and they are known as *Tschermak's criteria*. Table 11–1 presents five such criteria along with comments about the relative frequency of their use in experimental work. All these methods require constant fixation on a designated object (Ogle, 1950).

In all methods based directly on thresholds, the horopter locus is located by some measure of central tendency. For example, by using

Table 11–1. Horopter Criteria of Tschermak (1942) and Ogle (1950)

Criterion or Commonly Used Description(s)	Physiological Basis and Psychophysical Methods Applied by Investigators	Frequency of Use in Published Studies
"Center of the region of binocular single vision," or diplopia threshold horopter	Diplopia detection—methods of limits	Rarely
"Common visual direction," nonius, or dichoptic vernier horopter	Nonius or dichoptic vernier direction matching—method of adjustments (could also be method of limits)	Occasionally
"Apparent frontoparallel plane," "geodesic of visual space," or visual reference plane	Stereoscopic depth matching (according to Ogle, 1950)—method of adjustments	Most frequently
"Maximum stereoscopic sensitivity" or stereo displacement threshold horopter	Stereopsis thresholds—method of limits	Never systematically
"No stimulus to fusional eye movements" or zero stimulus to fusion horopter	Absence of fusional eye movements—none have been used	Never

the criterion of center of the region of bioncular single vision, a measurement of the proximal and distal diplopia thresholds is made, and
the average of these two angular thresholds is designated a horopter
point. Figure 11–1 shows the geometry of this measurement. The distance d_n between the horopter point and the bisector of the interpupillary line can be determined by finding the average binocular subtense
angle:

$$\frac{\alpha + \alpha'}{2} = \frac{2a/d_n + 2a/d_f}{2} = \frac{2a}{d_h} \tag{11–1}$$

where $2a$ is the interpupillary distance, d_n the distance from c to n, and
d_f the distance from c to f. This can be written as

$$d_h = 2\frac{d_n d_f}{d_n + d_f} \tag{11–2}$$

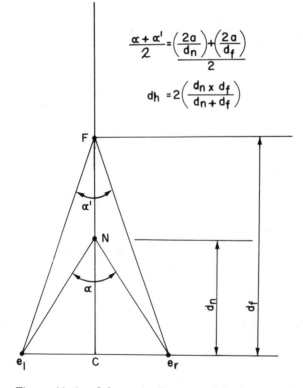

Figure 11–1.   Schematic diagram of the binocular subtense angles α and α' of
points N and F, respectively, the proximal and distal diplopia
limits of Panum's space.

which is an example of a harmonic mean, the reciprocals of which form an arithmetic progression (Rosenbach and Whitman, 1951). Since this criterion is based on the diplopia limit, we can consider the size of the diplopia threshold as an index of its possible precision. So the diplopia threshold horopter has an accuracy of about ±1 arcminute at the foveae given the data of Woo (1974) and ±7 arcminutes at a peripheral angle of 6° given the data of Ogle (1950).

The common visual direction horopter is also known as the *nonius horopter*. According to Bishop (1975), the name *nonius* is derived from the sixteenth-century Portuguese mathematician Nunez, and the name *vernier* from the Frenchman who subsequently improved on the original invention. Figure 11–2A shows the nonius apparatus of Ogle (1950). This is a grid nonius, and the view of the rods as seen by the subject is shown in Figure 11–2B. Note that the full extent of only half of each is seen by one eye; the other half is broken into a grid pattern and presented to the opposite eye. This viewing situation is also called *dichroptic* because different objects are presented separately to the two eyes. Polarizing material also can be used to construct a horopter apparatus (Flom, 1957). Such arrangements allow the subject to make vernierlike alignments of each rod while maintaining fixation on the

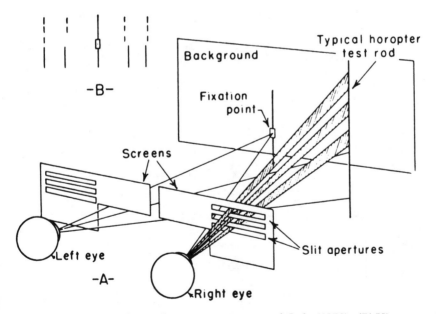

Figure 11–2. (A) The grid nonius apparatus of Ogle (1950). (B) View seen by a subject (Reprinted by permission).

central rod. The judgments are binocular in the sense that the subject is matching visual directions of one eye with those of the other eye. Once the upper and lower halves have been positioned so as to appear to form an unbroken line, the rod lies on the horopter locus and no further analysis is required. Since these measurements are based on vernier sensitivity, we can expect to determine corresponding points with an accuracy of about ±4 arcseconds at the foveae and ±5 arcminutes at a peripheral angle of 6° (LeGrand, 1967).

The apparent frontoparallel-plane (AFPP) criterion is by far the most popular with investigators of binocular vision, apparently because it produces a locus that is reported to be rather more stable from day to day and because it seems to require the least amount of training of subjects. Furthermore, peripheral settings are reported to be much easier to make, and subjects feel much more confident about the accuracy of their performance with this criterion than with the nonius criterion (Ogle, 1950).

The subject is asked to set the rods, like those illustrated in Figure 11–3, so that they "lie in a plane which is parallel to your face." As an alternative, they can be told to set the rods so that each is "at the same distance." Curiously, Ogle (1950) reported that either instruction produces results that are virtually identical to those of the other. Ogle suggested that this indicates that both settings are based on stereoscopic depth matches. However, Shipley and Rawlings (1970) disagreed. Using these two criteria, they found noticeable differences.

Stereopsis thresholds can be used to determine the horopter in the same way as diplopia thresholds. Tschermak (1942) called this *maximum*

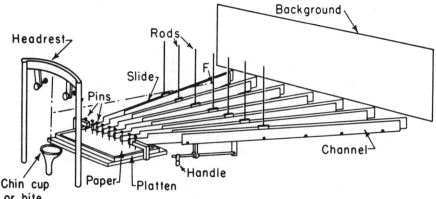

Figure 11–3. The apparent frontoparallel-plane apparatus of Ogle (1950, reprinted by permission).

stereoscopic sensitivity. However, no systematic studies of the horopter using this method exist. (However, see Blakemore, 1970.) We would expect an accuracy of about 5 arcseconds at the foveae and ±25 arcseconds at a peripheral angle of 6° (Hirsch and Weymouth, 1948; Ogle, 1950).

No reports have been found on zero stimulus to fusion horopters. The main problem with applying this criterion is achieving the necessary accuracy in objective measurement of eye movements. Robinson (1963) devised a system of measurement using a search coil in an alternating magnetic field. The coil is fitted to a haptic contact lens, and attains an accuracy of 20 arcseconds. While this device might be perfected to allow measurements of such a horopter, no one has completely developed the technique, apparently because of the problem of contact lens slippage. At any rate, the limit of accuracy of any such method would be due to the amplitude of the very fine high-frequency tremors, somewhere between ±17.5 arcseconds and ±1 arcminute (Alpern, 1969).

ASSUMPTIONS ABOUT THE HOROPTER

Each of these criteria operates under at least one important assumption. Some are listed in Table 11–2. Every method is subject to the assumption

Table 11–2. Some Assumptions Associated with Tschermak's and Ogle's Criteria

Criterion	Assumption
Diplopia—threshold	Horopter locus lies at the angular midpoint between the crossed-disparity and uncrossed-disparity diplopia thresholds (Woo, 1974)
Nonius	The fact that the fixation rod is the only object seen binocularly produces a testing situation equivalent to the whole field's being seen binocularly (Ogle, 1950)
AFPP	"Depth matching" directly locates the horopter locus (Ogle, 1962)
Stereo sensitivity	Horopter locus lies at the angular midpoint between the two (crossed and uncrossed) stereoscopic thresholds (Blakemore, 1970)
Zero fusion	Horopter locus produces zero stimulus to fusional eye movements (Ogle, 1950)

that underlies all thresholds and their application to human performance. In addition, reducing limits to a single point operates on the assumption that the horopter lies at the angular midpoint. This kind of difficulty can be met by simply redefining the horopter as a region in space that allows the test object to move without its displacement being detected (Walls, 1952). Yet, this may obscure a fundamental issue regarding fusional eye movements and corresponding points: Does stimulation of corresponding points produce any kind of signal for the eyes to move? Certainly, it would be surprising if this were the case. However, fixation disparity may represent the result of just such a slip.

Horopters can take two different forms. Using limits produces a horopter with a depth aspect. This is sometimes called the *physiological horopter* because it is based on a limit of accuracy of the visual system. The point form is sometimes called the *mathematical horopter*, because a numerical process is applied to determine a central locus (Walls, 1952). The major limitation in reducing horopters to a single locus by this method is usually that it ignores the real distal-proximal differences in sensitivity (Woo and Reading, 1978).

The assumption associated with the nonius is a form of an important question concerning binocular vision: Is binocular vision of the same nature when only one object in the field is viewed with both eyes as when a whole group of objects is seen binocularly (Ames et al., 1932)? Judging from experiences with anomalous correspondence (see Chapter 14), sometimes the amount of binocular information can alter visual directions (Mallett, 1973). Furthermore, the work of Julesz (1971) suggests that the normal binocular system may react differently depending on the amount of binocular disparity information present (see Chapters 7 and 8).

HOROPTER RESULTS

The results of studies using the AFPP criterion show that the horopter's shape changes rather dramatically with changes in fixation distance (see Figure 11–4). The curvature of the surfaces is always less than that of the Veith-Mueller circle, and the apparent frontoparallel plane coincides with the objectvie frontoparallel plane at a particular distance known as the *abathic distance* (Ogle, 1950).

Figure 11–5 shows that the AFPP plots for various alterations in magnification cause the settings to swing around the object of regard toward the eye that is looking through the magnifying lens (Ogle, 1950). Figures 11–6 and 11–7 illustrate the basis for this kind of rotation. For simplicity, the AFPP is pictured at the abathic distance, and corre-

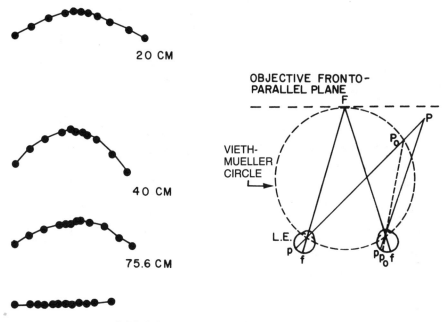

20 CM

40 CM

75.6 CM

609.6 CM

Figure 11–4. Raw data plots of horopter points taken using the apparent frontoparallel-plane criterion at different fixation distances (Ames et al., 1932).

sponding points are set at equal angles. Figure 11–6 shows how this plane appears tilted by introducing a size lens before one eye (Ogle, 1950). Figue 11–7 indicates how this surface must be positioned to appear frontoparallel to a subject wearing a size lens.

Figure 11–8 illustrates the unique geometric situation associated with asymmetric convergence. When the eyes switch fixation from F in the midsagittal plane to F' in any other plane, they converge an unequal amount. While the movement is accomplished according to Hering's law of equal innervation (Alpern, 1969), the eyes assume a final position in which the left eye has a larger convergence angle than the right eye. In this figure, P' is the objective frontoparallel plane, and N' is the normal to a line connecting F' and the bisector of the interpupillary line. Using the AFPP method under these circumstances produces some ambiguity. Does the subject set it in a plane that approaches the objective frontoparallel plane P, or is there a shift in her or his response behavior that amounts to an interpretation of the AFPP as equivalent to a normal to the egocentric visual direction N? Ogle's (1950)

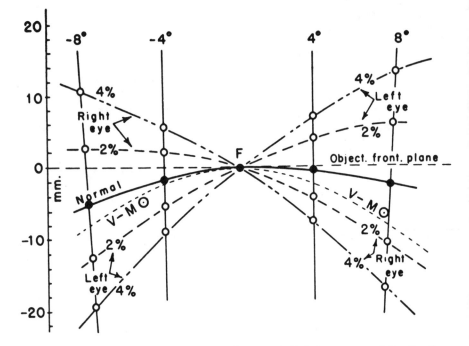

Figure 11–5.   Rotation of the apparent frontoparallel plane around the fixation point, caused by induced aniseikonia (Reprinted by permission from Ogle, 1950).

results suggest that the AFPP swings toward N, but only by half the required amount (Amigo, 1967).

Comparisons of data using the AFPP and the nonius led to the conclusion that the AFPP measures something other than a horopter (Ogle, 1962; Shipley and Rawlings, 1970). Certainly, the AFPP is based on some kind of relationship with corresponding points. However, it may be a remote and complicated association. Shipley and Rawlings (1970) call it a *geodesic of visual space*. A geodesic is the shortest distance between two points in any particular form of space. In euclidean space it is a straight line. In visual space it has a constant negative curvature. Luneburg (1947) was able to simulate the AFPP by taking an objective frontoparallel plane and transforming it to a particular noneuclidean visual space. The form of the space chosen was known as *Lobachevski's hyperbolic space* (see Chapter 15). This choice was based on the results of alley experiments, as discussed in Chapter 5. However, for most purposes it is sufficient to treat the apparent frontoparallel plane as a visual reference plane associated with, but not identical to, the horopter

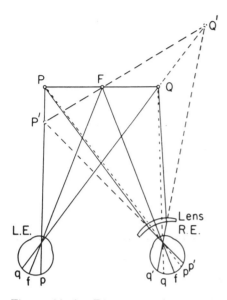

Figure 11–6.   Distortion of an objective frontoparallel plane caused by magnification of the horizontal meridian in the right eye (Reprinted by permission from Ogle, 1950).

that is important in the perceptions that occur in the presence of aniseikonia (see Chapter 13).

The nonius method produces the smallest scatter of data because it is based on vernier thresholds, which are incredibly fine ones. Furthermore, this method directly matches corresponding lines of sight. Experts have concluded that the nonius is the only completely valid form of horopter (Ogle, 1962; Shipley and Rawlings, 1970). Studies of the nonius horopter led to the rediscovery of the phenomenon of fixation disparity. By connecting data points to either side of the object to be fixated with a straight line, an estimate of fixation disparity can be made (Ogle, 1950). Figure 11–9 shows plots of nonius data for three different fixation distances (Ames et al., 1932) and indicates rather less change in shape as fixation distance is changed.

The fact that longitudinal horopter data do not lie on the Vieth-Mueller circle is known as the *Hering-Hillebrand horopter deviation*. Its existence is proof that corresponding points are arranged in an asymmetric fashion. Since a part of the change in horopter shape with fixation distance is due to this uneven distribution, the introduction of the Hering-Hillebrand horopter deviation allows us to assess what portion of the shape change is due to this arrangement and what portion is not.

Figure 11–4 shows that for horopter points to the right of the

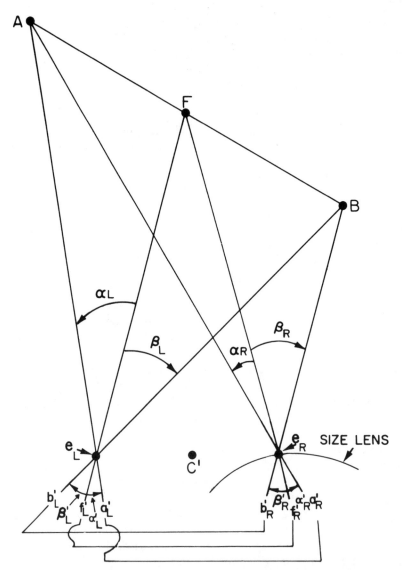

Figure 11–7. The positioning of two objects, *A* and *B*, so that the apparent
              frontoparallel-plane criterion is met while viewing with a hori-
              zontal meridionial magnification before the right eye.

midsagittal plane, the nasal angles of the right eye are larger than the
corresponding temporal angles of the left eye. This suggests that nasal
angles are underestimated, as predicted from the Kundt type of par-

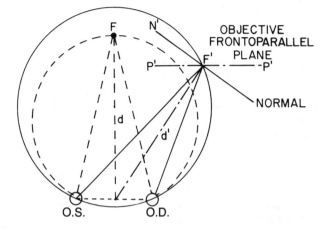

Figure 11–8.   Geometry of asymmetric convergence, showing Vieth-Mueller circles and the normal (N'), and frontoparallel (P') planes through F' (Ogle, 1950).

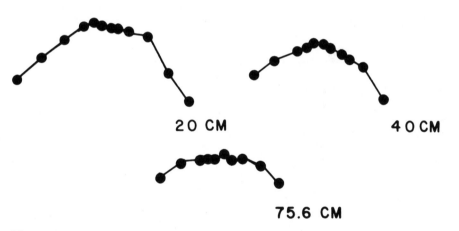

Figure 11–9.   Raw data plots of horopter points taken given the nonius criterion at different fixation distances (Ames et al., 1932).

tition results. Further, the nasal retina should have inferior resolution characteristics. We should also expect to find larger areas of spatial summation in the nasal retina and fewer crossed optic nerve fibers. That such differences may be quite small simply would illustrate how sensitive a measure the horopter really is.

ANALYSIS OF HOROPTER DATA

So far, comparisons have been based on inspection of raw data. Some were quite obviously different, others not so obviously different, and still others looked very much alike. When such a situation occurs, help can be sought by resorting to some process that facilitates arriving at a correct decision. Statistics serves such a function in many numerical domains (Winer, 1962), for it helps the investigator to reach the correct choice if it is fairly applied.

For the horopter, a method of analysis is needed to distinguish when two sets of data are really different. Perhaps such an analysis will lead to a further understanding of the cause of these differences.

Ogle (1932) described a method of analysis that is particularly well suited to applications of the principles of binocular vision to the problems of aniseikonia (see Chapter 13). He wished to express any given horopter plot in terms of two parameters: the relative curvature of the horopter locus and its asymmetry with regard to the midsagittal plane. He assumed that plots could be described by a conic section. Figure 11–10 illustrates this.

He chose to specify the conic's curvature relative to the curvature of the Veith-Mueller circle by a constant called H, where

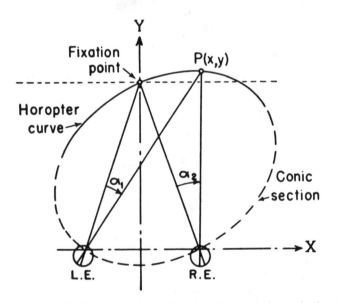

Figure 11–10. A conic section constructed through the fixation point and P, a point on the horopter (Ogle, 1950).

$$H = \cot \theta_1 - \cot \theta_2 \qquad\qquad (11\text{--}3)$$

which is the difference in the reciprocals of the tangents of the two lateral angles θ subtended by the fixation point, the entrance pupils, and a point on the horopter. Here H is a numerical value that specifies the deviation of a horopter point from the Veith-Mueller circle; It is a quantification of the Hering-Hillebrand horopter deviation (Ogle, 1932).

Then Ogle expressd the general equation for conic sections (Hill and Linker, 1951) in terms that are easy to measure: H, as defined above; $2a$, the interpupillary distance; d, the distance from the bisector of the interpupillary line to the fixation point; x, the distance between the horopter point and the midsagittal plane; and y, the distance between the horopter point and the bisector of the interpupillary line. The general form for conics then becomes

$$x^2\left(\frac{2a - Hd}{2a}\right) + y^2\left(\frac{2d + Ha}{2d}\right) - y\left(\frac{d^2 - a^2 + Had}{d}\right) -$$
$$\left(\frac{2a^2 + Had}{2}\right) = 0 \qquad\qquad (11\text{--}4)$$

If $H = 0$, then $\theta_1 = \theta_2$, and Equation (11–5) reduces to

$$x^2 + y\left(\frac{d^2 - a^2}{d}\right) - a^2 = 0 \qquad\qquad (11\text{--}5)$$

which is the equation for the Vieth-Mueller circle expressed in these same conveniently measured terms (Ogle, 1932).

Since $H \neq 0$, and since the equation for conics shown above is somewhat complicated, Ogle worked out generalized horopter forms in terms of the relationship among H, $2a$, and d. Figure 11–11 shows that when $H = 2a/d$, the horopter will be a straight line, which is the abathic distance condition; when $H > 2a/d$, the horopter is a hyperbola; when H is between $2a/d$ and 0, it is an ellipse; and when $H = 2a/d$, it is a parabola (Ogle, 1932).

Asymmetry is treated by considering rotations of the conic around a vertical axis through the fixation point such as occur in aniseikonia. Starting with the definition of H, we can rewrite it as

$$H = \frac{1}{\tan \theta_1} - \frac{1}{\tan \theta_2} \qquad\qquad (11\text{--}6)$$

which is

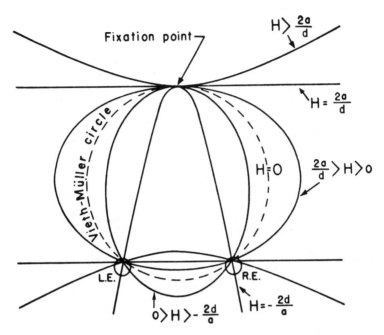

Figure 11–11. Various conics resulting as the parameter H assumes different values, in terms of the ratio of $2a$, the interpupillary distance, to d, the fixation distance (Reprinted by permission from Ogle, 1950).

$$H = \frac{\tan\theta_2 - \tan\theta_1}{\tan\theta_1 \tan\theta_2} \tag{11-7}$$

Rewriting and dividing by $\tan\theta_1$ yield

$$\frac{\tan\theta_2}{\tan\theta_1} - 1 = H\tan\theta_2 \tag{11-8}$$

Since Equation (11–8) is linear, we can express the ratio of $\tan\theta_2$ to $\tan\theta_1$ as the y value and $\tan\theta_2$ as the x value. Ogle called the ratio of the tangents R, and it can be found from

$$R = \frac{1+z}{1-z} \tag{11-9}$$

where

$$z = \frac{x^2 + (y - B)^2 - A}{2Axy} \tag{11-10}$$

and

$$A = \frac{d^2 + a^2}{2d} \qquad B = \frac{d^2 - a^2}{2d} \qquad (11\text{–}11)$$

Obviously, all such calculations are performed most easily by a programmable calculator or small computer.

Following computation, the data can be plotted on a cartesian coordinate system, and they lend themselves to a reasonably good straight-line fit (Miles, 1948). The y intercept is called R_o. It will be greater than 1.00 if the left-eye image is larger than the right-eye image (Ogle, 1950). Here R_o is an index of the difference in ocular image size or the amount of aniseikonia in the horizontal meridian. More generally, Ogle's operational equation for the analysis of horopter data becomes

$$R = H \tan \theta_1 - R_o \qquad (11\text{–}12)$$

The idea is to facilitate comparisons of horopter data by summarizing information into two terms: H, the slope of the best-fitting straight line, and R_o, the aniseikonia index. This is a quantification for the purpose of making comparisons. The analysis was developed originally to study horopters in patients with aniseikonia, and it does this handily, as witnessed by inspection of the data plotted in Figure 11–12 and anaylzed in Table 11–3. The changes in R_o produced by uniocular magnification are predicted rather well. *Percentage of magnification* is defined by the following equation (Ogle, 1950):

$$m\% = 100(M - 1) \qquad (11\text{–}13)$$

where M is magnification, defined as the ratio of the subtense angles (Fincham and Freeman, 1974). Note that the slope H is constant.

Figure 11–13 shows how H changes as a function of fixation distance. It shows H values for nonius and AFPP data on the same three subjects. Also plotted are the locus of the objective frontoparallel plane and the Vieth-Mueller circle. Clearly H changes much more for the AFPP than for the nonius. However, the AFPP locus seems to parallel the objective plot rather closely. For these three subjects, the abathic distance is slightly larger than 6 m (Ames et al., 1932).

Shipley and Rawlings (1970) were the first to have systematically applied another form of analysis. They felt that Ogle's analysis might not show important information about changes in individual pairs of corresponding points because it reduces horopter data to just two numbers. They suggested that a point-by-point analysis, such as can be provided for in an analysis of binocular disparity for each horopter point, should show much more about the nature of corresponding points.

The method involves finding the binocular disparity between angles formed at the two eyes for each datum point and a point on the

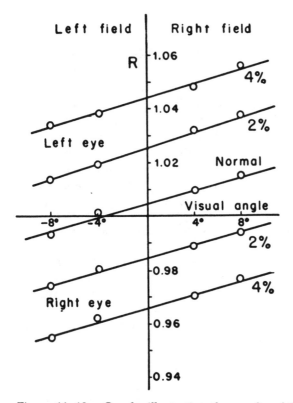

Figure 11–12.   Graphs illustrating the results of Ogle's H and R_o analysis (Reprinted by permission from Ogle, 1950).

Vieth-Mueller circle. By using binocular subtense angles, a computational simplification in the original method can be realized (Reading, 1980). Figure 11–14 illustrates the various angles involved in both forms of this analysis. The difference between α and α' is calculated for each data point. Then these are plotted on a cartesian coordinate system in which the ordinate is disparity in arcminutes and the abscissa is visual direction in degrees. Values on the ordinate greater than zero indicate that the nasal retinal angles are greater than the temporal ones (θ and θ' in Figure 11–14) whereas values less than zero indicate the opposite relationship.

Figure 11–15 shows the results of this form of analysis applied to the raw data plotted in Figure 11–5 and analyzed by Ogle's method, as shown in Figure 11–12. Size lenses were worn by a subject (R.D.H.) while making four-point AFPP settings (Ogle, 1950). In this figure, the star represent plots of the disparity for the objective frontoparallel plane

Table 11–3. Horopter Data and Analysis

| | Mean Settings (mm) | | | |
| | Visual Directions (degrees) | | | |
Magnification	−8	−4	+4	+8
4% O.D.	+10.43	+5.73	−7.70	−16.66
2% O.D.	+2.26	+2.06	−4.20	−10.43
0	−5.35	−1.86	−0.16	−2.10
2% O.S.	−12.70	−5.60	+4.26	+6.46
4% O.S.	−19.50	−9.00	+7.26	+13.70

| | R values | | | | |
Magnification	−8	−4	+4	+8	R_o
4% O.D.	0.9545	0.9612	0.970	0.9758	0.9655
2% O.D.	0.9732	0.9795	0.9885	0.9937	0.9837
0	0.9934	1.0005	1.0096	1.0150	1.0046
2% O.S.	1.0136	1.0196	1.0325	1.0374	1.0258
4% O.S.	1.0332	1.0387	1.0478	1.0560	1.0439

Source: Ogle (1950).

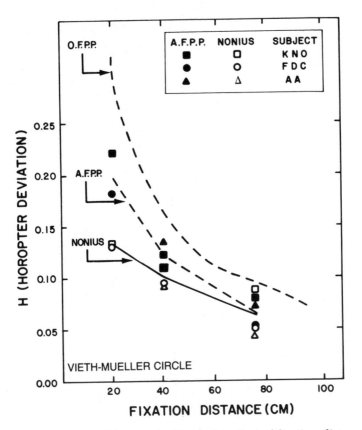

Figure 11–13. Changes in *H* as a function of fixation distance. Lines are best fit, by inspection (Reprinted by permission from Ogle, 1950).

(OFPP). In contrast to the results of Ogle's *H* and R_o analysis, the horopter disparities indicate that the AFPP undergoes some asymmetric changes with induced size differences and that these magnification changes also cause small amounts of fixation disparity. For visual directions to the left of the midsagittal plane, the closest match between the experimentally determined points and the objective frontoparallel plane occured when a 2 percent overall magnifier was worn before the right eye of the subject. To the right of the midsagittal plane, the best approximation to this reference plane occurs when the subject wore no size lenses. The loci for the various magnifications appear tilted in the direction predicted by the geometric effect, but show asymmetric distributions and cannot be accurately predicted from the no-size lens locus (see Chapter 13).

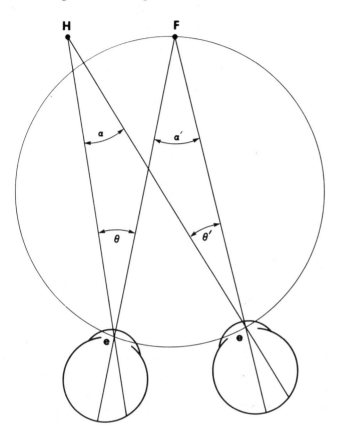

Figure 11–14. The angles involved in binocular disparity analysis of horopter
              data (Reading, 1980).

Figure 11–16 presents data on another subject (A.A.) given the
diplopia limit criterion. The geometric means of these limits are included
as the best available estimate of the horopter locus. Fixation disparity
also appears to be present in this plot.

Figure 11–17 shows a disparity analysis of data on the same subject
with the AFPP criterion with no prism in place before the eyes and with
5 prism diopters of base-in prism and 5 prism diopters of base-out
prism. A comparison of the analysis presented in Figure 11–16 with
that in Figure 11–17, in which the zero prism locus is adjusted to the
same level of fixation disparity as the geometric midpoint of the diplopia
limits, indicates that base-in prism seems to force a vergence change
which approaches or exceeds the proximal diplopia limits at − 12° and
− 8° of visual direction. Base-out prism produces a steeply curved locus

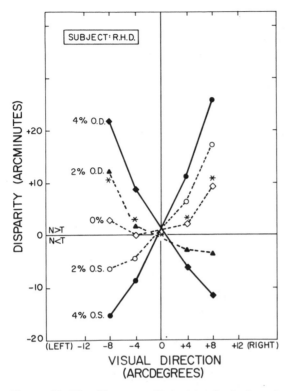

Figure 11–15.   Horopter disparities for induced anseikonia (Reading, 1980).

that approaches the distal diplopia limits at $-12°$, $-8°$, $+8°$, and $+12°$. All the loci are asymmetric with regard to the midsagittal plane, except the base-out points. The base-in locus approximates the objective frontoparallel plane for peripheral points to the right only. None of the three approach this reference plane for peripheral points to the left. Furthermore, prism alters fixation disparity, but only slightly (Reading, 1980). These plots suggest that the subject may have possessed a noncomitant oculomotor deviation and perhaps a form of anomalous correspondence (Reading, 1980). The potential for a manifest deviation was suggested by the description of the ocular characteristics: the subject was corrected for aniseikonia and had a large cyclorotary oculomotor deviation (Ames et al., 1932).

The application of disparity analysis to horopter data suggests that all methods can detect fixation disparity and aniseikonia and are subject to alterations owing to forced vergences.

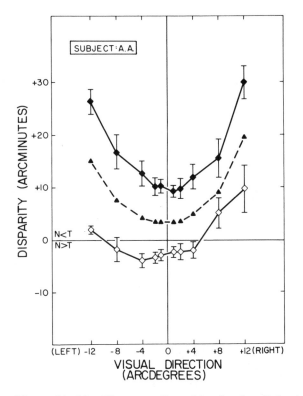

Figure 11–16.   Horopter disparities for the diplopia limits horopter (Reading, 1980).

STABILITY OF CORRESPONDING POINTS

Perhaps the most important issue concerning the nature of corresponding points is the fixity of the relationship. It is a question of some clinical importance since alterable points imply that it may be possible to train any particular set of points to correspond that might give a patient comfortable vision and perhaps some form of binocular function. Stability implies a rather more conservative approach as to the expectancies of such results (Ogle, 1950). The question arises from an inspection of raw horopter data plots taken at various fixation distances. To eliminate that portion of this shape change which results from the uneven distribution of corresponding points, Ogle used the value of H. He reasoned that if H was constant, then the points were stable. He found that H was constant, using the AFPP and altering the uniocular mag-

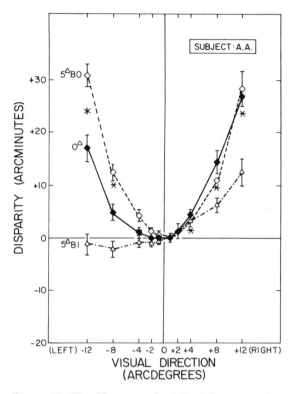

Figure 11–17. Horopter disparities by using the apparent frontoparallel plane
and prism (Reading, 1980).

nification. However, the nonius H changed slightly over that range of
distances in which accommodation and convergence were active. Therefore, Ogle suggested that perhaps this apparent instability in the nonius
horopter was due to some other factors associated with the near reflex.

Ogle was convinced that eye position was not important because
he considered that the nonius horopter was essentially unchanged in
asymmetric convergence.

Hallden (1956) and others have reported on the nature of some
optical factors that might be involved. These include a tilting of the
crystalline lens during accommodation, an alteration in the angle λ, and
an increase in the significance of the displacement of the nodal point
from the center of curvature of the retina with decreasing test distance.
Contraction of the ciliary muscle is known to produce traction on the
retina. If this force is uneven, then the retina will be differentially
stretched and the horopter will undergo a change in shape (Miles, 1975).

Flom and Eskridge (1968) used an experimental method which can show how important these other factors are in changing the horopter shape. Using afterimges, first the authors determined the sensitivity of their subjects to different degrees of physical misalignment of after-images, viewed monocularly at 100 cm. Later they had the subjects perform a series of nonius horopter settings. Once the two parts of the target were set in nonius alignment, they induced a new afterimage, which was then viewed at both 600 and 10 cm. All three of their subjects reported that the two components, a real target and an afterimage, appeared vernierly aligned or only slightly misaligned. It was the judgment of the authors that the misalignments reported were less than the sensitivity as previously determined. The technique bypasses all the optical factors previously mentioned and indicates that horopter shape changes are not due to instability of the corresponding points themselves. However, judgments involving afterimage locations are difficult to make.

Figure 11–18 presents the disparity plots of nonius data with different viewing distances (Ames et al., 1932). These show esofixation disparity and small changes in shape with changes in distance. To evaluate the meaning of these changes, the fixation disparity has been equalized and the probable error of measurement added to produce

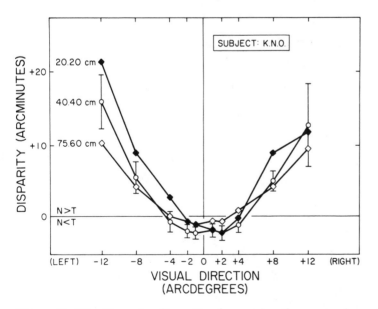

Figure 11–18. Horopter disparities from using the nonius horopter at various fixation distances (Reading, 1980).

Figure 11–19 (Reading, 1980). To a first approximation, the nonius horopter appears invariant at the different distances tested for this subject (K.N.O.). This statement is based on the fact that most points fall within or near 1 mean deviation of one another. However, a few points fall outside this permissible scatter, and these are usually associated with the 20.2-cm fixation distance. Therefore, being more conservative, we might say that only at rather small fixation distances does the horopter show anything approaching a significant alteration in shape or a hint of a slight instability. The data of Shipley and Rawlings (1970) show a similar stability for 2- and 3-m testing distances. At 1 m, all the points are approaching displacement by a significant amount. Figure 11–20 shows disparity plots for horopter data taken with and without a +2.12-d addition. Equating fixation disparity and allowing for measurement error indicate that no significant change has resulted. This suggests that the optical and mechanical factors associated with accommodation are really quite small.

Linksz (1954, p. 945) redefined the horopter as ". . . the sum of corresponding points of fixation as the eyes turn under a constant angle of convergence." To measure such a moving-eye horopter requires that the subject be trained to perform versional eye movements to a series of peripheral points without allowing a change in vergence to take place.

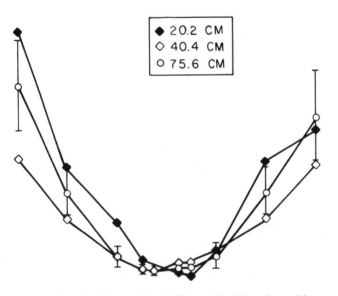

Figure 11–19. Disparities in Figure 11–20 replotted by equalizing fixation disparities and adding mean deviations (Reading, 1980).

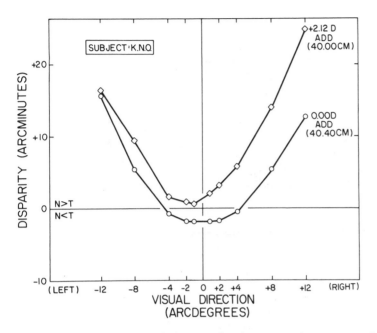

Figure 11–20.   Horopter disparities for the nonius horopter with and without a near add (Reading, 1980).

Shipley and Rawlings (1970) applied this concept to the collection of horopter data. For this study, they used upper and lower segments of a physically aligned central vertical light, viewed using polarizers, which they required the subject to keep in nonius alignment as he or she scanned to the left or the right. The peripheral target was adjusted by changing its distance so that throughout the final scan the formerly central target was always seen in nonius alignment. They reported that several hours of training were necessary before the subjects gained confidence in their judgments. They did not monitor eye position by any objective means. The upper graph in Figure 11–21 compares fixed- and moving-eye horopters for one subject. The generally close agreement indicates that corresponding points do not change with these kinds of eye movements unless the test distance is closer than about 1 m. At this distance they reported differences approaching a significant level. The lower part of Figure 11–21 indicates data for another subject, T.S., who had aniseikonia. They concluded that this plot indicated that the subject also manifests anomalous correspondence.

Shipley and Rawlings attributed the differences found at near fixation to the slippage of successive lines of sight as the eyes turn. This

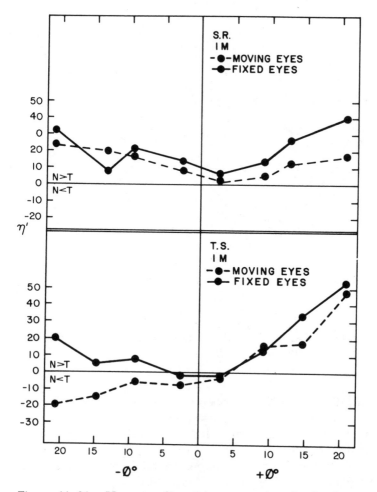

Figure 11–21. Horopter disparities comparing the fixed-eye nonius and the moving-eye nonius (Reprinted by permission from Shipley and Rawlings, 1970).

forms arcs, whose centers are known as *signing centers* (Fry and Hill, 1962). Figure 11–22 shows their application of the Fry-Hill concept to this problem. For example, a change in fixation from P_2 to P_3 produces the indicated slip of the primary lines of sight around arcs with centers at r, the sighting centers. This increases the actual angles of rotation, which in turn increases convergence in asymmetric gaze. It tends to correct for the discrepancy between the locations of the centers of projection and of rotation (see Chapter 5). What remains as different between moving- and fixed-eye horopters at these distances they attributed

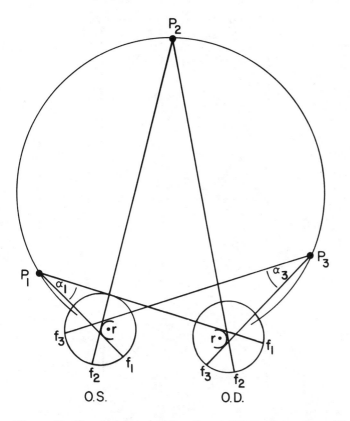

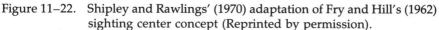

Figure 11–22.   Shipley and Rawlings' (1970) adaptation of Fry and Hill's (1962)
                sighting center concept (Reprinted by permission).

to a slight demagnification effect for the nasal versus the temporal
retina, as previously discussed (see also Chapter 14).

Another consequence of this demagnification occurs in aniseikonia. For a patient with a smaller image in the right eye, to the right
side, where the nasal retina of the right eye and the temporal retina of
the left are corresponding, the horopter should show an accentuated
tilt. To the left, it should be diminished. Figure 11–23 shows that this
is the case for the fixed-eye nonius horopter of subject T.S. who needed
a 2 percent overall size lens before the right eye to equalize the size
and shape of the ocular images.

Horopter data can be interpreted in another way. If nasal points
are subject to an additional demagnification associated with convergence (McCready, 1965), and if the egocenter is located about 10.5 cm
behind the interpupillary line, then a recoupling is required and these

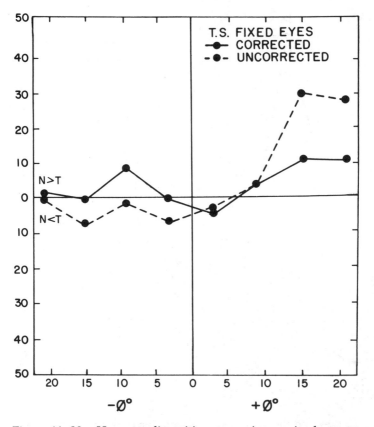

Figure 11–23. Horopter disparities comparing nonius horopter with and without correction for aniseikonia (Reprinted by permission from Shipley and Rawlings, 1970).

points are instable under such circumstances (Jones, 1974). Such a physiological zoom mechanism accounts for accommodative convergence micropsia. This phenomenon produces a reduction in apparent size and distance during forced convergence of the eyes and is also known as the *Silo effect* (Alpern, 1962).

Bourdy (1972) also believed that these points are alterable. She suggested that retinal directional values depend on receptor orientation. An asymmetric distribution of these and differing unilateral components of fixation disparity allowed her to account for the change in horopter shape with changes in fixation distance (Bourdy, 1972, 1978). We have already seen that the Stiles-Crawford effect influences chromostereopsis (see Chapter 8).

However, in referring to the analysis of horopter data presented in Figure 11–19, it would seem that these points only appear to shift over a range no larger than about 6 arcminutes at a peripheral angle of 12°. While this change may be significant, its magnitude is rather modest. Perhaps this apparent leeway in coupling is another phenomenon unique to Panum's area.

OVERVIEW

The horopter allows for a study of the relationship of corresponding points. It offers a sensitive measurement based on differences between the characteristics of the nasal and temporal retinas. The most precise and direct way to determine the horopter is by the nonius method.

Other methods are also available. Of those used experimentally, the diplopia threshold horopter seems to be most closely and simply related to the actual corresponding-point locus, provided that nasal and temporal differences are taken into account.

The apparent frontoparallel plane is a useful reference plane. It is quite sensitive to fixation disparities, forced vergence changes, and differences in uniocular image sizes.

Corresponding points show some hint of undergoing a recoupling at extremely short fixation distances. This may not be due entirely to a real instability, but rather the result of other factors changing in association with the near reflex. At any rate, the changes are rather small.

REFERENCES

Alpern, M. (1962), "Types of movement," *The Eye*, vol. 3, Academic, New York, 63–151.

Alpern, M. (1969), "Types of movement," *The Eye*, vol. 3, Academic, New York, 65–174.

Ames, A., Ogle, K. N., and Gliddon, G. H. (1932), "Corresponding retinal points, the horopter, and the size and shape of ocular images," *Journal of the Optical Society of America*, 22, 575–631.

Amigo, G. (1967), "The stereoscopic frame of reference in asymmetric convergence of the eyes," *Vision Research*, 7, 785–799.

Bishop, P. O. (1975), "Binocular vision," *Adler's Physiology of the Eye*, Mosby, St. Louis, 558–613.

Blakemore, C. (1970), "The range and scope of binocular depth discrimination in man," *Journal of Physiology*, 211, 599–622.

Boucher, J. A. (1967), "Common visual direction horopters in exotropes with anomalous correspondence," *American Journal of Optometry*, 44, 547–572.

Bourdy, C. (1972), "Directionnalité optique des recepteurs retiniens et points correspondants," *Vision Research*, 18, 445–451.

Bourdy, C. (1978), "Horoptere—vernier et couleur," *Vision Research*, 18, 445–451.

Fincham, W. G. A., and Freeman, M. H. (1974), *Optics*, Butterworth, London, 171–172.

Flom, M. C. (1957), "The empirical longitudinal horopter in anomalous correspondence," Ph.D. thesis, University of California, Berkeley.

Flom, M. C., and Eskridge, J. B. (1968), "Changes in retinal correspondence with viewing distance," *Journal of the American Optometric Association*, 39, 1094–1097.

Fry, G. A., and Hill, W. N. (1962), "The center of rotation of the eye," *American Journal of Optometry*, 39, 581–595.

Hallden, U. (1956), "An optical explanation of Hering-Hillebrand's horopter deviation," *Archives of Ophthalmology*, 55, 830–835.

Hill, M. A., and Linker, J.B. (1951), *Brief Course in Analytics*, Holt, New York, 135–148.

Hirsch, M. J., and Weymouth, F. W. (1948), "Distance discrimination, II, Effect on threshold of lateral separation," *Archives of Ophthalmology*, 39, 325–332.

Jones, R. (1974), "On the origin of changes in the horopter deviation," *Vision Research*, 14, 1047–1049.

Julesz, B. (1971), *Foundations of Cyclopean Perception*, Chicago University, 142–269.

LeGrand, Y. (1967), *Form and Space Vision*, Indiana University, Bloomington, 216–218.

Linksz, A. (1954), "The horopter: An analysis," *Transactions of the American Ophthalmological Society*, 41, 877–946.

Luneburg, R. K. (1947), *Mathematical Analysis of Binocular Vision*, Princeton University, Princeton.

McCready, D. W. (1965), "Size-distance perception and accommodation-convergence micropsia—A critique," *Vision Research*, 5, 189–206.

Mallett, R. F. J. (1973), "Anomalous retinal correspondence," *British Journal of Physiological Optics*, 28, 1–10.

Miles, H. J. (1948), *First Year of College Mathematics*, Wiley, New York, 473–477.

Miles, P. W. (1975), "Errors in space perception due to accommodative retinal advance," *American Journal of Optometry and Physiological Optics*, 52, 600–603.

Ogle, K. N. (1932), "Analytical treatment of the longitudinal horopter," *Journal of the Optical Society of America*, 22, 665–728.

Ogle, K. N. (1950), *Researches in Binocular Vision*, Saunders, Philadelphia, 18–55, 64–68, 200–215, 243–302.

Ogle, K. N. (1962), "The problem of the horopter," *The Eye*, vol. 4, Academic, New York, 325–348.

Reading, R. W. (1980), "A disparity analysis of some horopter data," *American Journal of Optometry and Physiological Optics*, 57, 815–821.

Robinson, D. A. (1963), "A method of measuring eye movement using a scleral search coil in a magnetic field," *IEEE Transactions in Bio-Medial Electronics*, BME 10, 137–145.

Rosenbach, J. B., and Whitman, E. A. (1951), *Essentails of College Algebra*, Ginn, Boston, 162–170.

Shipley, T., and Rawlings, S. C. (1970), "The nonius horopter," *Vision Research*, 10, 1225–1299.

Tschermak, A. (1942), *Introduction to Physiological Optics*, Charles C Thomas, Springfield, Ill., 148–210.

Walls, G. L. (1952), "The common sense horopter," *American Journal of Optometry*, 29, 460–477.

Winer, B. J. (1962), *Statistical Principles in Experimental Design*, McGraw-Hill, New York.

Woo, G. C. S. (1974), "Temporal tolerance of the foveal size of Panum's area," *Vision Research*, 14, 473–480.

Woo, G. C. S., and Reading, R. W. (1978), "Panum's area explained in terms of known acuity mechanisms," *British Journal of Physiological Optics*, 32, 30–37.

12

NEURAL ASPECTS OF BINOCULAR VISION

> There is something fascinating about science. One gets such wholesale returns of conjecture out of such a trifling investment of fact.
>
> *Mark Twain*

SINGLE-CELL NEUROPHYSIOLOGY OF BINOCULAR VISION

Considerable progress has been made since the techniques of electrophysiology have been applied to the study of the visual processes. With microelectrodes placed in the geniculate and visual cortex, the electrical activity of single neurons can be isolated and their response properties investigated. Figure 12–1 is a schematic diagram of the experimental arrangement used by Pettigrew (1972), the discoverer of disparity cells. By this method, he and others have been able to study the binocularly activated cells in the visual cortex of cats and occasionally monkeys. The animal is immobilized and positioned in front of a back-projection screen. Moving lines of light are projected onto this screen while the microelectrode picks up the neuron's responses. These responses are amplified and displayed on an oscilloscope and presented via a loudspeaker. The responses also are sent to an analyzer which counts the number of spikes of electrical activity across the extent of the field.

Of the millions of cells in the visual cortex, only as many as a hundred or so can be studied in any one animal at one time. Furthermore, the activity of adjacent cells cannot be determined. Nevertheless,

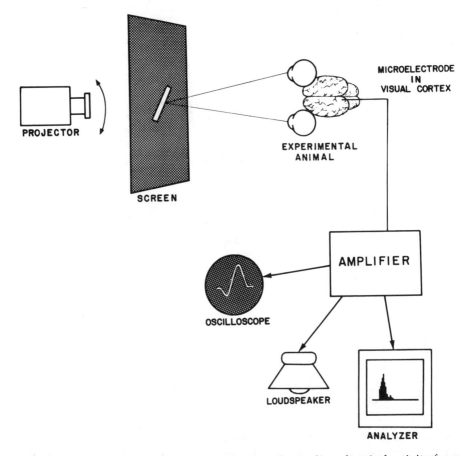

Figure 12–1.   Schematic diagram of method of recording electrical activity from single cells in the visual cortex (adapted from Pettigrew, 1972).

a good deal of progress has been made by applying these techniques to the study of binocular vision.

Yet, because of its complex structure, the cortex still contains many mysteries (Hubel, 1979). A recent technique of dying neural tissue with a substance that changes color with changes in cell membrane potential has been developed (Hartline, 1979). Application of this to the visual cortex will eventually allow exploration of whole regions to discover how the firing of one cell influences its neighbors.

BINOCULAR SUPPRESSION AND PRECORTICAL INTERACTIONS

The evidence for the existence of efferent, or centrifugal, optic nerve fibers in the mammalian visual system is less than compelling (Brindley, 1970). Polyak (1941) reported finding in the optic nerve and retina of chimpanzees fibers that could not be identified with any retinal cell bodies. Furthermore, Wolter and Liss (1956) found what appeared to be viable optic nerve fibers in humans who had undergone enucleations years before. However, these surviving fibers may belong to a certain type of centripetal or afferent cells that also survive extensive periods of light deprivation in cats and monkeys (Chow, 1973).

Flashing a light into the left eye of a cat affects the discharges at the optic chiasma to subsequent flashes presented to the right eye (Haft and Harman, 1967). The time characteristics of this inhibitory process suggest that the mechanism is a central-to-peripheral connection and not interretinal. Only in frogs have fibers running between the two retinas been functionally demonstrated (Shortess, 1963).

The anatomy of the lateral geniculate nucleus is decribed briefly in Chapter 10. Cutting the optic nerve causes incomplete atrophy in contralateral layers 1, 4, and 6 and ipsilateral layers 2, 3, and 5 (Brindley, 1970). While the cells of one lamina usually are considered to be isolated from those of other laminae, electron microscopy has shown some short axon cells that could mediate a form of binocular interaction in the cat (Brindley, 1970).

Electrical stimulation of the optic nerve produces presynaptic inhibition between two optic tract components from corresponding points (Sanderson et al., 1969). Postsynaptic inhibition has been demonstrated also in single cells of the geniculate (Suzuki and Kato, 1966). Inhibition consists of decreasing the rate of neuronal discharge by preconditioning the opposite optic nerve with electric shock or stimulating the contralateral eye with light (Bishop and Davis, 1953).

Photic stimulation also has been utilized, and it demonstrates that cells in the main laminae of the dorsal nucleus do have binocular fields. The field in the nondominant eye is of the exact size and position to correspond to the surrounding portion of the receptive field of the cell in the dominant eye and usually is purely inhibitory (Sanderson et al., 1969).

So far, geniculate-based interactions appear to be somewhat incidental to the binocular effects found more centrally (Bishop, 1973). Nevertheless, such activity could form an electrophysiological basis for some binocular suppression effects distal to the visual cortex, as suggested in Chapter 3.

BINOCULAR SUMMATION IN THE VISUAL CORTEX

As previously mentioned, many of the simple cells in the cat and complex cells in the monkey are binocular. Figure 12–2 shows a binocular cell that is equally influenced by either ipsilateral or contralateral light stimulation. When both eyes are stimulated together, a larger number of action potentials are generated. This cell demonstrates a form of binocular summation, since its binocular response produces 10 spikes of electrical activity, whereas stimulating only one eye or the other produces 4 spikes (Hubel and Wiesel, 1962). Such a response is called *binocular facilitation.* Pettigrew et al. (1968) found that almost all simple cells studied in the visual cortex of the cat showed complete binocular summation or binocular facilitation when the excitatory components of the receptive fields in each eye were activated by a light stimulus of the optimum size, shape, and position that was moving at an optimum speed and frequently in an optimum direction. These fields also exhibit reciprocal inhibition if the excitatory region of one is stimulated at the same time as the inhibitory region of the other. See Figure 12–3.

BINOCULAR DISPARITY CELLS

In addition to the other properties of receptive fields, single cortical cells respond maximally to a particular binocular disparity. Figure 12–3 shows the response histograms of a cell that yields its largest output when the two fields are precisely superimposed, which occurs at a distance equivalent to the point of binocular fixation. As the position of one field is shifted by prism displacement, the number of spikes per second diminishes until the two fields are completely separated. At that point, and for further increases in separation, the responses are identical to those recorded monocularly (Bishop, 1973).

Therefore, we can say that such cells have a rather precisely defined position in space, relative to the object of regard, at which binocular summation or facilitation occurs; a region in which binocular suppression takes place; and a boundary beyond which all binocular interactions cease. Bishop (1973) noted that such responses fine-tuned an optimum disparity for each cell. Barlow et al. (1967) found that these cells in the cat visual cortex corresponded to a wide range of spatial locations. In other words, different units are encoding objects at various

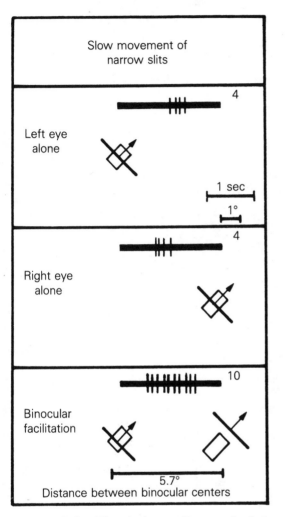

Figure 12–2. Electrical recordings and relative receptive field locations illustrating binocular facilitation (adapted from Barlow et al., 1967).

distances from the fixation point. The existence of the binocular disparity cells is the first step in establishing a neurophysiological basis for stereopsis.

In this study and that of Nikara et al. (1968), fields are mapped out on a tangent screen at different locations from their actual position during binocular fixation. This is done because the animal is anesthetized and the eyes assume a divergent position. Furthermore, the eyes undergo residual nonconjugate driftings. Therefore, the raw data re-

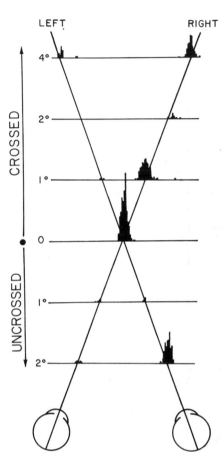

Figure 12–3. Responses from a single cell to different amounts of binocular disparity (adapted from Bishop, 1973).

quire some amount of correction to bring the two component fields into the relative position that they would most likely assume in an alert, binocularly fixating animal. Correction is accomplished by referring receptive field location to anatomic landmarks, by projection ophthalmoscopy (see Chapter 2), by monitoring spurious eye movements and making the necessary corrections, and by using certain statistical techniques (see cited papers for further details).

Blakemore (1970b) found that the columns of constant orientation preference, as discussed in Chapter 10, can be further divided into constant-depth and constant-direction columns. In a constant-depth column, all neurons have the same preferred orientation and binocular disparity ($\pm 0.5°$). Visual directions for these units vary over a range of about 4° to 5°. However, direction columns show a wide range of binocular disparities ($\pm 2.6°$) among the constituent cells and a somewhat reduced direction scatter, a 3.5° range.

Joshua and Bishop (1970) found that the range of binocular disparities increased as retinal eccentricity increased. Furthermore, more and more cells are found in these regions that respond best to objects located closer to the animal than the reconstructed objective fronto-parallel plane.

A NEURAL THEORY OF THE HOROPTER

Joshua and Bishop (1970) have taken the similarities between the characteristics of binocular disparity cells and the psychophysical form of the horopter as the basis for formulating a neural theory. They suggested that for any visual direction, the peak of the distribution of the number of cells with a given optimum response to a given disparity defines the horopter point. See Figure 12–4. In this figure, both disparity and direction distributions are shown. According to their theory, Panum's area is likely to extend over that region defined by 2 standard deviations, although this is, of necessity, a somewhat arbitrary choice. That both distance and direction are important to the theory is illustrated by points a and b. Point a represents the number of cells having the crossed binocular disparity value, which is 1 standard deviation from the peak of the 0° visual direction disparity distribution. Point b is at the peak of the 20° right visual direction distribution, and it represents the same number of cells as point a. If direction were not included in these considerations, b would be seen as diplopic, which is not the case.

Joshua and Bishop (1970) predicted the shape of the horopter locus by noting that any correction of receptive field locations used to simulate bifixation overshifted the fields of one eye, indicating that most are in register at a closer distance than the simulated fixation point itself. The amount of overshift increases with eccentricity. See Figure 12–5. Figure 12–6 shows the results of using such a process to construct a horopter for the cat. However, Shipley and Rawlings (1970) suggested that, based on the reported density of nasal versus temporal optic nerve fibers in the cat, the horopter should show considerably larger curvature than the Vieth-Mueller circle or, for that matter, than the plots based on the data of Joshua and Bishop.

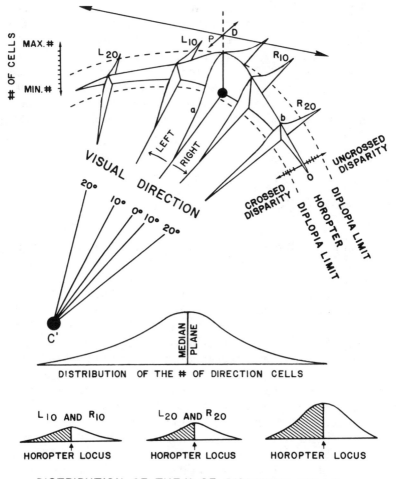

Figure 12–4.   Distribution of direction and disparity cells. The peak of the
distribution of the direction cells has been adjusted to illustrate
the need to consider both direction and disparity in constructing
a binocular theory based on the neural theory of the horopter.

DEVELOPMENT OF DISPARITY CELLS

Pettigrew (1974) studied the development of disparity cells in the cat.
Prior to the fourth postnatal week, he found that the neurons in area
17 responded equally to spot and line-shaped light stimulation of the
retina and were insensitive to binocular disparity. By the fifth week,

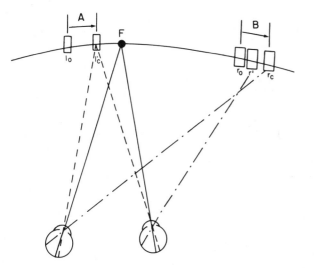

Figure 12–5. A shift of the receptive field for the left eye through distance A
brings it into register with that of the right eye. A similar shift
through B produces a crossed-disparity position (adapted after
Bishop, 1973).

these cells showed preferences for line stimuli of particular orientations
and responded differentially to changes in binocular disparity. Figure
12–7 illustrates the development of disparity cells. Furthermore, he
reported that kittens raised with both eyes sutured shut failed to show
any increase in the selectivity of these responses with age.

Apparently, the development of stereopsis, which is mediated by
binocular disparity cells, requires normal binocular experience during
the early period following birth. Perhaps the reports of gross stereopsis
in humans with residual heterotropias of a congenital origin represent
the results of a partial development of these cells.

MIDLINE STEREOPSIS

Figure 12–8 is a diagram of a human visual system in which the optic
chiasma was severed sagittally as a result of a bicycle accident (Blakemore, 1970a). Midline stereopsis is gone for objects such as B, in the
figure, that fall on nonfunctional regions of the retinas. However, A is
still perceived as closer than F because of the connections through the
splenium of the corpus callosum. Figure 12–9 shows what happens
when the callosal connections are completely severed. Here stereopsis

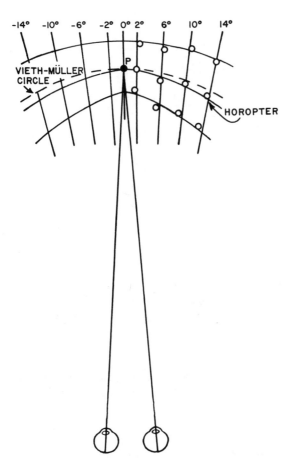

Figure 12–6. By using the process illustrated in Figure 12–5 and determining
the physical location of intersection for a number of receptive
fields, a horopter for the cat can be constructed (Joshua and
Bishop, 1970).

along the midsagittal plane is eliminated because it depends on this
central pathway (Mitchell and Blakemore, 1970).

In addition to callosal hookups, function along the median plane
is served by the overlapping and intermingling of nasal and temporal
optic nerve fibers around the vertical meridian through the center of
the foveae. Thorson et al. (1969) estimated that the size of this region
of overlap was about 0.6° in humans, based on a certain functional
criterion.

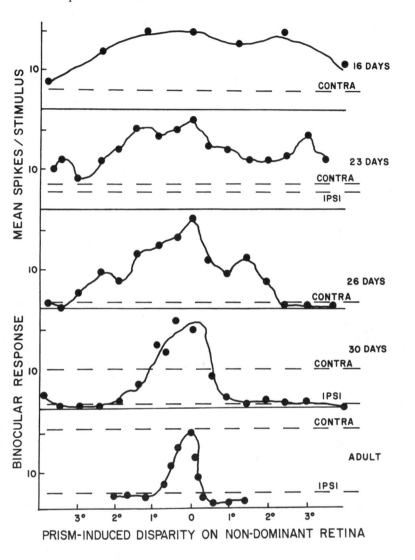

Figure 12–7.   Development of disparity cells in the kitten. Dashed lines indicate the levels of contralateral and ipsilateral monocular responses (Pettigrew, 1974).

EXTRASTRIATE SPATIAL FUNCTIONS

Ablation, restricted to one region of the occipital cortex on one side of
the medial surfaces of the calcurine fissure, produces a homonymous

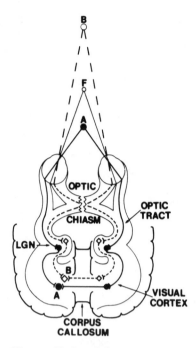

Figure 12–8.   Schematic diagram of the human visual system with the optic
               chiasma completely severed in the sagittal plane (Reprinted by
               permission from Blakemore, 1970a).

hemianopia that splits the macula. Weiskrantz et al. (1974) studied such
a case and found that the patient could accurately reach out and touch
objects in the affected field. The patient could also differentiate among
orientations of lines, discriminate different symbols, and initiate fixational eye movements in the correct direction. Measurement of separation acuity indicated a resolution threshold (75 percent correct) of 85
arcminutes at an eccentricity of 8°, 48 arcminutes on the affected side
and 35 arcminutes (at the same eccentricity) on the normal side. Despite
these visual performances, the patient had no awareness of visual function in the affected area. Thus conventional perimetry, based on subjective responses, may not yield the salient information about residual
function following retinochiasmal damage. These authors term this
phenomenon "blind sight."

     Humphrey (1974) reported the behavior of a rhesus monkey years
after virtually total removal of the striate cortex. This monkey could
operate in a fashion that appeared essentially normal with regard to
almost all spatially mediated behavior.

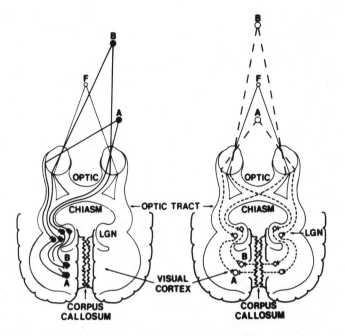

Figure 12–9. Schematic diagram of the human visual system with the corpus callosum completely severed (Reprinted by permission from Mitchell and Blakemore, 1970).

However, removal of the parietal cortex affects saccadic eye movement control, visual judgments of space, learning, and memory (Yin and Mountcastel, 1977; Brindley, 1970; Horel and Misantone, 1976).

Such visual performances in the absence of area 17 suggest that the geniculate may project fibers directly to areas 18 and 19, although no anatomic evidence exists for this (Polyak, 1957). Visual activity following removal of the parietal lobe demonstrates that other areas of the cortex are involved in the processing of spatial information (Mishkin, 1966). It may suggest also that this structure receives projections from the superior colliculus and so give evidence for the function of two separate visual systems (Schneider, 1969).

RECORDING ELECTRICAL ACTIVITY ON THE SKULL SURFACE

The visually evoked response (VER) is a specialized form of electroencephalography. It reflects cerebral potentials caused by adequate stimulation of the visual system (Regan, 1972). These indices of neural activity of a large number of cells are recorded by placing electrodes in good electrical contact with the scalp. Signals are amplified and averaged, as mentioned previously.

These responses are subject to a number of extraneous variables, including the effects of habituation, adaptation, attention, and so forth (Monnier, 1975). The technique also suffers from a number of problems, the most relevant of which involve day-to-day variability and differences among subjects. Its principal advantage is that it allows for the study of certain visual processes in humans. VER is believed to be the result of the electrical activity of the visual cortex that is generated in response to stimulation of the visual system [see Regan (1972) for a discussion of its origin].

As with single-cell studies, the information produced is indicative rather than detailed, seemingly reflecting the difficulties of working with very weak signals embedded in a background of considerable noise (Monnier, 1975).

Figure 12–10 is a schematic diagram of electrode placement and signal processing. It includes pictures of the electrogram (ERG) and the visually evoked response (VER). Recording the VER while stimulating the visual system binocularly and monocularly allows comparisons of the results in terms of differences in resulting electrical activity.

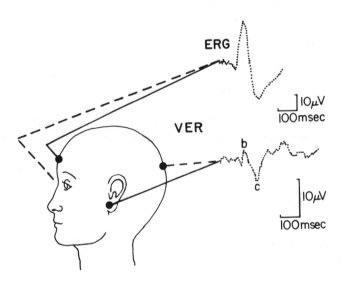

Figure 12–10.   Schematic diagram of approximate electrode placement and waveforms for the visually evoked response and the electroretinogram (Monnier, 1975).

BINOCULAR RIVALRY AND THE VISUALLY EVOKED RESPONSE

Figure 12–11 illustrates the pattern reversal of the recordings during binocular rivalry (Cobb et al., 1967). The rivalry trace, shown in rows 2 and 4, corresponds very closely to the monocular traces in rows 1 and 3, if we make allowances for noise and sampling fluctuations. Furthermore, these electrical responses are time-linked to the subject's

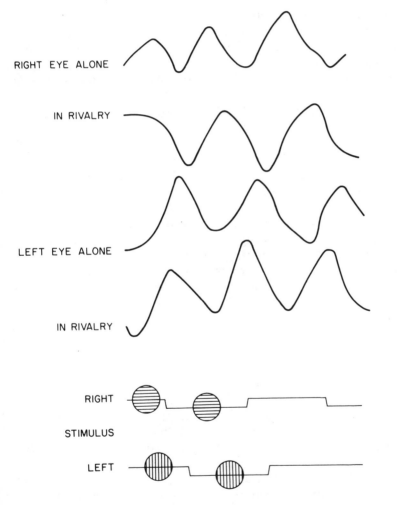

Figure 12–11.   Visually evoked response traces during binocular rivalry (Cobb et al., 1967).

reports of the suppression phase of rivalry, as shown in rows 5 and 6. Lawwill and Biersdorf (1968) found changes in both latency and amplitude of the VER during the suppression phase.

BINOCULAR SUMMATION AND THE VISUALLY EVOKED RESPONSE

The data of Harter et al. (1974) demonstrate binocular summation of the amplitudes of selected portions of the VERs for three out of four subjects. Perry et al. (1968) found that the binocular VER was 8 to 43 percent larger than the average of the two monocular VERs. Ciganek (1970) found a 40 percent binocular gain in response to bright flashes and a 100 percent binocular gain for dim flashes. The 40 percent figure is close to the results expected, based on psychophysical studies of binocular interactions at photopic levels. The 100 percent gain in dim light exceeds psychophysical values found for the binocular absolute detection threshold (see Chapter 4).

BINOCULAR FUSION AND THE VISUALLY EVOKED RESPONSE

Figure 12–12 indicates that the peak amplitude of the component which occurs 270 ms after stimulus onset is attenuated when the eyes are presented with triangle of differing orientation. This wave is present when the triangles have a similar orientation or during monocular viewing. Therefore, while this component may be an indicator of some electrical activity associated with fusion, it also may represent some other cortical function (Kawasaki et al., 1970).

BINOCULAR DISPARITY AND THE VISUALLY EVOKED RESPONSE

Figure 12–13 displays averaged VERs for gratings presented dichroptically and binocularly. These patterns are shifted back and forth before the eyes so as to continue to elicit cortical responses (Fiorentini and Maffei, 1970).

   If one of the gratings in the binocular presentation has a spatial frequency slightly different from the other, a binocular disparity is created. These data indicate that the amplitude of the VER changed as a

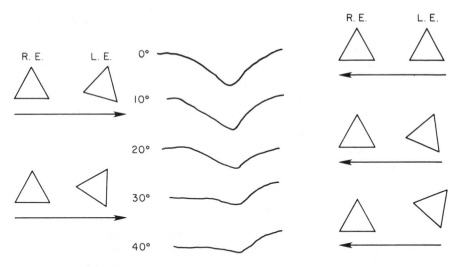

Figure 12–12.   VER responses as the orientation of a triangle is changed in one eye during binocular viewing (Kawasaki, Hirose, and Jacobson, 1970).

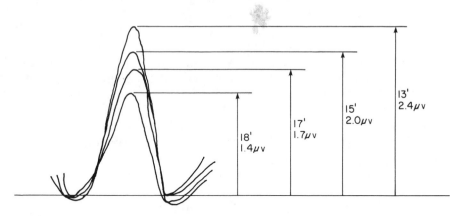

Figure 12–13.   VER responses, in microviolts, to various amounts of binocular disparity, in arcminutes (Fiorentini and Maffei, 1970).

function of changes in large binocular disparity. However, the lowest amplitudes appear to have occurred with no disparity and when the disparity was over 18 arcminutes. From around 13 to 18 arcminutes of binocular disparity, the amplitude (in microvolts) decreased. If we assume this is so, we are still left with the questions of amplitude changes between 0 and 13 arcminutes.

Regan and Spekreijse (1970) measured the binocular VERs, using alternating random-dot patterns displaying binocular disparities of 10, 20, and 40 arcminutes. They went to great lengths to avoid artifacts resulting from electrical activities potentially associated with eye movements, vertical disparities, and image movement. They found no correlation between amplitude and disparity. Some additional studies are needed to resolve these differences.

STRABISMUS, AMBLYOPIA, AND THE VISUALLY EVOKED RESPONSE

Studies of VERs of patients having the various forms of amblyopia have been done recently (Franceschetti and Burian, 1971). For that form associated with esotropia, Levi and Walters (1977) showed that a linear analysis of the VER waveform from the amblyopic eye is attenuated in the high-spatial-frequency range. Using psychophysical techniques for determining threshold contrast sensitivity, Hess and Howell (1977) identified two types of strabismic amblyopia. Both kinds show attenuation of sensitivity for high spatial frequencies. One type also has decreased contrast sensitivity in the low-spatial-frequency range. Levi and Walters (1977) also recorded this low-frequency loss, using the VER. Lennerstrand (1978) attempted to correlate changes in the binocular VER amplitude relative to the monocular VER amplitude with the threshold of stereopsis, as measured by using the Institute for Perception test. Wanger and Nilsson (1978) found that patients with microtropia fail to show binocular summation of the VER, and two of their subjects showed a prolonged latency when the amblyopic eye was stimulated.

The amblyopia associated with anisometropia produces reductions in the monocular VER that are very similar to those obtained in normals, when targets are viewed through defocusing lenses (Levi and Walters, 1977). White and Hansen (1975) showed that the binocular VER is sensitive to monocular blur and color. The latter effect amounts to less binocular summation for red colors than for blue ones. However, the use of blue light produces complex changes in the waveform.

FREQUENCY ANALYZERS

As suggested in evaluating the VER in amblyopia, the visual system appears to process information by using a series of spatial frequency analyzers (Campbell and Robson, 1968). The data of Regan (1972) show two different points of saturation of VER amplitudes as a function of increasing contrast, expressed as percentage of modulation. When stimulation is at low temporal frequencies, the VER increases with percentage of modulation up to about 20 percent. Beyond this point, there is a reduction in amplitude. At higher temporal frequencies, the largest recorded amplitude occurs at 90 percent modulation, the limit set by the apparatus. This fact confirms that the visual system also contains subsystems sensitive to different temporal frequencies (see Chapter 4).

Regan pointed out that in the lower-frequency domain, the point of saturation can be shifted to lower contrast by increasing the field size. Therefore, in this range, saturation is determined by the absolute amplitude of the neural signal. In the higher range, the saturation point is unaltered by changes in field size but is sensitive to luminance differences. Regan believed this to indicate that these high-temporal-frequency components have been processed by mechanisms distal to the final common pathway.

DISPARITY ADAPTATION

If a person stares at a pattern of alternate light and dark bars long enough, it seems to fade away. That is, the apparent contrast decreases slowly as the pattern is viewed for long periods. Measurements of contrast sensitivity following such adaptation show that the threshold contrast is elevated (Blakemore and Campbell, 1969). This adaptation can be transferred between the two eyes. That is, adapting one eye and testing the other also show an elevation in contrast threshold.

Presenting the adapting grating at a certain binocular disparity causes an increase in contrast thresholds for gratings presented at the same level of binocular disparity. Figure 12–14 presents some data that show this (Blakemore and Hague, 1972). This figure shows the change in threshold only over a range of 20 arcminutes of binocular disparity. The original data include a larger range and show that the binocular curve cycles upward again on both sides, at a point that corresponds to the angular gap of the next bar in the grating.

Felton et al. (1972) reported that their stereoanomalous subjects showed no disparity adaptation at all, even when the adapting grating and the test grating were presented at disparities for which the subject could correctly repond. Levi et al. (1979) found that the contrast adaptation effect did transfer normally in an anisometropic amblyopic subject.

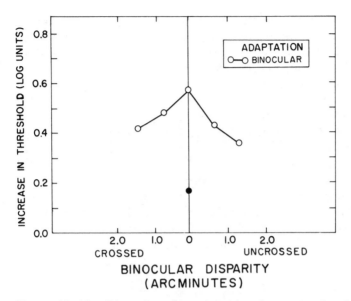

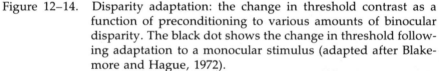

Figure 12–14. Disparity adaptation: the change in threshold contrast as a
function of preconditioning to various amounts of binocular
disparity. The black dot shows the change in threshold following adaptation to a monocular stimulus (adapted after Blakemore and Hague, 1972).

INFORMATION PROCESSING AND THE VISUAL CORTEX

Based on some of the facts presented, it can be suggested that the visual
cortex processes information by means that resemble Fourier transforms
(Pollen et al., 1971). The visual cortex contains units that are sensitive
to differing regions of both the spatial and temporal spectra.

Figure 12–15 shows the response characteristics of two different
kinds of retinal ganglion cells, called *sustained* (also known as X *cells,*
or *type I cells)* and *transient* (also known as Y *cells,* or *type II cells).* The
sustained cells repond continuously only to low temporal frequencies
and have a high spatial-frequency upper limit, or cutoff. However, the
transient cells respond only to contrast variations with brief periods of
electrical activity and have low spatial and high temporal cutoff points.

Figure 12–16 illustrates the distribution of these cells across the
retina and the effect of defocusing. Cells with these characteristics also
have been found in the lateral geniculate nucleus, superior colliculus,
and visual cortex of the cat (Ikeda and Wright, 1974).

A third kind of response has been identified. These other cells are

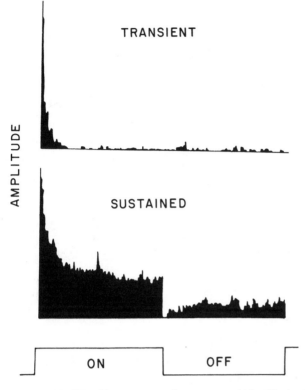

Figure 12–15.   Responses of two types of cells in the visual pathways (Reprinted by permission from Ikeda and Wright, 1974).

called *suppressed-by-contrast cells* (also know as *W cells*). They have large, unstructured fields and respond to overall luminance changes. In cats, the fibers project to both the ipsilateral and the contralateral superior colliculus (Cunningham and Murphy, 1978). Table 12–1 summarizes much of this information about the characteristics and possible functions of these cells.

The hierarchy of organization of the visual cortex demonstrates that the processing of information proceeds until a reconstruction of the exterior world is accomplished. One of the most economical ways to accomplish this is by analyzing brightness distributions into a series of sine waves of varying amplitude, frequency, and phase. Subsequent synthesis of this information produces a very accurate and complete reconstruction of the scene (Cornsweet, 1970).

Although it is not entirely clear what advantages are derived by arranging cells of similar characteristics in columns, Hubel and Wiesel

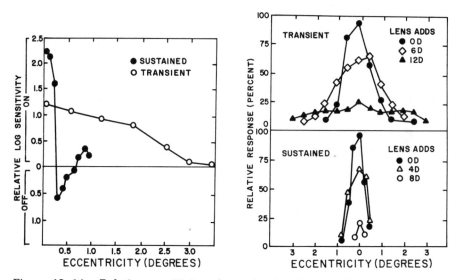

Figure 12–16.   Relative sensitivity of sustained and transient cells at various
                 retinal locations and changes in responses of these cells caused
                 by various amounts of defocus (Reprinted by permission from
                 Ikeda and Wright, 1974).

(1979) suggested that it may be best to arrange for multidimensional
attributes to be projected onto a two-dimensional surface. Position on
the cortex determines visual direction and depth. Columns exist for
orientation preference, ocular dominance, and maybe even fine spatial
frequencies and temporal discriminations.

The processing of stereopsis also uses these different-frequency
components. Julesz (1971) demonstrated that stereopsis results from
pattern matching of low, medium, and high spatial frequencies. However, his terminology seems to be relative since Levinson and Blake
(1979) and Schumer and Ganz (1979) reported that stereopsis frequency
analyzers are sensitive to only the low end of the spatial frequency
range. Furthermore, Hess (1978) found that a strabismic amblyope
showing a low-spatial-frequency loss is also stereoblind.

Random-dot stereograms can be employed to show that this spatial
frequency analysis takes place before the perception of stereopsis. The
processing of stereopsis precedes form recognition, if we assume a serial
order to the handling of information in the visual cortex (Julesz, 1971).

STEREOPSIS IN ANIMALS

Behavioral techniques have been applied to a variety of animals to see
whether they can respond to binocular disparity. Stereopsis has been

Table 12–1. Characteristics and Functions of Cell Types

Category	A	B	C	D
Location in visual field	Central	Peripheral	Peripheral	Central
Cell type	Sustained (X)	Transient (Y)	Transient (Y)	Suppressed by con-trast (W)
Fiber type	Slow tonic	Fast phasic	Fast phasic	Slowest
Destiny	Cortex	Cortex	Superior colliculus	Superior colliculus
Characteristics detected	High spatial and low temporal frequencies	Low spatial and high temporal frequencies	Movement	Null motion
Functions	Direction and dispar-ity discrimination	Saccades and tem-poral discrimination	Fixation reflex	Pursuit eye move-ments
Examples	Fine acuity, stereop-sis, and fusion	Fixation-registered, gross acuity, stereo, and fusion	Fixation-unregis-tered	Pursuit unregistered

Source: Modified after Ikeda and Wright (1974).

demonstrated in toads (Collett, 1977), falcons (Fox, et al., 1977), cats, (Fox and Blake, 1971), and monkeys (Bough, 1970).

The threshold for these animals, or any others, has been measured only occasionally. For the cat, it is about 2 arcminutes (Packwood and Gordon, 1975). Sarmiento (1975) measured the stereoscopic threshold for two macaques. Applying the 75 percent correct-response criterion to graphs of his data indicates thresholds of about 2 and 5 arcseconds. Certainly, this large apparent difference between the stereo sensitivity of these two animals would indicate that many neural features of the cat need direct corroboration by using monkeys before a wholesale application to human vision is completed.

REFERENCES

Barlow, H. B., Blakemore, C., and Pettigrew, J. D. (1967), "The neural mechanism of binocular depth discrimination," *Journal of Physiology*, 193, 327–342.

Bishop, P. O. (1973), "Neurophysiology of binocular single vision and stereopsis," *Handbook of Sensory Physiology*, vol. VII/3, Springer-Verlag, Berlin, 256–305.

Bishop, P. O., and Davis, R. (1953), "Bilateral interaction in the lateral geniculate body," *Science*, 118, 241–243.

Blakemore, C. (1970a), "Binocular depth perception and the optic chiasm," *Vision Research*, 10, 43–48.

Blakemore, C. (1970b), "The representation of three-dimensional visual space in the cat's striate cortex," *Journal of Physiology*, 209, 155–178.

Blakemore, C., and Campbell, F. W. (1969), "On the existence of neurons in the human visual system selectively sensitive to orientation and size of retinal images," *Journal of Physiology*, 203, 237–260.

Blakemore, C., and Hague, B. (1972), "Evidence for disparity detecting neurons in the human visual system," *Journal of Physiology*, 225, 437–455.

Bough, E. W. (1970), "Stereoscopic vision in the macaque monkey; A behavioral demonstration," *Nature*, 225, 42–44.

Brindley, G. S. (1970), *Physiology of the Retina and Visual Pathway*, Williams & Wilkins, Baltimore, 90–132.

Campbell, F. W., and Robson, J. (1968), "Application of Fourier analysis to the visibility of gratings," *Journal of Physiology*, 197, 551–556.

Chow, K. L. (1973), "Neuronal changes in the visual system following visual deprivation," *Handbook of Sensory Physiology*, vol. VII/3, Springer-Verlag, Berlin, 599–614.

Ciganek, L. (1970), "Binocular addition of the visually evoked responses with different stimulus intensities in man," *Vision Research*, 10, 479–487.

Cobb, W. A., Morton, H. B., and Ettlinger, G. (1967), "Cerebral potentials evoked by pattern reversal and their suppression in visual rivalry," *Nature*, 216, 1123–1125.

Collett, T. (1977), "Stereopsis in toads," *Nature*, 267, 349–351.

Cornsweet, T. M. (1970), *Visual Perception*, Academic, New York, 312–364, 387–398.

Cunningham, T. J., and Murphy, E. H. (1978), "Ontogeny of sensory systems," *Handbook of Behavioral Neurobiology*, Plenum, New York, 39–71.

Felton, T. B., Richards, W., and Smith, R. A. (1972), "Disparity processing of spatial frequencies in man," *Journal of Physiology*, 225, 349–362.

Fiorentini, A., and Maffei, L. (1970), "Electrophysiological evidence for binocular disparity detectors in human visual system," *Science*, 169, 208–209.

Fox, R., and Blake, R. R. (1971), "Stereoscopic vision in the cat," *Nature*, 233, 55–56.

Fox, R., Lehmkuhle, S. W., and Bush, R. C. (1977), "Stereopsis in the falcon," *Science*, 197, 79–81.

Franceschetti, A. T., and Burian, H. M. (1971), "Visually evoked responses in alternating strabismus," *American Journal of Ophthalmology*, 71, 1292–1297.

Haft, J. S., and Harman, P. J. (1967), "Evidence for central inhibition of retinal function," *Vision Research*, 7, 499–501.

Harter, M. R., Seiple, W. H., and Musso, M. (1974), "Binocular summation and suppression," *Vision Research*, 14, 1169–1180.

Hartline, F. F. (1979), "Biological application of voltage sensitive dyes," *Science*, 203, 992–994.

Hess, R. (1978), "Interocular transfer in individuals with strabismic amblyopia; A cautionary note," *Perception*, 7, 201–205.

Hess, R. F., and Howell, E. R. (1977), "The threshold contrast sensitivity function in strabismic amblyopia: Evidence for a two-type classification," *Vision Research*, 17, 1049–1055.

Horel, J. A., and Misantone, L. J. (1976), "Visual discrimination impaired by cutting temporal lobe connections," *Science*, 193, 336–338.

Hubel, D. H. (1979), "The brain," *Scientific American*, 241, 44–53.

Hubel, D. H., and Wiesel, T. N. (1962), "Receptive fields, binocular interaction, and functional architecture in the cat's visual cortex," *Journal of Physiology*, 160, 106–154.

Hubel, D. H., and Wiesel, T. N. (1979), "Brain mechanisms of vision," *Scientific American*, 241, 150–162.

Humphrey, N. K. (1974), "Vision in a monkey without striate cortex," *Perception*, 3, 241–255.

Ikeda, H., and Wright, M. (1974), "Is amblyopia due to inappropriate stimulation of the 'sustained' pathway during development?" *British Journal of Ophthalmology*, 58, 165–173.

Joshua, D. E., and Bishop, P. O. (1970), "Binocular single vision and depth discrimination, receptive field disparities for central and peripheral vision and binocular interaction in peripheral units in cat striate cortex," *Experimental Brain Research*, 10, 389–416.

Julesz, B. (1971), *Foundations of Cyclopean Perception*, University of Chicago, 90–102.

Kawasaki, K., Hirose, H., and Jacobson, J. H. (1970), "Binocular fusion, effect of breaking on the human visual evoked response," *Archives of Ophthalmology*, 84, 25–28.

Lawwill, T., and Biersdorf, W. S. (1968), "Binocular rivalry and visual evoked responses," *Investigative Ophthalmology*, 7, 378–385.

Lennerstrand, G. (1978), "Binocular interaction studied with visual evoked responses (VER) in humans with normal or impaired binocular vision," *Acta Ophthalmologica*, 56, 628–637.

Levi, D. M., Harwerth, R. S., and Smith, E. L. (1979), "Humans deprived of normal binocular vision have binocular interactions tuned to size and orientation," *Science*, 206, 852–854.

Levi, D. M., and Walters, J. W. (1977), "Visual evoked responses in strabismic and anisometropic amblyopia: Effects of check size and retinal locus," *American Journal of Optometry and Physiological Optics*, 54, 691–698.

Levinson, E., and Blake, R. (1979), "Stereopsis by harmonic analysis," *Vision Research*, 19, 73–78.

Mishkin, M. (1966), "Visual mechanisms beyond the striate cortex," *Frontiers in Physiological Psychology*, Academic, New York, 93–119.

Mitchell, D. E., and Blakemore, C. (1970), "Binocular depth perception and the corpus callosum," *Vision Research*, 10, 49–54.

Monnier, M. (1975), *Functions of the Nervous System*, Elsevier, Amsterdam, 260–640.

Nikara, T., Bishop, P. O., and Pettigrew, J. D. (1968), "Analysis of retinal correspondence by studying receptive fields of binocular single units in cat striate cortex," *Experimental Brain Research*, 6, 353–372.

Packwood, U., and Gordon, B. (1975), "Stereopsis in normal domestic cat, Siamese cat, and cat raised with alternate monocular occlusion," *Journal of Neurophysiology*, 38, 1485–1497.

Perry, N. W., Childers, D. G., and McCoy, J. G. (1968), "Binocular addition of the visual evoked response at different cortical locations," *Vision Research*, 8, 567–573.

Pettigrew, J. D. (1972), "The neurophysiology of binocular vision," *Scientific American*, 227, 84–95.

Pettigrew, J. D. (1974), "The effect of visual experience on the development of stimulus specificity by kitten cortical neurons," *Journal of Physiology*, 237, 49–74.

Pettigrew, J. D., Nikara, T., and Bishop, P. O. (1968), "Binocular interaction on single units in cat striate cortex: Simultaneous stimulation by single moving slit with receptive fields in correspondence," *Experimental Brain Research*, 6, 391–410.

Pollen, D. A., Lee, J. R., and Taylor, J. H. (1971), "How does the striate cortex begin the reconstruction of the visual world?" *Science*, 173, 74–77.

Polyak, S. L. (1941), *The Retina*, University of Chicago, 338–342.

Polyak, S. L. (1957), *The Vertebrate Visual System*, University of Chicago, 446–510.

Regan, D. (1972), *Evoked Potentials in Psychology, Sensory Physiology, and Clinical Medicine*, Clarendon Press, Oxford, 234–249.

Regan, D., and Spekreijse, H. (1970), "Electrophysiological correlate of binocular depth perception in man," *Nature*, 225, 92–94.

Sanderson, K. J., Darian-Smith, I., and Bishop, P. O. (1969), "Binocular corresponding receptive fields of single units in the cat dorsal lateral geniculate nucleus," *Vision Research*, 9, 1297–1303.

Sarmiento, R. F. (1975), "The stereoacuity of macaque monkey," *Vision Research*, 15, 493–498.

Schneider, G. E. (1969), "Two visual systems," *Science*, 163, 895–902.

Schumer, R., and Ganz, L. (1979), "Independent stereoscopic channels for different extents of spatial pooling," *Vision Research*, 19, 1303–1314.

Shipley, T., and Rawlings, S. C. (1970), "The nonius horopter," *Vision Research*, 10, 1225–1299.

Shortess, G. K. (1963), "Binocular interaction in the frog retina," *Journal of the Optical Society of America*, 53, 1423–1429.

Suzuki, H., and Kato, E. (1966), "Binocular interaction at cat's lateral geniculate body," *Journal of Neurophysiology*, 29, 909–920.

Thorson, J., Lange, G. D., and Biederman-Thorson, M. (1969), "Objective measurement of the dynamics of a visual movement illusion," *Science*, 164, 1087–1088.

Wanger, P., and Nilsson, B. Y. (1978), "Visual evoked responses to pattern-reversal stimulation in patients with amblyopia and/or defective binocular functions," *Acta Opthalmologica*, 56, 617–626.

Weiskrantz, L., Warrington, E. K., Sanders, M. D., and Marshall, J. (1974), "Visual capacity in the hemianopic field following a restricted occipital ablation," *Brain*, 97, 709–728.

White, C. T., and Hansen, D. (1975), "Complex binocular interaction in the visual evoked response," *American Journal of Optometry and Physiological Optics*, 52, 674–678.

Wolter, J. R., and Liss, L. (1956), "Zentrifugale (antidrome) Nervenfasein immenschlichen Sehnerven," *Albrecht von Graefes Archiv fur Ophthalmologie*, 158, 1–7.

Yin, T. C. T., and Mountcastle, V. B. (1977), "Visual input to the visuomotor mechanism of the monkey's parietal lobe, *Science*, 197, 1381–1383.

13

VISUALLY GUIDED BEHAVIOR AND ANISEIKONIA

I don't quite hear what you say, but I beg
to differ entirely with you.
Augustus DeMorgan

VISUALLY GUIDED BEHAVIOR

As mentioned earlier, the study of human performance is a complicated subject. It can be approached by the behavioral paradigm of fixing as many variables as possible, varying one or two inputs, and observing the output, that is, the observable performance (Brindley, 1970). Then statistics is applied to establish that any emerging cause-and-effect relationship is not due to chance (Winer, 1962). Of course, other phenomena associated with the human sensory systems do not necessarily lend themselves to expression as numerical entities. For these, introspection or simple observation is all that is currently available (Brindley, 1970).

Because of the complexity of the nervous system, conclusions derived from all such studies should be subject to confirmation by other means. Since these means are not always available, such information remains vulnerable to revision by future advances in the technology of science or to contradiction by other behavioral studies using superior experimental designs. Certainly, studies should be required that independently confirm certain findings before some of this information is used in a clinical setting.

Nevertheless, it is appropriate to look at selected aspects of localization, ocular dominance, and visually guided behavior to round out our discussion of binocular vision.

A WALKING EXPERIMENT

One consequence of Cyclopean projection can be studied by measuring the path taken by a subject asked to walk toward a distant object. Bailey (1957) studied this behavior, using three normal binocular subjects, a one-eyed subject, two strabismic subjects with normal correspondence, and four strabismic subjects with anomalous correspondence. The study was conducted on an open playing field, and each subject was asked to walk to a target located 1000 yd away. After the subject walked about 50 yds, deviation in path direction was measured.

Normal subjects operating binocularly walked on nearly straight paths. Then these and other subjects were tested monocularly by using a pinhole goggle to restrict the field of view. This monocular measurement was used to ascertain whether errors increased substantially when one eye or the other was used for sighting. If this were so, it might imply that such individuals usually project from a master eye.

Normals, using the pinhole goggle and viewing monocularly with their preferred eye, walked paths that were within 0.5° of the straight line connecting the starting point and the distant goal. This performance was about as good as for binocular walking without pinholes. When they used their nonpreferred eye, the error was about 1°. The one-eyed subject performed at a level of accuracy equal to that for the normal preferred-eye subject.

The two strabismic subjects with normal correspondence performed as well as the normal preferred-eye group when they used their preferred eye but made much larger errors with the other eye. Thus such individuals localize from the center of the entrance pupil of their preferred eye in these situations. When using either eye, the four strabismic subjects with anomalous correspondence performed only slightly worse than the normal nonpreferred-eye group. This suggests that anomalous correspondence is either a crude form of binocular projection or an alternating, somewhat imprecise, monocular projection (see Chapter 14).

Such studies are perplexing because they seem to indicate that normals using the preferred eye performed equally well binocularly and monocularly. This could suggest that normals also project from the preferred, or dominant, eye under such circumstances.

BINOCULAR CENTER OF PROJECTION

Fry (1961) proposed an experimental procedure for more directly mea-suring the location of the binocular center of projection. His method is based on two assumptions: that the center lies in a plane parallel to the median plane and that the visual angles between any two points in the field of view are equal to the physical angles. Figure 13–1 shows a sketch of the apparatus. The subject fixated $\overline{P}$ and brought a finger up from below an opaque surface to locate the image P' of a second object P. Figure 13–2 shows how this information is used to locate C', the binocular center of projection.

Bailey (1958) used a method based on these principles, but he located the second object so that it was seen as diplopic. Figure 13–3 shows his experimental arrangement. Here the subject located both images, P_R and P_L. By using Fry's assumptions, the angles are scaled off to produce an intersection at the binocular center of projection. Unfortunately, the data presented by Bailey show considerable variabil-ity from trial to trial and from day to day, which is characteristic of most absolute localizations based on diplopic images (Reading, 1971).

BINOCULUS

Charnwood (1949) suggested a more pragmatic approach to locating the center of binocular projection. He assumed that it was located some-

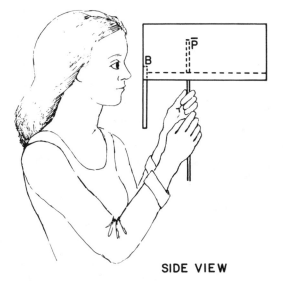

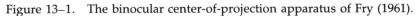

SIDE VIEW

Figure 13–1.   The binocular center-of-projection apparatus of Fry (1961).

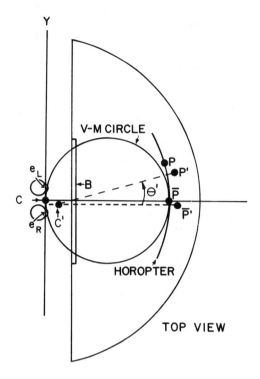

Figure 13–2.   Top view of Fry's apparatus shows how the locations of $\bar{P}'$ and
                P' are used to locate C', the binocular center of projection (Fry,
                1961).

where along the interpupillary line. Figure 13–4 illustrates his measurement method. The subject was positioned so that two distant beads
A and B, suspended from above by fine threads, appeared to be aligned
when viewed with both eyes open. Also suspended above the subject,
but out of the field of view, was a plumb bob that served as a marker.
A camera recorded the subject's final position of alignment.

Charnwood found that most subjects centered themselves so that
the plumb line fell close to a plane bisecting the interpupillary line.
Introducing a defocusing lens of 1-D power before one eye caused a
shift in the alignment position to a plane passing through the entrance
pupil of the opposite eye. This position also could be shifted by introducing neutral density filters before one eye or the other (Francis and
Harwood, 1951).

Charnwood (1949) suggested that these shifts in alignment position reflected shifts in ocular dominance brought about by altering the

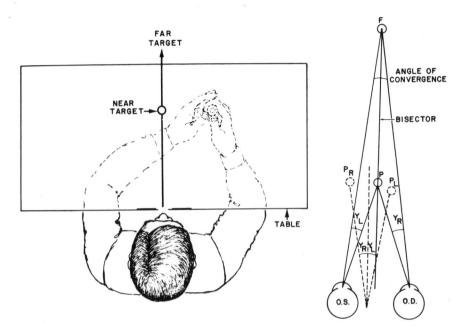

Figure 13–3.   Apparatus used by Bailey (1958) to locate the binocular center of projection with diplopic images.

stimulus strength to one eye or the other. Fry (1961) criticized this approach as forcing the subject to choose a point for alignment. Fry said that if you explain the test to the subjects, they could align, at will, on either eye, either ear, the nose, or anything else. Furthermore, Blank (1959) believed that the point did not have any location in physical space. However, since Charnwood was interested in ocular dominance as it related to clinical practice, and since almost all tests for dominance are more or less subject to such criticisms, the method is still of some interest.

OCULAR DOMINANCE

We have seen that single cells in the visual cortex show a range of ocular dominances (see Chapter 10). In terms of human behavior, this issue takes the form of inquiring into the existence and significance of the master-eye concept as well as its relationship to handedness, speech patterns, and human development.

Walls (1951b, p. 387) defined dominance as consisting of ". . .

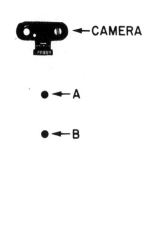

Figure 13–4.   Method of locating the binoculus used by Charnwood (1949).

any sort of physiological preeminence, priority, or preferential activity of one member of any bilateral pair of structures in the body." Gazzaniga and LeDoux (1978) studied subjects with split brains and concluded that the cortex was originally plastic as to laterality. Hemispheric specialization occurred concurrently with the development of language abilities, usually in the left inferior parietal lobe. Then, the later-developing visual-motor center, called *manipulospatial* by these investigators, developed in the right inferior parietal lobe. The left hemisphere also could function for manipulospatial tasks, but not as accurately as its counterpart.

The usual problems manifested in cross dominances are believed to be motor coordination difficulties, apparently brought on by secondary changes in dominance forced on the individual by environmental and cultural conditions (Beaumont, 1974).

In vision, the significance of dominance is much less straightforward. For example, Walls (1951b) listed 25 separate criteria for determining ocular dominance that have been used at one time or another. These have been slightly condensed, combined, and somewhat regrouped, and they are presented in Table 13–1.

Usually, clinicians do one of three things to determine dominance: ask the patients whether they are right- or left-handed, ask which eye they use to aim a rifle or similar monocular sighting devices, or perform some test for sighting or directional dominance. The classifications used are usually strong, weak, mixed, and uncertain. Often this information is utilized in the theory of prescribing in cases involving anisometropia with low-grade amblyopia. According to Borish (1975), where acuities cannot be equalized, the dominant eye should receive the clearer image.

Purely sensory dominances may or may not correlate with other forms, which are sensory-motor by their very nature (Walls, 1951b). Directional dominances are both sensory and motor and should be the most useful for general application. However, Mallett (1969) used a form of motor dominance, as indicated by fixation disparity measurements, to determine which eye's corrective lens would receive the compensating prism component. Correlative dominances may be the least reliable and valid form of all. Beaumont (1974) concluded that no relationship exists between the various forms of ocular dominance and handedness.

Using the visually evoked response (VER), Perry et al. (1968) found that the amplitude was greater when recorded by electrodes placed on the scalp above one hemisphere than when recorded from the other. However, they found no correlation between this and sighting dominance. Kaushall (1975) found that the left hemisphere appeared more dominant in binocular rivalry, whereas the right hemisphere dominated for binocular brightness matchings. He reported that the uncrossed pathway dominates the crossed pathway for rivalry, but not for brightness. Lennerstrand (1978) noted a trend toward an accentuation of VER dominance in the presence of amblyopia. Cohen and Duckman (1975) reported that amblyopia was more likely to develop in the nondominant sighting eye.

Loss of function in the master eye usually produces a rather profound disturbance in locomotion, but with time most monocular patients seem to be able to function quite adequately (Wernick, 1980). Cerebral damage to the left inferior parietal lobe can cause loss of verbal identification of visually presented objects, but normal manipulospatial performance. Right inferior lobe damage results in awkward manipulospatial behavior, but normal verbal identification (Gazzaniga and LeDoux, 1978).

Table 13–1. Ocular Dominances

Group 1: General Sensory Dominances

---

1. The eye whose image is seen more frequently in binocular rivalry
2. The eye having the better visual acuity
3. The eye that has the "more substantial-seeming image" in physiological diplopia
4. The eye whose afterimage persists longer
5. The eye whose image is less readily ignored, as in monocular microscopy

---

Group 2: Directional Dominances

---

1. The eye with which one sights
2. The eye with which the subject notices less jump in an alternate cover test
3. The eye whose occlusion elicits a greater feeling of uneasiness or unsteadiness, as in locomotion
4. The eye whose image undergoes less motion during changes in fixation from a far target to a near one (see Hering's lateral-shift effect below)

Group 3: Motor Dominances

---

1. The eye that fixates centrally in the presence of fixation disparity, heterophoria, or heterotropia
2. The eye that continues to fixate at distances within the near point of convergence

---

Group 4: Correlative Dominances

---

1. The eye before which one holds a card to read
2. The eye on the side of the dominant hand

Source: Modified after Walls (1951b).

HERING'S LATERAL-SHIFT EFFECT

Figure 13–5 is a diagram of a stimulus arrangement used by Hering (as reported by Ogle, 1962a). The subject initially fixates the distant target. At a signal, the near target, which is presented on the primary

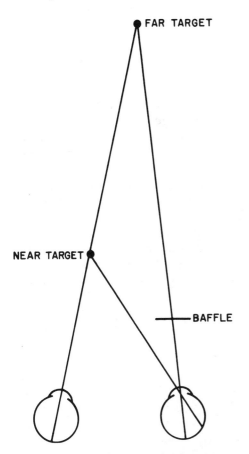

Figure 13–5.   Arrangement of objects and baffles used to demonstrate Hering's lateral-shift effect (Ogle, 1962a).

line of sight of the left eye, is illuminated and the subject is asked to fixate this target. A baffle prevents the right eye from viewing the far target. Since both targets are located on the primary line of sight of the left eye, the innervation for convergence and that for leftward version will cancel for the left eye and sum for the right, as illustrated by the objective measurement of eye position recorded by Alpern and Ellen (1956).

Ogle reported that left-eye-dominant subjects see no movement or lateral shift of the near target's image. Right-eye-dominant subjects see the near target shift to the left. Mixed dominant patients see less movement. Ogle (1962a) reported that the dominance determined by this means was in agreement with that determined by a sighting test for 7 of 10 subjects tested.

DOMINANCE AND RIGIDITY

Humphriss (1969) examined a wide age range of subjects, using the amount of plus lens power that induces a blur in one of the ocular images of sufficient magnitude to cause the subject to perceive a shift in the apparent color of an acuity chart, viewed through complementary colored filters (see Chapter 3). When more defocusing was needed to induce a breakdown of color fusion for one eye than for the other, he called this a demonstration of rivalry dominance. He found an age trend that runs from no dominances in a group of subjects 10 to 20 years old to strong dominances for a group of subjects 46 to 50 years old. He related this to a rigidity hypothesis which, in effect, said that some people were more determined or persevering than others and that the proportion of these increased with age.

STATION POINT

Jones (1979) also performed walking experiments and reported that the results gave a reasonably good confirmation of the hypothesis that the egocenter, called the *station point* by Jones, was located some 10 cm back of the interpupillary line. Thus it was located at the axis of rotation of the head and body. He commented that such a location accounted for accommodative convergence micropsia and implied that perceptual stability during eye movements must be accomplished by a centrifugal process.

OCULAR DOMINANCE AND THE BINOCULAR CENTER OF PROJECTION

Beyond those practical instances cited earlier, ocular dominance may have little to do with human behavior. To judge from the length of the list of possible dominance tests in Table 13–1, perhaps a great many different phenomena demonstrate dominance. Furthermore, the use of more and more different tests of dominance on a group of patients would indicate that most individuals should be classified as mixed. Employing the Hering lateral-shift effect may be the most useful means of classifying dominance in terms of its significance in spatial vision.

The results of such a test seem to indicate that binocular localizations are organized around a point which can be located at one entrance pupil or the other, or any place in between, for a given individual. Nevertheless, the significance of its particular location in a given subject seems to be somewhat obscure.

PRISM DISTORTIONS

Prism prescriptions are an important dimension in the correction of oculomotor imbalances (Borish, 1975). The main effect is intended to be alleviation of fusional stress, but sometimes an important sensory side effect is caused by the inherent optical distortions. It is well known that patients wearing base-out prism for the first time describe the floor as appearing to slope away, as if they were standing on the top of a hill, whereas base-in prism gives the impression of being in a recess, or at the bottom of a valley. Objective frontoparallel planes appear concave to the observer wearing base-out prism and convex to the observer wearing base-in prism (Waters, 1952).

Ogle (1952) listed the optical factors involved as changing angular magnification in the base-apex meridian, increasing curvature of the images of straight lines at right angles to the base-apex meridian, and altering angular magnification at right angles to the base-apex line with changing lateral angles. See Figure 13–6. Fortunately, some of these effects become less noticeable with longer and longer wearing time. This suggests partial adaptation to these distortions (Welch, 1978). Rarely does this exceed 40 percent of the value necessary to totally eliminate perception of these effects (Slotnick, 1969). By selecting the proper base curve of the lenses, some distortions can be eliminated or minimized (Ogle, 1952).

SPATIAL DISPLACEMENTS AND INVERSIONS

Today most investigators agree that the visual system predominates over the other senses (Welch, 1978). Because the visual input is so easily transformed by optical devices, the usual experiment has consisted of putting on some inverting or displacing appliances and reporting impressions of how things look and experiences of trying to perform various tasks such as reading, walking, and flying airplanes.

A very simple demonstration of performance changes with optical displacement illustrates most of the major points involved in the relationship between vision and motor activity. For example, the subjects

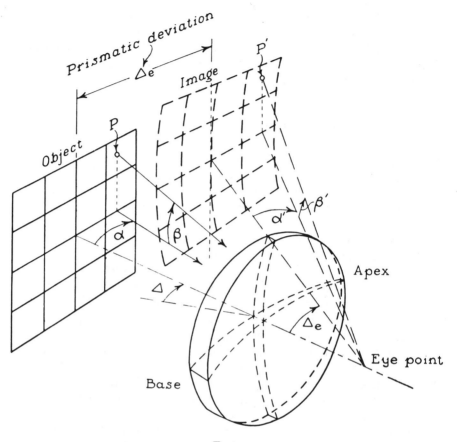

Prism

Figure 13–6. Illustration of the image distortions caused by an ophthalmic prism (Reprinted by permission from Ogle, 1952).

wear prisms before both eyes with the base of each directed to the left. Now, if the subjects quickly reach for a nearby object, they will miss it by moving the arm and hand too far to the right. As the hand approaches the apparent position of the object, the sense of touch will not signal an error; but eventually the subjects can see that the hand is going to miss the target. That is, an error in the position sense has occurred, and it is corrected by visually guiding the hand to the correct location. After several such trials the subjects correct the arm and hand movements so that they move directly, and without error, to the physical object. They have learned that the motor response has to be modified in order to directly reach out and touch the object (Welch, 1978).

The time between the start and the end of the searching movements is spoken of as the *adaptation period*. After removal of the prisms, the subject initially makes the opposite error, reaching too far to the left. This aftereffect is usually referred to as *readaptation* (Howard and Templeton, 1966).

The fact that visual location of the object viewed through the prism has not altered the local signs is demonstrated by eliminating the view of the hand and arm, called *eliminating the error signal* (Harris, 1974). Control theory calls this eliminating the feedback loop, or creating an open-loop system. This simply means that the error signal is unavailable to the subject. Interposing an opaque screen, such as a tabletop, between the object and the hand accomplishes this separation. Then responses show no adaptation or systematic shift from trial to trial and no readaptation after the prisms come off. Thus displacement of visual information does not result in a modification of local signs, but can result in a modification of the position sense (Hay and Goldsmith, 1973).

That the visual system directly predominates over the vestibular system has been demonstrated by Melvill Jones and Gonshor (1975). They fitted subjects with Dove prisms before both eyes, oriented so that the motion of an object moving from right to left produced apparent motion from left to right. The visual reversal caused a reversal in the direction of the vestibular nystagmus after 10 days of adaptation. This amazing plasticity apparently means that the subject is best served by the coordination of the optokinetic and vestibular reflexes. It is surprising that this adaptation can take place, even in adult subjects.

We have seen how malleable binocular depth judgments are (see Chapter 8). Wallach et al. (1963) estimated that viewing a rotating von Hornbostel cube[1] through a telestereoscope produced a 20 percent adaptation after 10 min of viewing. This is not a total surprise, since stereopsis is a relative depth cue which depends on other information to produce a sensation of absolute distance. As mentioned earlier, under circumstances in which the absolute depth cue conflicts with binocular disparity information, not only does the stereopsis depth match shift, but also it suffers a loss of sensitivity. Perhaps this represents an override of fine stereopsis; then these results would be due to a gross form of binocular function, and the adaptation would amount to only a shift between these two components and not anything like a change in correspondence, as is frequently implied.

Another popular approach is to place inverting devices before the two eyes and study the behavior of subjects while they perform all kinds of tasks. Without going into great detail, it can be demonstrated that no alteration in local signs or corresponding points takes place (see, for example, Walls, 1951a; Howard and Templeton, 1966; Welch,

1978). Walls (1951a) reported the results of an experiment involving some image inverters placed before the eyes of a monkey. She obtained instant adaptation by simply bending her head over and looking between her legs.

ANISEIKONIA

Although several issues of clinical importance regarding aniseikonia are discussed, the main purpose here is to briefly describe some functional aspects of aniseikonia that extend several of the principles of binocular vision in the normal subject. In no way can this kind of treatment be considered thorough and exhaustive.

This does not mean that the issue is unimportant. It is one of the most extensively studied phenomena in visual science. Following exultation at its discovery, aniseikonia received unprecedented support for lavish research and development activities (Burian, 1948). Then it entered into a period of rather extensive use and finally reached a stage of rather complete clinical neglect (Halass, 1966), its status today. Certainly, aniseikonia was not what some early workers claimed: ". . . as important a refractive anomaly as astigmatism." Nevertheless, it is a successful form of treatment for some patients (Bannon, 1954).

For those interested in a more complete treatment, see Ogle's (1950) pioneering book, Bannon's (1954) clinical manual, and the review article of Halass (1966).

Clinical Attributes

Aniseikonia is a fabricated word. It is created from the Greek words that mean unequal images (Lancaster, 1938). It is defined as the relative difference in size and/or shape of the ocular images (Cline et al., 1980). The term *ocular* is used in order to cover its possible causes, including a maldistribution of corresponding points and a result of the optical correction of anisometropia. The former cause is called *essential aniseikonia;* the latter is known as *induced aniseikonia* (Eskridge, 1958).

Essential aniseikonia can be due to an innate, anatomically distorted map of corresponding elements, a developmentally modified distribution, or a modification of the output from the visual system to the higher neural processes (Eskridge, 1958). Induced aniseikonia occurs at the rates listed in Table 13–2 (Borish, 1975).

Estimates of its incidence in the general population can be approximated from the studies of Burian (1943a). Table 13–3 shows his

Table 13–2. Induced Aniseikonia

Nature of Anisometropia	Corrected by Spectacle Lenses (%/D)	Corrected by Contact Lenses (%/D)
Refractive	1.5	0.25
Axial	0.25	1.50

Source: Borish (1975).

Table 13–3. Results of Burian (1943a) on Incidence of Aniseikonia in Three Selected Groups

Amount of Aniseikonia (%)	Flight Cadets (%)	College Students (%)	Clinical Patients (%)
0 to 1	100	70	36
1 to 2	0	23	55
Over 2	0	7	9

results. Perhaps something less than 1 percent of a patient population will require a size lens prescription, although this is pure conjecture.

Bannon (1954) tabulated the reported symptoms of aniseikonia sufferers, and these are presented in simplified form in Table 13–4.

OPTICAL CHARACTERISTICS OF MAGNIFICATION

Magnification effects of spectacle lenses have been classified by Ogle (1950) and others into two factors: shape and power. Because spectacle lenses are not truly thin lenses, a shape factor exists (Bennett and Francis, 1962). It corresponds to the effect of adding a Galilean telescope, or afocal magnifier, to the power factor, which in turn corresponds to the magnification effects of a vergence altering thin lens. The formulas are as follows:

$$M_s = \frac{1}{1 - (t/n)F_1} \qquad \text{shape factor} \qquad (13\text{–}1)$$

$$M_p = \frac{1}{1 - hF_v} \qquad \text{power factor} \qquad (13\text{–}2)$$

Table 13–4.   Relative Frequencies of Symptoms Reported by Patients
with Aniseikonia

Frequency of Patients' Reports	Symptom
Most frequent (20 to 75 percent of cases studied)	Aesthenopia Headache
Less frequent (10 to 19 percent)	Photophobia Reading difficulties Nausea Motion sickness Diplopia Nervousness
Least frequent (less than 10 percent)	Vertigo General fatigue Persistent difficulties with space perception

Source: Bannon (1954).

$$M = M_s M_p \qquad \text{total magnification} \qquad (13\text{–}3)$$

$$m = \frac{t}{n}F_1 + hF_v \qquad \text{approximation} \qquad (13\text{–}4)$$

where

t = center thickness
n = refractive index
h = vertex distance
F_1 = front surface power
F_v = vertex power
M = magnification
m = percentage of magnification

In the approximation, Equation (13–4), t and h are expressed in centimeters. Otherwise [as in Equations (13–1) to (13–3)], all dimensions are in meters and diopters. See Bennett and Francis (1962) for more details.

THE HOROPTER AND ANISEIKONIA

We have seen how the presence of aniseikonia causes the objective frontoparallel plane to tilt around the fixation point, farther away to the side having the larger image. Setting this back to a position that appears frontoparallel causes the reference plane to swing to a position that is closer than the fixation point on this same side (see Chapter 11).

Figure 13–7 shows horopter disparities for the diplopic limit criterion on a subject wearing a 3 percent overall magnifier before the right eye (Reading, 1980). Figure 13–8 illustrates the effect on the nonius horopter disparities of having the subject wear a 1.5 percent overall magnifier before the right eye (Reading, 1980). Both figures are predictably asymmetric with respect to the fixation point. However, not

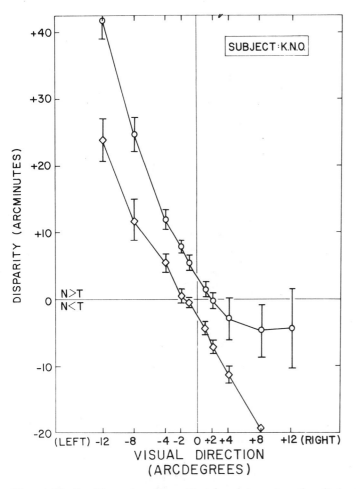

Figure 13–7. Horopter disparities for data using the diplopia limit criterion with a 3 percent overall magnifier before the right eye (Reading, 1980).

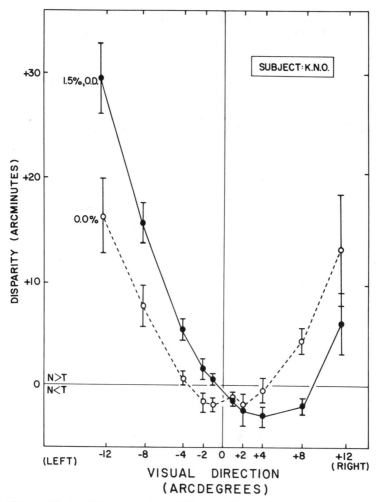

Figure 13–8.   Horopter disparities for data using the nonius criterion with a
1.5 percent overall magnifier before the right eye (Reading,
1980).

all shifts in horopter disparities can be predicted accurately from the
nonius data taken without magnifiers. Thus some of the translations
in the horopter, resulting from aniseikonia, may be caused by measurement error, spurious eye movements, or some sensory shift in correspondence. Certainly, a systematic study of these irregularities would
be most welcome, since if these changes are due to some sort of re-

coupling, aniseikonia may be more complicated than is usually believed (see Chapter 14).

CLASSIFICATION OF MAGNIFICATION DIFFERENCES

Aniseikonia can take several forms. If the object retains its shape but changes in size only, this is the result of an overall magnification. Aniseikonia also can result from both a shape and a size change. This form is known as *meridional*, since this magnification effect exists in only one meridian (Bennett and Francis, 1962). Magnifying only one meridian changes the apparent size in one dimension and produces a shape change.

There are three kinds of meridional magnification difference: one resulting from magnification in the horizontal meridian, called the *geometric effect*; one in the vertical meridian, called the *induced effect*; and the oblique meridional magnifications. The latter forms, treated as vectors, resolve into various amounts of magnification in meridians at 45° and 135° (Ogle, 1950). The geometric effect derives its name from the predictability of the distortions of binocular space as illustrated in Figures 11–6 and 11–7.

DEMONSTRATION OF SPATIAL DISTORTIONS

The best way to see the effects of these various distortions is to use a magnifier before one eye and binocularly view a leaf room. This is simply a rectangular room whose surfaces are covered with artificial leaves, artificial grass, or any such material that obscures the contours at its corners and the texture details of the walls, ceiling, and floor (Davis, 1959). One wall is left open, so that the subject can view the effects.

Figure 13–9 shows a schematic of the various distortions (Ogle, 1950). The topmost diagram shows either an overall, a geometric, or an induced effect, since the method does not permit differentiation. The two lower figures show distortions resulting from the two resolved forms of oblique magnifications.

INDUCED, GEOMETRIC, AND OVERALL EFFECTS

According to Ogle (1950), a magnifier oriented so that the meridian of magnification is vertical acts as if it were a horizontal magnification of

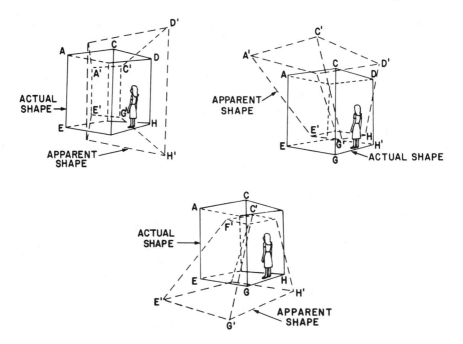

Figure 13–9.   Distortions in the appearance of a leaf room (Ogle, 1950).

the opposite eye. Therefore, vertical magnification induces a resultant tilt such as the one found when a real horizontal magnification change of the other eye occurs. Changes in the magnification of the vertical meridian produce only vertical disparities, and so no distortion of the stereoscopic perception of space should result (Ogle, 1950).

Figure 13–10 is a sketch of a tilting-plane apparatus (Ogle, 1950). The object plane consists of a glass plate covered with ink blotches of different size, to minimize perspective cues, and the angle of tilt is set by the subject so that the plane appears frontal. This angular setting is related to the magnification difference between the two eyes by

$$\tan \theta = \frac{M - 1}{M + 1} \frac{d}{a} \tag{13–5}$$

where θ = angle of tilt
  M = magnification difference
  d = test distance
  a = half the interpupillary distance

Bourdy (1960) measured the induced effect by using the tilting

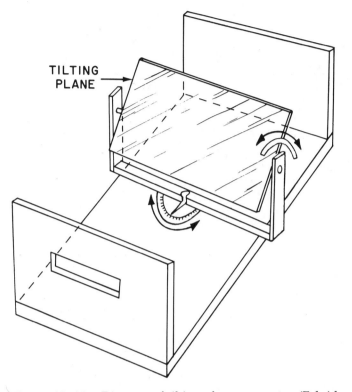

TILTING
PLANE

Figure 13–10.   Diagram of tilting-plane apparatus (Eskridge, 1958).

plane. Figure 13–11 illustrates her results. Both the induced and geometric effects caused an increasing tilt with increasing magnification up
to a point. Here, the curve saturated, because of either interference
from perspective cues or disruption of fusion, which tends to break
down at these large magnification values. Of course, this latter factor
did not prevent stereopsis from operating; it only degraded its sensitivity (Reading and Tanlamai, 1980). While Ogle (1950) reported that
the induced effect often produced a sigmoid-shaped curve, a part of
this roll-off effect might reflect an artifact owing to sampling error in
the presence of a degraded stereo sensitivity.

The induced tilt almost matched that due to the geometric effect
at small magnifications. Of course, it was a reverse tilt. Both effects
caused an increasing tilt with increasing fixation distance.

Figure 13–12 presents Bourdy's (1960) data for the overall effect.
This effect undergoes an extreme form of damping at the 300-cm fixation
distance. At 40 cm, the magnification of the right eye causes tilts iden-

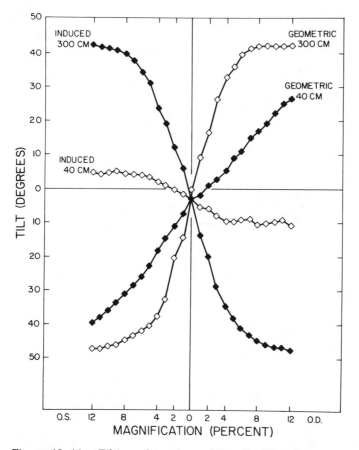

Figure 13–11.   Tilting-plane data of Bourdy (1960). For the data at a test distance of 300 cm, the solid dots indicate the induced effect. For
the 40-cm data, the solid dots indicate the geometric effect.

tical to those for the geometric effect, as shown in Figure 13–11. With
the lenses before the left eye, the resulting tilt for the overall effect is
less than for the geometric effect.

The way in which vertical disparities are involved in the induced
effect is indicated by using the apparent frontoparallel apparatus. Here,
the induced effect causes no horopter tilt unless two or more separate
markers are attached to one or more of the horopter rods. These spots
allow for the detection of vertical disparities, or at least vertical slips
are superfluous without them (Ogle, 1950).

The effect of an overall magnification difference between the two

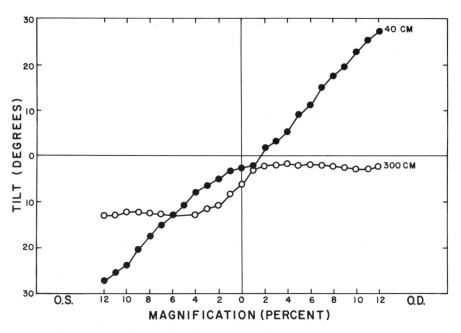

Figure 13–12.   Data illustrating the overall effect (Bourdy, 1960).

eyes has been judged as a partial cancellation of the geometric effect by the induced effect, to leave a net distortion that is a diminished geometric effect. Figure 13–12 shows some of Burdy's (1960) measurements.

Ogle's theory of the induced effect says that 'the vertical magnification sets off a compensatory mechanism in the opposite monocular perceptual system, which acts as an overall magnification of a magnitude necessary to cancel the vertical magnification difference. This does happen, but a net difference is left in this eye's horizontal meridian which produces the observed distortions. For example, a 3 percent axis 180 size lens before the left eye would induce nearly the equivalent of a 3 percent overall size change in the right eye's visual system. These two components tend to cancel, leaving the equivalent of almost a 3 percent horizontal effect on the right side (Ogle, 1938).

Ogle (1938) supported this theory by pointing out that one way to interpret changes in the shape of the AFPP with asymmetric convergence is in terms of the operation of such a compensatory mechanism. One eye receives a larger image owing to the difference in distance from any one object point to the entrance pupils of the two eyes. At near distance, all points off the median plane produce vertical disparities and require some form of compensatory mechanism to prevent them from producing an induced effect (Ogle, 1939).

Ogle (1938) suggested that this apparently induced change may be optical, as brought about by some kind of shift in position or orientation of the crystalline lens; functional, as by a change in the coupling between points; or perceptual, as attributable to the shape-constancy phenomenon.

CYCLOFUSION AND ANISEIKONIA

Torsional eye movements are best described as a wheellike rotation of the eye around an axis that coincides with the primary line of sight (Cline et al., 1980). These occur as conjunctive movements which are compensatory to changes in the position of the head with respect to the body (Alpern, 1969). These movements can be disjunctive when they occur in association with convergence, particularly if combined with elevation or depression (Allen, 1954). Such movements also can occur independently of all other forms of fusonal eye movements (Ogle and Ellerbrock, 1946).

The importance of cyclofusion here lies in its relationship to aniseikonia. Figure 13–13 shows a view seen through an obliquely oriented meridional magnifier. Notice that vertical and horizontal lines are displaced angularly, or scissored, toward the meridian of magnification. For example, with such magnifiers before both eyes, the situation is as also illustrated in Figure 13–13. The image of point B is displaced from the primarily vertical meridians on the two retinas in a temporal direction. This creates an uncrossed binocular disparity, which leads to the perception that this portion of the line is closer (Cibis, 1952).

These kinds of movements are described as very slow ones. The motor response lags the stimulus, and it takes some noticeable amount of time to reach anything like a match with a given cyclofusional stimulus, even if allowance is made for the usual final positional lag (Alpern, 1969). Thus initially a subject will see a vertical-line target tilted in depth, as described earlier. The tilt will decrease with time, and eventually if the stimulus is within the subject's cyclofusional amplitude, the target will appear to right itself. Sullivan and Kertesz (1978) indicated that a precise match between stimulus and final motor response is not required, since the brain has a compensatory mechanism that causes slightly misaligned targets to appear vertical.

Using a vertical line and a horizontal line, forming a cross, and viewing this through a meridional size lens, axis oblique, before one

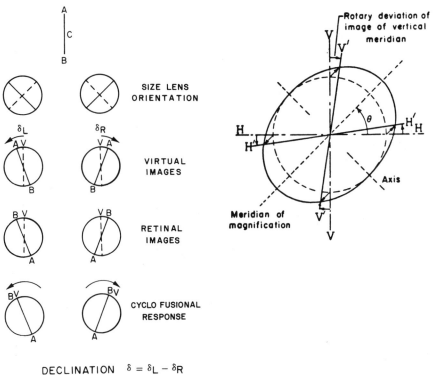

DECLINATION $\delta = \delta_L - \delta_R$

Figure 13–13.   View of horizontal and vertical lines through a meridional magnifier (right) and a vertical line and the resulting retinal image
locations and cyclofusional eye movements (left).

or both eyes, produce a situation in which cyclofusion would reduce
tilts of the vertical component but increase the disparity for the horizontal component. This tends to prevent cyclofusion, and the tilt of the
vertical component is a more obvious and permanent perception (Ogle,
1950).

Figure 13–14 presents data for a vertical-line target and an oblique
cross. The flatness of the data with the vertical-line object confirms that
tilts of such an object are compensated mostly by the activity of a
cyclofusional mechanism. For the oblique cross, no compensation by
movement of the eyes has occurred (Ogle, 1950).

Meridional magnification of the image of the right eye oriented at
axis 180° causes an oblique cross to appear to swing to the left. Magnification at axis 90° causes a swing to the right. If vertical lines are
added, because they act as stimuli for cyclofusion, oblique magnification

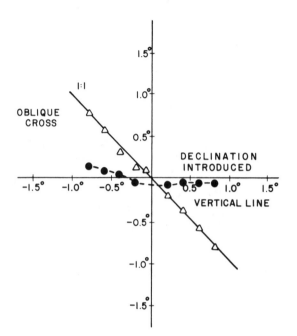

Figure 13–14. Tilting-plane settings for various amounts of oblique magnifi-
                cation using either a vertical-line object or an oblique-cross ob-
                ject (Ogle, 1950).

causes an apparent fore-and-aft tilt of the top and bottom of the oblique
cross, as predicted from the principles presented earlier (Ogle, 1950).
Therefore, a target containing both vertical lines and an oblique cross
allows differentiation of the three types of magnification. Such targets
are utilized in one form of eikonometry.

EIKONOMETRY

To correct aniseikonia, the most satisfactory approach involves direct
measurement. Then correction is made by neutralizing any differences
with appropriate afocal size lenses. If the measurement is based on a
null method, then the amount measured is the indicated correction
(Ogle, 1943).

    To measure aniseikonia, the device must achieve an accuracy of
something less than 1 percent. It should also differentiate among the
horizontal, vertical, and oblique forms and should be easily usable by
the clinician and the patient (Ogle, 1943).

While the leaf room, the tilting plane, and the horopter apparatus are all useful in demonstrating or measuring certain consequences of ocular-image size differences, each has the flaw of being somewhat limited as a diagnostic device. Clinically, special instruments called *eikonometers* are utilized. These are based on either direct comparison of the sizes of the two perceived images or distortions of stereoscopic space produced by aniseikonia.

Eikonometers have two components: a target and a set of variable magnifiers. Depending on the target configuration, these are known as the *direct-comparison eikonometer* and the *space eikonometer*. The theory and design of variable-magnification units have been described by Ogle (1950).

Figure 13–15 shows an arrangement of a variable-magnification unit and target used to directly compare the sizes of the perceived images (Ogle, 1943). Figure 13–16 shows the configuration for iseikonia, overall, axis 180°, and axis 90° conditions. This model does not measure oblique size differences, and judgments can be complicated in the presence of fixation disparity (Eskridge, 1958). The method depends on size

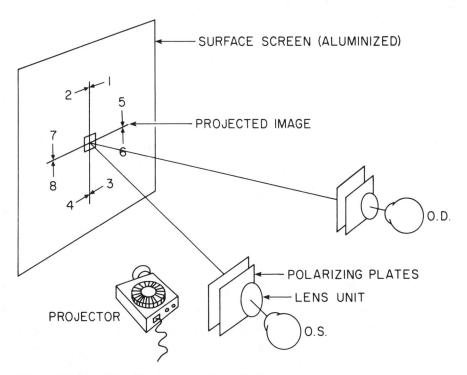

Figure 13–15. The direct-comparison eikonometer.

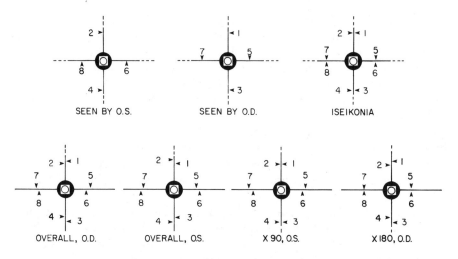

Figure 13–16.   Appearance of the direct-comparison eikonometer test objects: *top*, iseikonia; *bottom* (from left to right), overall, right eye larger; overall, left eye larger; geometric, left eye larger; and induced, right eye larger.

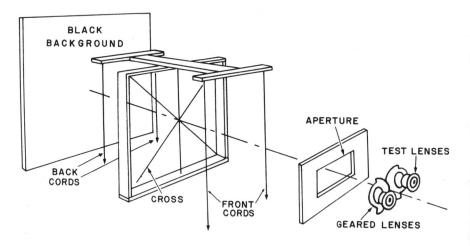

Figure 13–17.   The space eikonometer (Ogle, 1950).

judgments, and as previously discussed, this limits its accuracy to about 1 percent, although Ogle (1950) cited its accuracy as ±0.50 percent.

   Figure 13–17 is a representation of a space eikonometer. Figure 13–18 shows how the configuration produced by various magnification

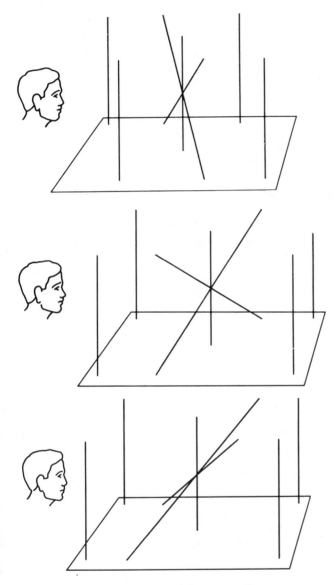

Figure 13–18.   Distortions of the space eikonometer test objects: *top*, geometric;
middle, induced; *bottom*, oblique (Bannon, 1954).

differences appears in the office model, which replaces real-depth targets with a photographic transparency viewed in projected depth. Ogle
(1950) reported that it had an absolute limit of accuracy of ±0.10 percent.

However, for most clinical purposes, the accuracy will range from about 0.25 to 0.75 percent (Bannon, 1954). Nevertheless, extrapolating from the data of Reading and Tanlamai (1980) and applying these to the design parameters of the office model of the space eikonometer (Ogle, 1950) indicate that the subject will need to possess a threshold of stereopsis smaller than about 59 arcseconds to see any distortions at all.

Furthermore, unless the subject's stereo threshold is about 16 arcseconds or less (75 percent correct-response criterion), the measurement error will exceed ±1.0 percent, a level commonly considered the lower limit of clinical significance. In addition, application of this instrument often requires several practice sessions to train some patients to make space judgments sufficiently accurate to arrive at a satisfactory size lens prescription (Bannon, 1954).

Space eikonometers utilize a slightly different approach to the measurement of oblique aniseikonia than was presented previously. This form is called *declination*, defined as the sum of the rotary deviations of the primary vertical meridians of the two retinas from the objective vertical, as indicated in Figure 13–13. Ogle's text should be consulted for further details.

SCREENING FOR ANISEIKONIA

Although various screening devices have been proposed, most lack the necessary sensitivity, and many involve projected-depth displays that are flawed by the fact that this tends to dampen stereoscopic perceptions (Halass, 1966).

Apparently, the stereograms prepared by photographing the space eikonometer targets displaying various amounts of magnification difference and viewing these in a standard stereo viewer may be the best available screening procedure based on stereoscopic perceptions (Cohen et al., 1957). However, such a system may have its own optical distortions, as do standard stereoscopes and even some screening cards (Sachsenweger, 1964).

Miles (1947) described a method of direct-comparison screening that involved two laterally separated point sources of light viewed through Maddox rods. While this technique, too, has limited accuracy, such methods may prove useful when a suitable eikonometer is not available. The interested reader should consult Halass (1966) for details of this and other screening devices.

ADAPTATION TO ANISEIKONIA

Burian (1943b) studied the effect of wearing an axis 90° size lens before one eye for 8 to 14 days. Three subjects participated, including Burian himself, and kept a diary of their impressions. Each day, once in the morning and again every evening, direct-comparison eikonometer readings, apparent frontoparallel plane settings, and tilting-plane measurements were made.

All three subjects noted the initial distortions of familiar surroundings. Burian found that this was more noticeable for near and steady fixation and was accompanied by headaches, asthenopia, irritability, and dyspepsia, but these symptoms were not strong enough to prevent the successful accomplishment of their usual work tasks. Burian commented that his surgical duties were discharged with no difficulty.

The symptoms subsided in severity with the passage of time, but they were always present during the experimental period. However, the subjective impression of distortions seemed to lessen and disappeared after 3 or 4 days. At the end, these reappeared and readaptation occurred (Burian and Ogle, 1945).

Adaptation to the induced effect has not been found to occur (Ogle, 1950), whereas the geometric effect showed a 50 percent reduction in space eikonometer settings over a 9-day period (Burian and Ogle, 1945). Steffler and Remole (1979) found that a 75 percent adaptation to a small amount of induced oblique magnification difference occurred over a period of 60 days.

Furthermore, at any time, when any of the subjects of these studies were asked to look at trees full of leaves or to walk into a field of tall grass, the impression of the distortions always returned. Whatever the nature of this adaptive process, it did not appear to alter the fundamental physiological relationship known as corresponding points. Apparently, the adaptive process is highly dependent on viewing constant and familiar carpentered surroundings (Ogle, 1950).

Nevertheless, adaptation is given as the reason that the essential form of aniseikonia usually does not cause any great difficulties. For example, Burnside and Langley (1964) took fundus photographs and measured the difference in the papillomacular distance in both eyes of a group of subjects. From this distance, using schematic eye values for the various ocular dimensions, they predicted the amount of horizontal aniseikonia that should be measured. Eikonometry performed on these same subjects showed that the measured values were considerably less than the predicted ones. Engel (1963) measured axial length and then performed eikonometry. He found a similar relationship. Both studies are generally considered to offer evidence that adaptation to essential aniseikonia does occur.

Despite the degree of adaptation to certain forms of aniseikonia, the reports that the distortions return every time the environment lacks monocular space cues imply that over reliance on adaptation may be dangerous to patients when they have to function in certain surroundings.

EYE MOVEMENTS AND ANISEIKONIA

Not everyone has been convinced that aniseikonia is a purely sensory anomaly. For example, Friedenwald (1936) asserted that size lenses really provided a partial compensation for an anisophoria. Ogle (1950) argued that this is not true because of the small amounts involved. For example, for a 20° shift of fixation, a patient with a 1 percent size difference would experience a slip of only about 0.2°, or 12 arcminutes. The magnitudes involved suggest an anisophoric fixation disparity, owing to differential prismatic effects of the lenses used to correct anisometropia, to aniseikonia, or to a real anisophoric deviation. At any rate, the resulting fixation disparity would be a kind of noncomitant oculomotor deviation and, as Shipley and Rawlings (1970) suggested, a form of anomalous correspondence, a topic we discuss in Chapter 14.

That there is an important oculomotor component associated with aniseikonia is hinted at by the suggestion of Charnwood (1950) that such patients frequently reacted favorably to prism incorporated into their spectacle prescriptions. Furthermore, a study of 25 patients with clinically significant aniseikonia showed that nearly all had oculomotor imbalances (Field, 1943). As previously mentioned, fixed-eye horopter data with induced size differences also show altered fixation disparity.

NOTE

1. The von Hornbostel cube is a skeleton wire cube which, when viewed monocularly, reverses as does the Necker cube. In the experiment described here, settings based on binocular disparity are altered by the presence of the periodically reversing empirical cues.

REFERENCES

Allen, M. J. (1954), "The dependence of cyclophoria on convergence, elevation, and the system of axes," *American Journal of Optometry*, 31, 297–307.
Alpern, M. (1969), "Types of movement," *The Eye*, vol. 3, Academic, New York, 65–174.

Alpern, M., and Ellen, P. (1956), "A qualitative analysis of horizontal movements of the eyes in the experiment of Johannes Mueller," *American Journal of Ophthalmology*, 42, 389–396.

Bailey, N. J. (1957), "Visual projection in walking experiments," *American Journal of Optometry*, 34, 360–376.

Bailey, N. J. (1958), "Locating the center of visual direction by a binocular diplopia method," *American Journal of Optometry*, 35, 484–495.

Bannon, R. E. (1954), *Clinical Manual on Aniseikonia*, American Optical, Buffalo, 1–119.

Beaumont, J. G. (1974), "Handedness and hemisphere function," *Hemisphere Function in Human Brain*, Elek, London, 89–120.

Bennett, A. G., and Francis, J. L. (1962), "Ametropia and its correction," *The Eye*, vol. 4, Academic, New York, 133–179.

Blank, A. A. (1959), "The Luneburg theory of binocular space perception," *Psychology: A Study of a Science*, McGraw-Hill, New York, 395—426.

Borish, I. M. (1975), *Clinical Refraction*, Professional, Chicago, 257–304, 440.

Bourdy, C. (1960), "Grandeur relative des images retiniennes et vision binocular de l'espace," *Revue D'Optique*, 39, 64–76.

Brindley, G. S. (1970), *Physiology of the Retina and Visual Pathway*, Williams & Wilkins, Baltimore, 132–138.

Burian, H. M. (1943a), "Clinical significance of aniseikonia," *Archives of Ophthalmology*, 29, 116–133.

Burian, H. M. (1943b), "Influence of prolonged wearing of meridional size lenses on spatial location," *Archives of Ophthalmology*, 30, 645–666.

Burian, H. M. (1948), "History of the Dartmouth Eye Institute," *Archives of Ophthalmology*, 40, 163–175.

Burian, H. M., and Ogle, K. N. (1945), "Aniseikonia and spatial orientation," *American Journal of Ophthalmology*, 28, 735–743.

Burnside, R. M., and Langley, C. (1964), "Anisometropia and the fundus camera," *American Journal of Ophthalmology*, 58, 588–594.

Charnwood, J. R. B. (1949), "Observations on ocular dominance," *The Optician*, 118, 85–86.

Charnwood, J. R. B. (1950), *An Essay on Binocular Vision*, Hatton, London, 73–88.

Cibis, P. A. (1952), "Faulty depth perception caused by cyclotorsion," *Archives of Ophthalmology*, 47, 31–42.

Cline, D., Hofstetter, H. W., and Griffin, J. R. (1980) *Dictionary of Visual Science*, Chilton, Radnor, 33, 673.

Cohen, H. L., Forman, M. Z., and Milan, R. H. (1957), "A qualitative and quantitative method for screening aniseikonia," *American Journal of Optometry*, 34, 184–196.

Cohen, S., and Duckman, R. H. (1975), "Ocular dominance and amblyopia," *American Journal of Optometry and Physiological Optics*, 53, 47–50.

Davis, R. J. (1959), "Empirical corrections for aniseikonia in preschool anisometropes," *American Journal of Optometry*, 36, 351–364.

Engel, E. (1963), "Incidence and magnitude of structurally imposd retinal image size differences," *Perception and Motor Skills*, 16, 377–384.

Eskridge, J. B. (1958), *Aniseikonia*, The Ohio State University, Columbus.

Field, H. B. (1943), "A comparison of ocular imagery," *Archives of Ophthalmology*, 29, 981–988.

Francis, J. L., and Harwood, K. A. (1951), "The variation of the projection centre with differential stimulus and its relation to ocular dominance," *Transactions of the International Optical Congress*, British Optical Association, 75–87.

Friedenwald, J. S. (1936), "Diagnosis and treatment of anisophoria," *Archives of Ophthalmology*, 15, 283–304.

Fry, G. A. (1961), "Eye-body coordination in the perception of space," *Transactions of the International Ophthalmic Optical Congress*, Crosby Lockwood, London, 16–33.

Gazzaniga, M. S., and LeDoux, J. E. (1978), *The Integrated Mind*, Plenum, New York, 45–76.

Halass, S. (1966), "Aniseikonia—A survey of the literature," *American Journal of Optometry*, 43, 505–523.

Harris, C. S. (1974), "Beware of the straight-ahead shift—A nonperceptual change in experiments on adaptation to displaced vision," *Perception*, 3, 461–476.

Hay, J. C., and Goldsmith, W. M. (1973), "Space-time adaptation of visual position constancy," *Journal of Experimental Psychology*, 99, 1–9.

Howard, I. P., and Templeton, W. B. (1966), *Human Spatial Orientation*, Wiley, New York, 367–418.

Humphriss, D. (1969), "The measurement of sensory ocular dominance and its relation to personality," *American Journal of Optometry*, 46, 603–614.

Jones, R. (1979), "Where is the visual egocenter?" presented at the annual meeting of the American Academy of Optometry, Anaheim, Calif.

Kaushall, P. (1975), "Functional asymmetries of the human visual system as revealed by binocular rivalry and binocular brightness matching," *American Journal of Optometry and Physiological Optics*, 52, 509–520.

Lancaster, W. B. (1938), "Aniseikonia," *Archives of Ophthalmology*, 20, 907–912.

Lennerstrand, G. (1978), "Binocular interaction studied with visual evoked responses (VER) in humans with normal or impaired binocular vision," *Acta Ophthalmologica*, 56, 628–637.

Mallett, R. F. J. (1969), "Fixation disparity in clinical practice," *Australian Journal of Optometry*, 52, 97–109.

Melvill Jones, G., and Gonshor, A. (1975), "A goal-directed flexibility in the vestibulo-ocular reflex arc," *Basic Mechanisms of Ocular Motility and Their Clinical Implications*, Pergamon, New York, 227–245.

Miles, P. W. (1947), "Factors in the diagnosis of aniseikonia and paired Maddox-rod tests," *American Journal of Ophthalmology*, 30, 885–897.

Ogle, K. N. (1938), "Induced size effect," *Archives of Ophthalmology*, 20, 604–623.

Ogle, K. N. (1939), "Relative sizes of ocular images of the two eyes in asymmetric convergence," *Archives of Ophthalmology*, 22, 1046–1067.

Ogle, K. N. (1943), "Association between aniseikonia and anomalous binocular space perception," *Archives of Ophthalmology*, 30, 54–64.

Ogle, K. N. (1950), *Researches in Binocular Vision*, Saunders, Philadelphia, 101–326.

Ogle, K. N. (1952), "Distortion of the image by ophthalmic prisms," *Archives of Ophthalmology*, 47, 121–131.

Ogle, K. N. (1962a), "Ocular dominance and binocular retinal rivalry," *The Eye*, vol. 4, Academic, New York, 409–417.

Ogle, K. N. (1962b), "Special topics in binocular spatial localization," *The Eye*, vol. 4, Academic, New York, 349–368.

Ogle, K. N., and Ellerbrock, V. J. (1946), "Cyclofusional movements," *Archives of Ophthalmology*, 36, 700–735.

Perry, N. W., Childers, D. B., and McCoy, J. G. (1968), "Binocular addition of the visual evoked response at different cortical locations," *Vision Research*, 8, 567–573.

Porac, C., and Coren, S. (1975), "Suppressive processes in binocular vision: Ocular dominance and amblyopia," *American Journal of Optometry and Physiological Optics*, 52, 651–657.

Reading, R. W. (1971), "The tracking of targets located outside of Panum's area," *British Journal of Physiological Optics*, 26, 217–227.

Reading, R. W. (1980), "A disparity analysis of some horopter data," *American Journal of Optometry and Physiological Optics*, 57, 815–821.

Reading, R. W., and Tanlamai, T. (1980), "The threshold of stereopsis in the presence of differences in magnification of the ocular images," *Journal of the American Optometric Association*, 51, 593–595.

Sachsenweger, R. (1964), *Stereokopische Taflen Zur Bestimmung der Aniseikonie*, Barth, Leipzig.

Shipley, T., and Rawlings, S. C. (1970), "The nonius horopter," *Vision Research*, 10, 1225–1299.

Slotnick, R. S. (1969), "Adaptation to curvature distortion," *Journal of Experimental Psychology*, 81, 441–448.

Steffler, D. J., and Remole, A. (1979), "Adaptation to spectacle induced meridional aniseikonia," University of Waterloo, Waterloo, Ontario.

Sullivan, M. J., and Kertesz, A. E. (1978), "Binocular coordination of torsional eye movements in cyclofusional response," *Vision Research*, 18, 943–949.

Wallach, H., Moore, M. E., and Davidson, L. (1963), "Modification of stereoscopic depth perception," *American Journal of Psychology*, 76, 191–204.

Walls, G. L. (1951a), "The problem of visual direction," *American Journal of Optometry*, 28, 55–83, 115–146, 173–212.

Walls, G. L. (1951b), "A theory of ocular dominance," *Archives of Ophthalmology*, 45, 387–412.

Waters, E. N. (1952), *Ophthalmic Mechanics*, Edwards, Ann Arbor, 50–57.

Welch, R. B. (1978), *Perceptual Modification*, Academic, New York.

Wernick, R. (1980), "One-eyed jacks, like the rest of us, aren't that wild," *Smithsonian*, 10, 63–71.

Winer, B. J. (1962), *Statistical Principles in Experimental Design*, McGraw-Hill, New York.

14

ANOMALOUS CORRESPONDENCE

> . . . when you have eliminated the impossible, whatever remains, however improbable, must be the truth.
>
> *Arthur Conan Doyle*

Strabismus has associated with it many anomalies that may contribute to its manifestation or may result from the deviation itself. These include amblyopia, abnormal suppression, eccentric fixation, and anomalous correspondence (Burian and von Noorden, 1974). Anomalous correspondence is a purely binocular phenomenon not yet treated in these discussions in a systematic way, and so it deserves some attention.

Anomalous correspondence is defined as the binocular condition in which stimulation of the two foveal centers gives rise to two separate visual directions (Cline et al., 1980). In other words, it violates Hering's law of identical visual direction (see Chapter 6). By implication, there exists an extrafoveal point in the deviating eye which, when stimulated along with the fovea of the fixating eye, will give rise to a common visual direction. In very simple terms, we can think of anomalous correspondence as the result of an apparent slip of corresponding points in the deviating eye to become recentered on some eccentric point (sometimes confusingly called the *false macula*). It is exclusively binocular in the sense that no shift in monocular local signs need occur. That is, the condition exists only if both eyes are open (Burian, 1951).

To diagnose its presence, it is necessary to demonstrate that the two primary lines of sight do not correspond. However, for a given set of test conditions, if a peripheral point is located in the deviating eye that corresponds to the fixating fovea, then several different relationships are revealed (Griffin, 1976). The angle of deviation of the primary line of sight from bifixation is called the *objective angle*, sometimes referred to simply as the *angle of deviation*. It is objective in the sense that the examiner determines it by some form of alternate cover test. The angle at which an object presented to the primary line of sight of the fixating eye superimposes on another object presented peripherally to the deviating eye constitutes the *subjective angle of squint*. It is subjective because the patient locates this angle by, for example, swinging the arms of a haploscopic device to position two targets so that they give rise to a common, but anomalous, visual direction (Alpern, 1969). Various measurement methods have been discussed, for example, by Griffin (1976).

In this context, anomalous correspondence is present when the objective angle is not equal to zero and the subjective angle is not equal to the objective angle, considering measurement error (Flom and Kerr, 1967). For example, if an objective angle measured by the alternate cover test indicates 4 prism diopters of right esotropia, then the measurement error should be no more than about ±2 prism diopters. If, on the same patient, the subjective angle is 2 prism diopters of right esotropia and the scatter of five settings has a range of ±2 prism diopters, then anomalous correspondence has not been demonstrated.

If the difference exceeds the measurement error, then anomalous correspondence is present and is classified as follows. *Harmonious* anomalous correspondence is present if the objective angle is not equal to zero and the subjective angle is equal to zero. It is called *unharmonious* if the objective angle is not equal to zero and the subjective angle is less than the objective, but different from zero. If the subjective angle is larger than the objective, then it is called *paradoxical* correspondence. It is also called paradoxical if the objective angle is, say, eso and the subjective angle exo, or vice versa. Table 14–1 summarizes this terminology. Often the difference in these two angles is spoken of as the *angle of anomaly* (Flom, 1957). Figure 14–1 is a schematic representation of some of these angles.

Characteristics

Flom (1957) summarized some of the various viewpoints about the cause of anomalous correspondence. These include considering it the result of a congenital anatomic defect that also causes the strabismus,

Table 14-1. Relationship among Objective Angle, Subjective Angle, and Angle of Anomaly

Correspondence Is Called:	Objective Angle* (prism diopters) (O)	Subjective Angle (prism diopters) (S)	Angle of Anomaly (A)
Normal	15 eso	15 eso	0
Anomalous and harmonious	15 eso	0	15
Anomalous and unharmonious	15 eso	10 eso	5
Anomalous and paradoxical #1	15 eso	30 eso	15
Anomalous and paradoxical #2	15 eso	15 exo	30

*Also called the angle of squint, or angle of deviation.

considering it a sensory adaptive process that is acquired after the onset of strabismus during the critical period, and asserting that it is really a lack of correspondence owing to a lack of simultaneous binocular perception.

In sharp contrast to these views are those of Morgan (1961), Boeder (1964), and Shipley and Rawlings (1970). Morgan considered that anomalous correspondence was the result of an anomaly in the innervational pattern to the extraocular muscles. He pointed out that all registered eye movements, such as versions, produce a change in the egocentric localization in normal subjects. In strabismus, the deviating eye reports a displacement of apparent positions with respect to the fixating eye via an innervational record. This innervationally generated shift produces an anomalous projection pattern.

Guillery and Kaas (1971, 1973) attempted to correlate the presence of albinism resulting from autosomal recessive inheritance in certain animals, such as the Siamese cat and the "white" tiger, with abnormal projections from the temporal retina to the contralateral lateral geniculate nucleus and convergent strabismus. Abnormal projections also have been mapped in the cortex of such animals (Shantz and LeVay, 1979). However, Rengstorff (1976) studied some 277 Siamese cats, using a telephotographic technique, and found that only 43 percent showed an apparent esotropia. Furthermore, 35 percent were apparently exotropic. He cautioned that since the anatomic location of the area centralis has not been studied in the Siamese cat, the deviation must be considered apparent. Further, he noted that the incidence of oculomotor de-

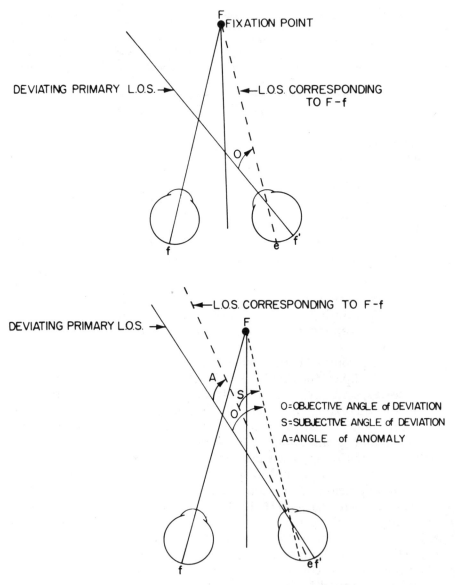

Figure 14–1.   Angular relationships involved in anomalous correspondence. The upper figure shows the harmonious form, while the lower one illustrates the unharmonious variety. (L.O.S. = line of sight.)

viations in other types of cats, dogs, or other animals with normal pathways had not been reported; yet his personal observations suggested that these, too, might show rather high incidences of apparent oculomotor deviations. Finally, he somewhat whimsically implied that the seemingly abnormal pathways of the Siamese cat may represent evidence for a form of "supercat." My personal observations indicate that sometimes the apparent oculomotor deviation is related to the excitement of our family cat [a Siamese, named Sasha, also observed by Mallett (1973)] such as occurs when she is presented with a morsel of turkey close to her nose. By some means, this seems to stimulate bilateral overconvergence. After all, both dogs and cats are reported to have a limited capacity of accurate convergence (Walls, 1942).

The lack-of-correspondence hypothesis is quite applicable to patients with large angles of deviation (Bagolini and Capobianco, 1965). Apparently, this group (about 40 or more prism diopters) adapts to the strabismus by abnormal suppression, and projection is purely monocular (Verhoeff, 1938). When stimuli are arranged to break through this suppression, these patients usually demonstrate normal correspondence (Flom, 1963).

While normal correspondence seems mostly rigid and mainly innate, sometimes the anomalous variety appears to be quite liable, so that stimulus parameters can be arranged to show the coexistance of both forms (Mallett, 1970). Usually, one form dominates. The degree of domination gives rise to a basis of grading the severity or depth of the anomaly. Burian (1951) pointed out that when a particular test was used that introduced a situation quite different from those usually encountered in the normal surroundings, the normal correspondence system tended to dominate. However, a test that produced the least "sensorial dissociation" (Bagolini, 1967) favored domination by the anomalous system. Table 14–2 presents the clinical scale of Bagolini and Capobianco (1965).

According to Hallden (1952), the large number of unharmonious forms found by the major amblyoscope is due to proximal convergence. He considered that true unharmonious correspondence was found only by using a projection test and that it occurred only following surgery or orthoptics. Paradoxical correspondence is also believed to result only after such treatments (Burian and von Noorden, 1974).

Flom and Kerr (1967) called attention to the importance of considering measurement error in grading anomalous correspondence. Since it is a phenomenon mainly associated with the smaller angle squints (Jampolsky, 1951), errors in measurement can confound these apparent distinctions. Additionally, they believed that different results on various tests could be accounted for by the presence of unsteady eccentric

Table 14–2.   Depth of Anomalous Correspondence according to
Bagolini and Capobianco (1965)

"Depth of Adaptation"	*Test in Order of Degree of "Dissociation"*
Least deeply adapted Most deeply adapted	1. Striated lenses 2. Polarized light projection 3. Major amblyoscope (troposcope) 4. Red lens test 5. Four-dot test 6. Afterimage test

fixation and changes in eye position. Johnston (1970) confirmed this idea and pointed out that variability in diagnosis also could occur as a result of change in fixation between the preferred and the nonpreferred eye, a change in the testing distance, and a change in the method used to determine the angle of anomaly.

Jampolsky (1951) implied that measurement errors could be reduced somewhat for small angle squints (less than 15 prism diopters) by using very small test objects in a troposcope. Furthermore, he reported that, in addition to the presence of an intransigent anomalous correspondence, such individuals manifested a binocular functional scotoma such as was reported by Taylor (1973) to occur in congenital esotropia.

Perhaps refined measurement techiques and the monitoring of eye position would show that the depth concept is a real one, at least in some instances. Certainly, Jampolsky's observations allow for the suggestion that the size of the deviation is an important parameter in determining the nature and fixity of this anomaly.

Sensory Aspects

Verhoeff (1940) used the timing of the physical onset of two lights, variously positioned in the binocular field, to demonstrate that the direction of an apparent motion, or phi phenomenon, could be reversed for a patient depending on bifixation or manifestation of 25 prism diopters of occasional exotropia. Often exotropes show an anomalous system when squinting and a normal one when bifixating. Furthermore, in constant monocular esotropia, Maraini and Santori (1967) found that forcing the patient to fixate with the usually deviating eye sometimes spontaneously reverted the correspondence to the normal form.

Reading (1972) studied binocular masking, using a normal and a strabismic subject (27 prism diopters of esotropia). This approach called for presenting a long-duration flash of light at a fixed intensity on the primary line of sight of the deviating eye and a short, variable-intensity test flash to the primary line of sight of the fixating eye. The long-duration light is called the *masking stimulus* since it elevates the detection threshold for the shorter test stimulus. Reading found that the anomalous correspondent showed suppression and a reduction in masking as a function of the time between the onset of the two flashes, presented separately to the two eyes. While spurious eye movements may have been involved, this finding may still suggest that anomalous correspondence sometimes represents a desensitized form of binocular perception, as implied (in Chapter 13) from the results of walking experiments and from reports of binocular functional suppression, presented above.

Mallett and Reading (1971) investigated some temporal and intensive stimulus parameters necessary to replace anomalous projection with the normal form by alternately flashing lights to two eyes in one subject with 30 prism diopters of esotropia. These lights were positioned at the objective angle and flashed at a rate of 1 to 9 Hz. When steady lights were used at this position, the subject reported diplopia. Between the 4- and 7-Hz flash rates, this perception changed to one of seeing the two images dance back and forth at a separation equal to the measurement error of the objective angle.

Both Williams (1974) and Lema and Blake (1977) found that binocular summation of suprathreshold stimuli was no better than that of the most sensitive eye in strabismic subjects.

THE HOROPTER IN ANOMALOUS CORRESPONDENCE

Early investigators considered measurements of the horopter on such patients most desirable. Because it had revealed so much about the nature of normal binocular function, the method might well have helped to sort out the true nature of this anomaly from what was otherwise a series of somewhat unrelated and seemingly contradictory observations. Nevertheless, actual measurements proved difficult, and it was only when Flom (1957) added an alternate flashing of the components of a nonius horopter apparatus that any horopter data on these subjects became available. He did not use any objective measurement of eye position. Furthermore, he reported rather exceptional improvements in the accuracy of peripheral nonius settings by using this flashing technique on normal subjects. Shipley and Rawlings (1970) could find no substantial differences between flashing- and steady-light nonius accuracy.

Figure 14–2 represents most features typical of Flom's (1957) raw data. The horopter locus is displaced rather far from the fixation point and sometimes shows an aniseikonic tilt. The most striking feature of many of his plots is a notch in the locus that always occurred in the region between the two primary lines of sight. Although this has come to be identified with the horopters of anomalous correspondence by Boucher (1967) and Johnston (1970), both of which also used a flashing-light nonius, Flom was not so sure that this feature was unique to this condition. He also found a notch in the raw data of a strabismic subject with normal correspondence (Flom, 1957).

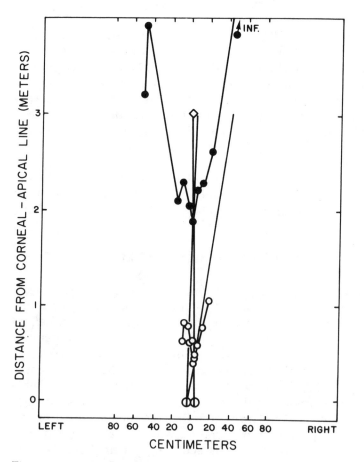

Figure 14–2. Plot of raw horopter data for one esotropic subject from Flom's (1957) study.

Mallett (1973) suggested that the rates of flashing used in all these studies were just right to convert the anomalous correspondence to the normal form. At any rate, Mallett's data from using a steady-light non-ius show no clear evidence of such a notch, nor do the data of Hallden (1973) or Bagolini and Capobianco (1965), who used another horopter criterion.

Bagolini and Capobianco (1965) attached small lights to horopter rods and had strabismic subjects (4 to 20 prism diopters of esotropia) determine diplopia limits while wearing striated lenses. This allowed the subject to notice the effect of any abnormal suppression, which apparently occurred only on rare occasions. Eye position was not measured. As previously mentioned, this indicated that Panum's space underwent considerable expansion. Undoubtedly, the reported irregularities in these data were due to the rather large measurement errors, which are characteristic of data taken on such subjects. Pasino and Maraini (1966) found essentially the same thing in a group of seven subjects with small angles (less than 6 prism diopters) of convergent strabismus.

Hallden (1973) presented horopter data for one anomalous subject (the angle of deviation was equal to 14 prism diopters of exotropia), using the subjective angle determinations across the binocular field of view, a form of the nonius criterion. His data are presented in Figure 14–3. The horopter is displaced only about 1° toward the subject, and a part of it is tilted toward the subject on the right with the right-eye fixation and toward the left with the left-eye fixation. The radii of the circles surrounding the x's represent 4 times the standard error of the mean of 16 to 22 settings. Hallden did not monitor eye position.

Mallett's (1973) data also show some asymmetry in certain regions of the binocular field. Using nonius projections, or subjective angles, provided by a modified synoptiscope, he found that the accuracy of the settings was no worse than about 9 arcminutes at a peripheral angle of 9°. Figure 14–4 shows his data. He did not measure eye movements by any systematic means.

Both Hallden and Mallett found fairly normal-looking horopters over at least a small portion of the binocular field. However, as Flom (1957) pointed out, even these are truly anomalous. Figure 14–5 illustrates horopter locations for normal correspondence in strabismus. Some of Boucher's (1967) results indicated that it was located behind the head of an exotropic subject demonstrating normal correspondence.

DISPARITY ANALYSIS

For these raw data, as with the horopter data for normals, analysis is difficult. Both Flom and Weymouth (1961) and Hallden (1973) suggested

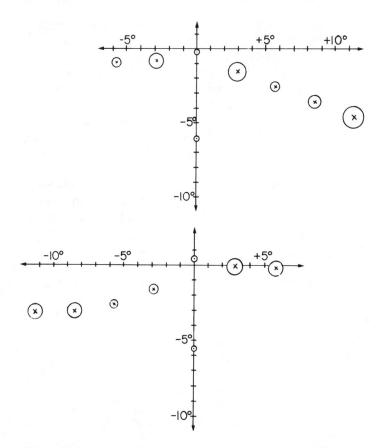

Figure 14–3.   A raw data plot for an exotropic subject (Reprinted by permission from Hallden, 1973).

methods of data reduction that were based on Ogle's H and R_o approach (see Chapter 11). Reading (1981) applied a simplified form of Shipley and Rawlings' disparity analysis to some of the available data.

Figure 14–6 presents horopter disparities for a subject that illustrate the effects of altering monocular fixation. These plots are the result of a disparity analysis of the data of Flom (1957). They seem to show a considerable shift in horopter disparities. While a part of this may be due to the presence of a noncomitancy and asymmetric convergence in strabismus, some of the irregularity may be due to spurious eye movements. For subject F.K., fixating with the left eye, apparently the horopter disparities are fairly regular, show an esodeviation, and have an aniseikonic tilt. Figure 14–7 shows horopter disparities from the data of Boucher (1967) in which an objective measurement of eye position

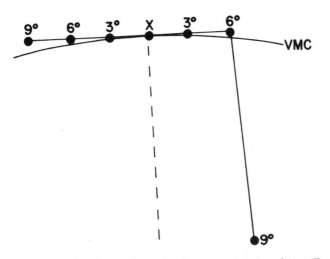

Figure 14–4.   A raw data plot for an esotropic subject (Reprinted by permission from Mallett, 1970, British Journal of Physiological Optics).

allowed the data to be partially corrected. This attempt at correction produces a more nearly normal disparity plot (Reading, 1981).

Figure 14–8 shows horopter data coverted to disparities for subjects with occasional esotropia. For bifixation, eye movements do not always appear to be such a large factor, since generally the resulting horopter disparities appear similar to those of a normal subject. Reading (1981) analyzed other data from the studies of Flom (1957) and Boucher (1967) and reported that bifixation did not always produce a completely normal-appearing plot, nor did the results of surgery or the application of prism.

The plots of Hallden and Mallett resemble those found for bifixation, or following correction of eye position, over at least a portion of the binocular field. Perhaps their subjects also achieved bifixation during some of these horopter measurements (Reading, 1981). Until more horopter data become available that are obtained under conditions in which eye position can be ascertained, the true form of the horopter in anomalous correspondence must remain somewhat uncertain.

ALTERATIONS OF CELL DISTRIBUTIONS

Figure 14–9 shows the distribution of cells responding maximally for various amounts of vertical disparity. The dotted distribution indicates the usual one found in normal cats. The solid one is for a kitten reared

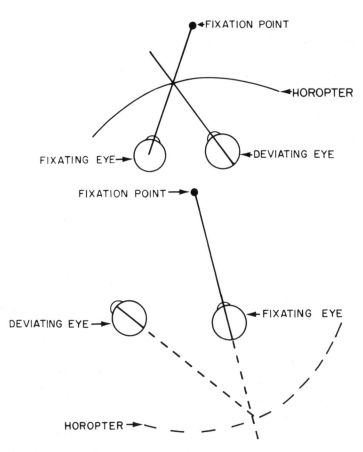

Figure 14–5.   Location of the horopter in strabismus with normal correspondence.

for 4 months while wearing 4 prism diopters of vertical prism (Shlaer, 1971). Although the sample size is quite small, this seems to indicate that slight alterations of habitual eye position or constant vertical fusional innervation, or both, causes a significant shift toward adaptation to the induced displacement. Furthermore, Shinkman and Bruce (1977) found that the orientation preference distribution could be altered in kittens raised while wearing goggles that produced 16° of cyclofusional disparity. Smith et al. (1979) found that kittens reared wearing 30 prism diopters, base in or base out, produced a dominance distribution altered to one of almost all monocular cells. Maffei and Bisti (1976) reported that surgically induced strabismus in kittens reared in the dark produced a similar dominance shift. This implies that the development of

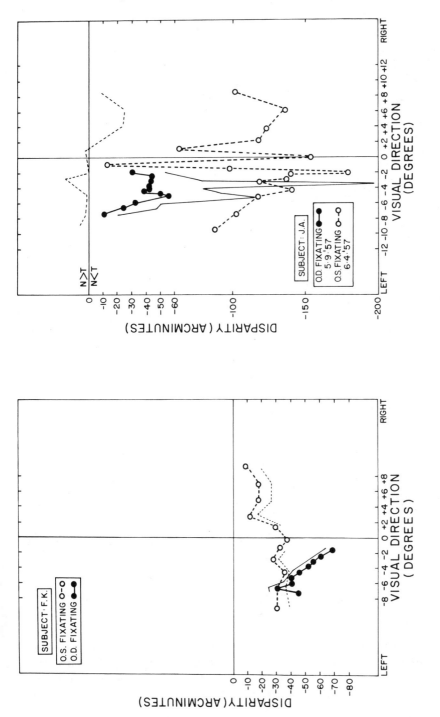

Figure 14-6. Horopter disparities illustrate the effect of altering monocular fixation (Reading, 1981).

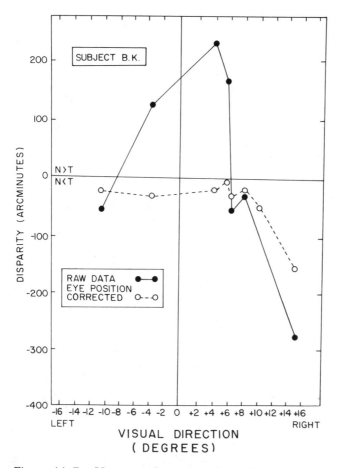

Figure 14–7.   Horopter disparities show the effect of correcting eye position (Reading, 1981).

binocular cells is an extremely complex process requiring a delicate sensory-motor balance (see also Chapters 10 and 12).

ANOMALOUS CORRESPONDENCE IN STRABISMUS, FIXATION DISPARITY, AND ANISEIKONIA

If anomalous correspondence is a sensory adaptation, then the extent to which the horopter appears as it does for normal subjects is an index of the success of this process. The reports reviewed here would seem to indicate that only sometimes does it approximate a somewhat equiv-

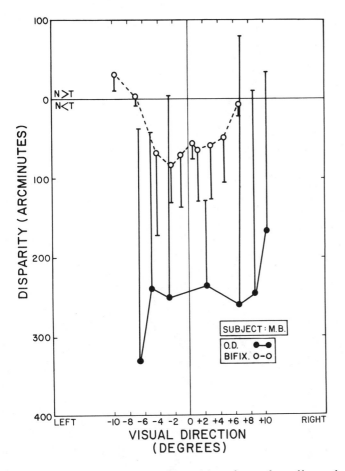

Figure 14–8. Horopter disparities show the effect of achieving bifixation (Reading, 1981).

alent condition to the normal, and then usually only over a small portion of the binocular field. Even then, eye movements may have produced this apparent regularity.

Based on some small samples, we could conjecture that at least some cases result from small displacements of the intersection of the primary lines of sight from the fixation point, or fusional stress, during the sensitive period. This could imply that the neurotropic destiny of some fibers developing from the retina back to the visual cortex could be disrupted or redirected (Sperry, 1951). The problem is the coexistance of the normal projection system, which can be demonstrated in many cases. Perhaps only a portion of the fibers is redirected. Although bi-

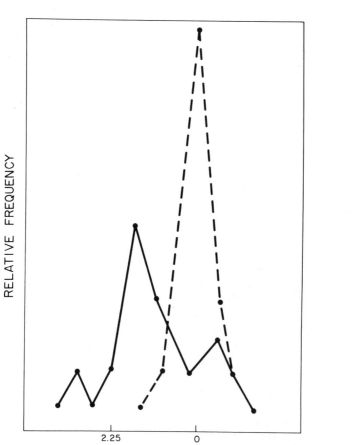

Figure 14–9.   Distributions of the number of cells responding maximally to vertical disparities (Shlaer, 1971).

furcation seems somewhat unlikely, Stone (1966) found branching of ganglion cell axons from a central strip 0.9° wide around the area centralis in the normal cat, and Cunningham (1976) reported an abnormally large number of these following early enucleation in the infant rat. As an alternative, these results might be produced by habituation of associative synaptic pathways which are not normally viable (Charnwood, 1950).

Actually, Morgan's (1961) motor innervation theory has much to recommend it. Anomalous Correspondence can be considered a motor adaptation process. For example, it explains monocular diplopia experienced by these patients following surgical correction or during orthoptic treatment as well as covariance of the objective angle and the angle of anomaly. It also explains how the Hering afterimage test can show that correspondence is normal when viewed in a dark room and anomalous when viewed in a lighted room full of visual details. By extension, it could account for the grades of the anomaly as assigned by Bagolini and Capobianco (Morgan, 1961).

This viewpoint extends the concept of anomalous correspondence to apply to all patients who indicate a slip between motor responses and corresponding points. Thus anomalous correspondence may well be an important factor not only associated with strabismus, but also occurring in cases of fixation disparity (see Chapter 7) and aniseikonia (see Chapter 13). Aniseikonia may be an etiological factor in precipitating manifest oculomotor deviation (Flom, 1957). In addition, the fact that almost all normals so readily adapt eye movement patterns to changes in the sensory array (Henson, 1978) may mean that the anomaly simply represents one manifestation of the extreme plasticity of the motor system.

Ikeda and Wright (1974) advanced a neural theory of amblyopia that also could account for anomalous correspondence. As noted in Chapter 12, there are at least three classes of ganglion cells, geniculate cells, and cortical cells. Table 12–1 shows their flow diagram, modified to apply to anomalous correspondence. For example, loss of categories A and B would result in anomalous correspondence.

Several authors have speculated about the anatomic level at which anomalous correspondence could take place. Walls (1951) suggested that anomalous correspondence was an attribute associated with a slip between the normal isomorphic relationship between areas 17 and 19. Johnston (1971) suggested that it was mediated between the hemispheres by the corpus callosum. Charnwood (1950) implicated the association fibers of area 17. Of course, it is also possible that the inferior parietal lobe is involved. We already discussed some of the behavioral evidence for the role of this neural region in at least some forms of spatial vision (see Chapters 12 and 13).

TREATMENT OF ANOMALOUS CORRESPONDENCE

When anomalous correspondence is present in a small angle squint, it is generally agreed that it is not amenable to alleviation by treatment (Jampolsky, 1951). In these cases, the eyes may appear straight enough for most purposes. Furthermore, although such cases do not represent complete cures (see Chapter 10), even with small functional scotomas, frequently they obtain a gross form of stereoscopic perception (Taylor,

1973). However, some reports of second-degree motor fusion may be no more than the result of a shift in the angle of anomaly (Maraini and Pasino, 1964). Vigorous orthoptic treatment of such cases only consolidates the anomaly (Mallett, 1970).

Anomalous correspondence in large angles of strabismus usually is mixed with abnormal suppression, and here the treatment strategy is to first eliminate the suppression and then grapple with the projection problem (Flom, 1963). Mallett (1970) suggested that about 8 prism diopters alternating between base-up and base-down on successive days frequently aided in establishing dominance of normal correspondence. Failing this, he suggested that prism be added until the original deviation was reversed, for example, from eso to exo. Exercises in which the eyes are alternately exposed to fusion targets at a rate between 4 and 7 Hz also may encourage the establishment of normal projection (Mallett, 1970). Surgery alone seems to convert gross deviations to microtropias, with only occasional instances of complete functional cures (Flom, 1963).

REFERENCES

Alpern, M. (1969), "Strabismus," *The Eye*, vol. 3, Academic, New York, 203–214.

Bagolini, B. (1967), "Anomalous correspondence: Definition and diagnostic methods," *Documenta Ophthalmologica*, 23, 346–398.

Bagolini, B., and Capobianco, N. M. (1965), "Subjective space in comitant squint," *American Journal of Ophthalmology*, 59, 430–442.

Boeder, P. (1964), "Anomalous retinal correspondence refuted," *American Journal of Ophthalmology*, 58, 336–373.

Boucher, J. A. (1967), "Common visual direction horopters in exotropes with anomalous correspondence," *American Journal of Optometry*, 44, 547–572.

Burian, H. M. (1951), "Anomalous retinal correspondence: Its essence and its significance in diagnosis and treatment," *American Journal of Ophthalmology*, 34, 237–253.

Burian, H., and von Noorden, G. (1974), *Binocular Vision and Ocular Motility*, Mosby, St. Louis, 214–275.

Charnwood, J. R. B. (1950), *An Essay on Binocular Vision*, Hatton, London, 85–88.

Cline, D., Hofstetter, H. W., and Griffin, J. R. (1980) *Dictionary of Visual Science* Chilton, Radnor, PA. 144–145.

Cunningham, T. J. (1976), "Early eye removal produces excessive bilateral branching in the rat: Application of cobalt filling method," *Science*, 194, 857–858.

Flom, M. C. (1957), "The empirical longitudinal horopter in anomalous correspondence," Ph.D. thesis, University of California, Berkeley.

Flom, M. C. (1963), "Treatment of binocular anomalies of vision," *Vision of Children*, Chilton, Philadelphia, 197–228.

Flom, M. C., and Kerr, K. E. (1967), "Determination of retinal correspondence, multiple-testing results and the depth of anomaly concept," *Archives of Ophthalmology*, 77, 206–213.

Flom, M. C., and Weymouth, F. W. (1961), "Retinal correspondence and the horopter in anomalous correspondence," *Nature*, 189, 34–36.

Griffin, J. R. (1976), *Binocular Anomalies—Procedures for Vision Therapy*, Professional, Chicago, 97–120.

Guillery, R. W., and Kaas, J. H. (1971), "A study of normal and congenitally abnormal retinogeniculate projections in cats," *Journal of Comparative Neurology*, 143, 73–100.

Guillery, R. W., and Kaas, J. H. (1973), "Genetic abnormality of the visual pathways in a 'white' tiger," *Science*, 180, 1287–1289.

Hallden, U. (1952), *Fusional Phenomena in Anomalous Correspondence*, Almquist and Wiksells, Uppsala, Sweden.

Hallden, U. (1973), "The longitudinal horopter in a case of concomitant strabismus with anomalous correspondence," *Acta Ophthalmologica*, 51, 1–11.

Henson, D. B. (1978), "Corrective saccades: Effects of altering visual feedback," *Vision Research*, 18, 63–67.

Ikeda, H., and Wright, M. J. (1974), "Is amblyopia due to inappropriate stimulation of the 'sustained' pathway during development?" *British Journal of Ophthalmology*, 58, 165–175.

Jampolsky, A. (1951), "Retinal correspondence in patients with small degree strabismus," *Archives of Ophthalmology*, 45, 18–26.

Johnston, A. W. (1970), "An analysis of clinical test results for anomalous correspondence," *Australian Journal of Optometry*, 53, 38–56.

Johnston, A. W. (1971), "Clinical horopter determination and the mechanism of binocular vision in anomalous correspondence," *Ophthalmologica*, 163, 102–119.

Lema, S. A., and Blake, R. (1977), "Binocular summation in normal and stereoblind humans," *Vision Research*, 17, 691–695.

Maffei, L., and Bisti, S. (1976), "Binocular interaction in strabismic kittens deprived of vision," *Science*, 191, 579–580.

Mallett, R. F. J. (1970), "Anomalous retinal correspondence—The new outlook," *Ophthalmic Optician*, 10, 606–624.

Mallett, R. F. J. (1973), "Anomalous correspondence," *British Journal of Physiological Optics*, 28, 1–10.

Mallett, R. F. J., and Reading, R. W. (1971), "Variations in the state of retinal correspondence with intermittent stimuli: A case study," *Ophthalmic Optician*, 11, 847–850.

Maraini, G., and Pasino, L. (1964), "Variations in the angle of anomaly and fusional movements in cases of small-angle convergent strabismus with harmonious anomalous correspondence," *British Journal of Ophthalmology*, 48, 439–443.

Maraini, G., and Santori, M. (1967), "Anomalous retinal correspondence and monolateral squint," *Ophthalmologica*, 153, 179–183.

Morgan, M. W. (1961), "Anomalous correspondence interpreted as a motor phenomenon," *American Journal of Optometry*, 38, 131–148.

Pasino, L., and Maraini, G. (1966), "Area of binocular vision in anomalous correspondence," *British Journal of Ophthalmology*, 50, 646–650.

Reading, R. W. (1972), "Binocular masking effect in a normal and an anomalous subject," *Journal of the American Optometric Association*, 43, 174–178.

Reading, R. W. (1981), "A disparity analysis of the anomalous correspondence horopter," *American Journal of Optometry and Physiological Optics*, 58, 372–377.

Rengstorff, R. W. (1976), "Strabismus measurements in the Siamese cat," *American Journal of Optometry and Physiological Optics*, 53, 643–646.

Shantz, C. J., and LeVay, S. (1979), "Siamese cat: Altered connections of visual cortex," *Science*, 204, 328–330.

Shinkman, P. G., and Bruce, C. J. (1977), "Binocular differences in cortical receptive fields of kittens after rotationally disparate binocular experience," *Science*, 197, 285–287.

Shipley, T., and Rawlings, S. C. (1970), "The nonius horopter," *Vision Research*, 10, 1225–1299.

Shlaer, R. (1971), "Shift in binocular disparity causes compensatory change in the cortical structure of kittens," *Science*, 173, 638–641.

Smith, E. L., Bennett, M. J., Harwerth, R. S., and Crawford, M. L. J. (1979), "Binocularity in kittens reared with optically induced squint," *Science*, 204, 875–877.

Sperry, R. W. (1951), "Mechanisms of neural maturation," *Handbook of Experimental Psychology*, Wiley, New York, 236–280.

Stone, J. (1966), "The naso-temporal division of the cat's retina," *Journal of Comparative Neurology*, 126, 585–600.

Taylor, D. M. (1973), *Congenital Esotropia: Management and Prognosis*, Stratton, New York.

Verhoeff, F. H. (1938), "Anomalous projection and other visual phenomena associated with strabismus," *Archives of Ophthalmology*, 19, 663–699.

Verhoeff, F. H. (1940), "Phi phenomenon and anomalous projection," *Archives of Ophthalmology*, 24, 247–309.

Walls, G. L. (1942), *The Vertebrate Eye*, Cranbrook, Bloomfield Hills, MI, 288–338.

Walls, G. L. (1951), "The problem of visual direction," *American Journal of Optometry*, 28, 55–83, 115–146, 173–212.

Williams, R. (1974), "The effect of strabismus on dichoptic summation," *Vision Research*, 14, 307–309.

15

BINOCULAR FUNCTION

To see a World in a Grain of Sand,
And a Heaven in a Wild Flower,
Hold Infinity in the palm of your hand,
And Eternity in an hour.

William Blake

DISPLAY OF THREE-DIMENSIONAL INFORMATION

The elementary principles of stereoscopy are presented in Chapters 7 and 9. Readers interested in greater detail should see Valyus (1962) and LeGrand (1967). Here we mention some of the other means of obtaining depth from two-dimensional images.

Holography produces three-dimensional reconstructions of objects by recording the spatial distributions of intensity and phase on a photographic plate. This process has been described in some detail, for example, by Schawlow (1968) and Fincham and Freeman (1974).

If a shutter such as that shown in Figure 15–1 is placed before the eyes and a motion-picture film contains alternate right and left views on successive frames, then rapid alternation between right and left views can be presented by synchronizing these (Valyus, 1962). This small delay between the presentations still allows for adequate stereopsis for most purposes (see Chaper 8). To avoid annoying brightness flicker, the rate of projection must be 4 times the normal (24 frames per second times 4).

Figure 15–2 shows how stereo effects can be achieved by using ground glass or a lenticular or prismatic screen. These all produce a displacement sufficiently large to channel separate views to the two eyes (LeGrand, 1967). The principal advantage of this display system is that it requires no special devices for viewing. In Russia, considerable

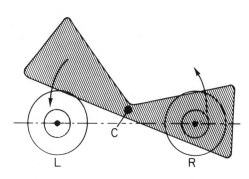

Figure 15–1. A shutter which pivots about C to alternately expose each eye to synchronized left and right views on successive frames of a movie film (Valyus, 1962).

development of this system for the display of motion pictures has been accomplished (Valyus, 1962).

A pseudobinocular effect can be obtained by viewing photographs, or other flat objects, with a lens of wide aperture and biconvex form. Such a device produces image distortions that are sufficiently different between the two eyes to create perceptible binocular disparities (Valyus, 1962).

Another depth effect, used in motion pictures, involves projecting images onto a curved panoramic screen. The images subtend angles that are greater than the size of the static visual fields. As long as motion of the camera taking the original pictures occurred, stereopsis is not missed and the scene is convincingly similar to viewing in the real world.

Stereoscopic views are utilized in science and technology to help visualize complex structures, as in crystallography, and to compare two separate views recorded at different times, as in astronomy and radiography. This method also is employed in making topographic maps from aerial photographs (Valyus, 1962). In optometry, it could be used to detect subtle changes in the ocular fundi.

MATHEMATICAL THEORIES OF BINOCULAR VISION

Figure 15–3 shows plan outlines of a series of wall configurations which, when viewed with the head fixed from points L and R, all look conventional, that is, right-angled and plane-surfaced, as with the usual room (Luneburg, 1950). The design of such rooms and their construction

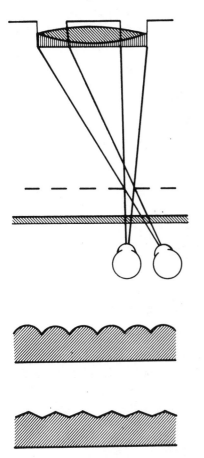

Figure 15–2. Several methods of channeling separate components of an image formed by a lens to the two eyes. This can be done by using a striped screen *(top)*, a prismatic surface *(middle)*, or a lenticular surface *(bottom)* (LeGrand, 1967).

by Ames (1955) introduced a mathematician named Luneburg to the problems of binocular space perception.

We will attempt to present Luneburg's theory in as nonmathematical a fashion as possible and so borrow heavily from the excellent description of Charnwood (1950). Those who wish a more mathematically rigorous treatment should consult the original works (Luneburg, 1947, 1950), some subsequent developments by Blank (1959), and the summary of experimental evidence by Graham (1965).

For these congruent rooms to be visually equivalent, they must

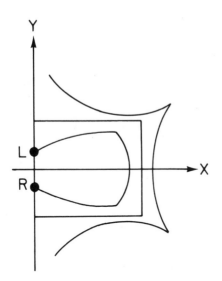

Figure 15–3.   Outline of configurations known as *Ames congruent rooms* (Reprinted by permission from Luneburg, 1950).

share the same line element. A *line element* is the metric of a particular
manifold or set of points and is the rule of measurement that applies
to the collection of these points or space. For example, in euclidean
space the line element is

$$ds^2 = dx^2 + dy^2 + dz^2 \qquad (15\text{--}1)$$

For points at a finite distance, the term *geodesic* is used. A geodesic is
the shortest line segment joining two points in the manifold or set.
Again, for euclidean space, this is a straight line, or

$$s = \int \sqrt{dx^2 + dy^2 + dz^2} \qquad (15\text{--}1)$$

assumes a minimum value (Luneburg, 1947).

Most people operate in surroundings and in a fashion that approximates euclidean space (Fry, 1950). However, since earth is more
or less a sphere, its geometry is different. The geodesics here are great
circles. Maps provide us with two-dimensional projections of this
sphere, but they always distort some things. For example, the projection
of a sphere onto a cylinder with its axis coincident to the axis through
the poles (known as Mercator projection) represents features at the
equator satisfactorily, but distances are greatly exaggerated and shapes
considerably distorted at the poles (Charnwood, 1950).

The foregoing illustrates the concrete existence of geometries other than euclidean. Another way to say this is simply that the world is not flat. For a sphere, the geodesic, or metric, is (Charnwood, 1950)

$$ds^2 = dx^2 + (\sin^2 x)\, dy^2 \qquad (15\text{--}3)$$

Because the phenomena of size and shape constancy can exist only in a particular form of noneuclidean space known as the *space of constant negative curvature*, Luneburg (1950) selected this for his transformations from physical (euclidean) to visual space (a riemannian space known as *hyperbolic* in form). Its metric (Luneburg, 1947) can be written as

$$ds^2 = \frac{1}{\sinh O(\gamma + \mu)} (O^2\, d\gamma^2 + d\phi^2 + \cos^2\phi\, d\theta^2) \qquad (15\text{--}4)$$

where γ is binocular parallax, ϕ is binocular latitude, θ is binocular elevation, and O and μ are personal constants. Figure 15–4 illustrates this coordinate system. Taking the intergal of this equation, we can transform parallel lines in physical space to diverging curves in visual space. Likewise, objective frontoparallel planes become curved, as described in Chapters 6 and 11.

According to Charnwood (1950), the process of binocular space perception can be described as the solving of Equation (15–4). In general, the solution will be unique, but the constants must be provided from some nonvisual source, perhaps from the visual association centers. The overall process, then, could be an integration of the perceptual equivalents of depth and position of individual points or local elements. The constants provide for a unique solution that may be quite different than the physical configuration, as illustrated by Ames' congruent rooms.

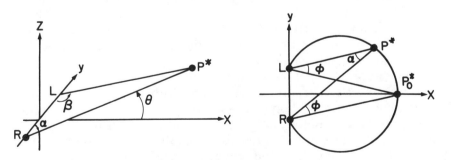

Figure 15–4. Coordinate system of Luneburg (1950, reprinted by permission).

REQUIREMENTS OF ANY THEORY OF BINOCULAR VISION

Tschermak listed eight fundamental facts that must be accounted for by any theory (Charnwood, 1950). Rephrased and modified slightly from those in Charnwood's report, they are as follows:

1. Externalization of sensations and their egocentric organization
2. Lack of permanent constancy in apparent direction of components of a physical object
3. Failure of impressions to exactly correspond to the geometric positions of stimuli
4. Reference of impressions from the two eyes to one common egocentric point
5. Phenomena of corresponding points and stereopsis resulting from binocular disparity, independent of eye movements
6. Displacement of the center of rotation from the center of projection
7. Modification of localization of retinal meridians produced by inclining the head
8: Phenomenon that objects fixed in physical space appear to be at rest and objects moving appear to move, regardless of the motion of the observers or their eyes

We can elaborate on local sign theory to encompass many of these requirements. For example, we can say that it is an intrinsic feature of all the major senses to relate the organism to the external world. That is, a signal that is within comes to be associated with, or projected toward, its external stimulus from the location of the body image. This, of course, explains nothing.

As suggested by Luneburg, the local-sign relationship is an ordering of points with an external scale factor required for any particular set of localizations. Because of the nature of this relationship, constancy can be broken, and a one-for-one relationship between objects and percepts does not always exist.

The displacement of the rotation center from the projection center, modifications of localization of meridians with the head tilted, and correct perception of motion all seem to require some cooperation between sensory and motor processes. Undoubtedly, this relationship is quite complex. Apparently it is mainly innervational processes that keep the sensory house in order and which can also significantly alter egocentric localizations.

The purely binocular phenomena of fusion, corresponding points, and stereopsis have caused several people to speculate about how such a system might work.

BINOCULAR MODELS

Barany proposed the anatomic schema illustrated in Figure 15–5 (Fry, 1953). It is well established that the axons of corresponding ganglion cells synapse with cells in the lateral geniculate that are in register. Barany proposed that the axons of these geniculate cells also synapse in registry, in layer IVc for contralateral fibers and layer IVa for ipsilateral fibers. The cells then interact with the corresponding synapse and, to a lesser degree, noncorresponding synapses across the span of layer IVb. This latter layer is called the *stripe of Gennari* of the visual cortex.

Verhoeff (1902) proposed that the nature of this interaction could be described by assigning algebraic numbers to each of the points on the two retinas (see Figure 15–6). Note that the two foveae are assigned the value of zero; temporal points, negative values; and nasal points, positive values. In this schema, we can define the horopter as those points that sum to zero, as is the result of processing for object points F and H. Crossed-disparity detection results when two cortical points sum to a positive value, and uncrossed disparity is detected when they sum to a negative value, as for object points A and A'. For a point off the median plane, for example for S, s_R and s_L equal $+2$.

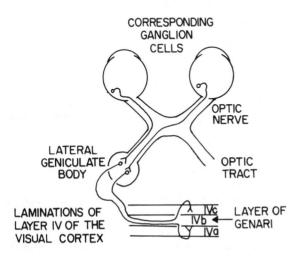

Figure 15–5.   Barany's schema to explain the physiology of corresponding points (Fry, 1953).

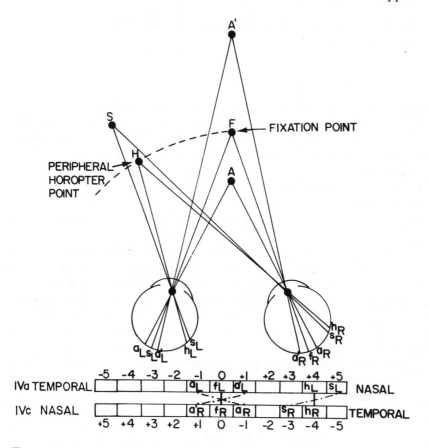

Figure 15–6. An algebraic model of binocular function (Verhoeff, 1902).

The figure can be elaborated to represent a similar arrangement which allows for the Panum-area phenomenon, stereopsis, and so on. It could account for a phenomenon reported by Verhoeff (1902) and illustrated by free-fusing Figure 15–7. Note that the thin vertical line in the middle figure "corresponds" with the thick vertical line in the left-hand portion of the figure. Yet this thick line bypasses the thin one to combine, or fuse, with the thick, slanted, "noncorresponding" line *a* in the binocular percept. In Verhoeff's schema, this would mean that the corresponding-point interaction has been weakened by decreasing the stimulus strength of one of the pair and allowing a stronger non-corresponding-point interaction to override it. Similar temporal effects could account for the Pulfrich stereophenomenon.

Charnwood (1950), in his excellent book on binocular vision, pre-

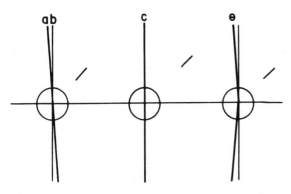

Figure 15–7. Stereogram used to illustrate the overriding of correspondence by altering stimulus strength (Verhoeff, 1902).

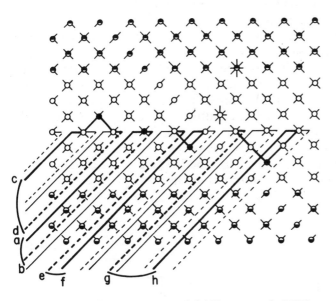

Figure 15–8. A computer model (Charnwood, 1950).

sented what must be one of the earliest examples of the application of information theory to vision. He was a clinical investigator steeped in neuroanatomy and clinical practice, as well as a peer of the British realm, a first-class automotive mechanic, and an innovative race car designer (Bryant 1956). His model is shown in simplified form in Figure 15–8. He started by considering the histology of the visual cortex. While the figure does not exactly reflect this, the diagonal lines correspond to the geniculate axons. He suggested that the stereopsis could result from the processing of information by a computing machine that meets two conditions: some way of keeping the signals paired and two in, one out. In this representation, incoming messages *a* and *b* yield zero disparity and so represent a horopter point. Messages *c* and *d* represent the processing by such a computer for an uncrossed disparity; *e* and *f*, that for a crossed disparity; and *g* and *h*, that for a larger crossed disparity.

Charnwood suggested that one way the pairing process might occur is by time-gaiting or having singles sent off in pairs at intervals. If the messages exchange members of the pairs so that, *e* and *h*, and *f* and *g*, are now paired, then they wind up at the points shown as stars in Figure 15–8. Since some time is lost at each junction or synapse, the greater the disparity, the longer it takes before a junction at one cell or point occurs. After this happens, the model has a specific output and so maps out three-dimensional space.

Charnwood suggested that this was an oversimplification and that various degrees of complexity could be added to make the model conform more and more to the histological structure of the cortex. In so doing, the model also could be made to account for such things as the Pulfrich stereophenomenon, Panum's space, and Panum's limiting case. Certainly such a model has an enduring elegance which is directly derived from its simplicity.

Dodwell (1970) developed a whole series of models along the lines used by Barany, Verhoeff, and Charnwood. The one we consider here features locking elements, as indicated in Figure 15–9. These elements

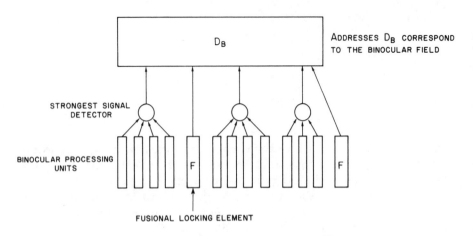

Figure 15–9.   A model that includes fusional aspects (Dodwell, 1970).

establish the fusion of the various disparities. According to Dodwell, disparity information is handled by the binocular processing units which function very much as described by Charnwood in his model. This resultant, then, is the input for the strongest signal detector that, in turn, competes for addresses or positions within D_B which represent a map of the whole binocular field. This model indicates that stereopsis can be processed at several different stages, as suggested by Julesz (1971). Dodwell said that it also incorporated features that handle suppression and rivalry.

Marr and Poggio (1979) proposed a computational theory of stereopsis. They suggested that each image was filtered at each different orientation by four separate spatial frequency analyzers whose characteristics have been reported by Wilson and Bergen (1979). Each is about two octaves wide, and the spatial area of operation of each filter increases with increasing eccentricity. At any one location two types occur, one showing relatively sustained responses and the other exhibiting relatively transient responses, as discussed in Chapter 12.

The interplay of excitation and inhibition in each unit's receptive field produces zero crossings of its sensitivity function, which roughly correspond to the position of edges in the optical image. Marr and Poggio's model calls for a matching of these zero crossings in the two images over an area equivalent to the excitatory center of the receptive field. Julesz and Spivack (1967) referred to this as *local stereopsis* (see Chapter 8).

This stage achieves correspondence, which is stored in a dynamic buffer. The larger units control vergence eye movements, which bring successively different sets of objects and their binocular disparities into the matching range of the smaller units. In this way, an overall percept is built up in the dynamic buffer, the site of *global stereopsis*. Unlike Julesz' (1963) computer model or dipole model (Julesz, 1971), this one is reported to correctly predict many of the features of binocular vision by using both random-dot patterns and conventional contours in projected or real space. However, it does predict a size for Panum's space that is considerably larger than that found by Woo (1974). Nevertheless, Schor and Tyler (1980) considered that such an expansion could happen if only the lower spatial frequencies were involved.

It would seem that the matching problem required to establish correspondence presented in this computational model also could be solved by the methods suggested by Verhoeff (1902) and Charnwood (1950). That is, the system could be a time-gated device. This seems to require that responses generated by one of the monocular systems have a larger magnitude, a form of dominance, and that each system have an asymmetric latency difference map across each retinal surface (Reading and Woo, 1972). Such features are present in the human visual system (see Chapter 8).

Figure 15–10 is a flow diagram that combines some of the features suggested by these various models. It is a simplification of a model by Skavenski and Hansen (1978) with some modifications. This figure presents a simplified schema of some of the interrelationships between sensory and motor activities. Stimulation of diffuse detectors initiates a gross form of fusion and stereopsis. If an obstacle prevents the reduction of disparity to a level that falls into the range of the specific detector, or if the two components of the pair are of sufficiently different stimulus strength, then a selector comes into operation to produce abnormal suppression.

If attention is not directed to a particular remote object, then only stereopsis from double images results. With time, the latter sensation fades owing to the Troxler effect. Given that the two images are of essentially equal quality and the mechanism is fully operational, disparities are reduced to a low level by fine fusional processes which allow for fine stereo perceptions. If a difference exists, or if the fine mechanism is faulty, then an alternator produces a suppression and/ or rivalry.

MODELS IN GENERAL

Modeling is a fascinating process. Here we make no claim for completeness. However, sufficient leads have been presented to allow the interested reader to explore this kind of intellectual tinkering. Most models express more about the biases of the modeler than about the

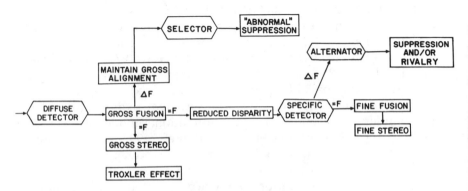

Figure 15–10. A sensory motor model of binocular function.

processes simulated. Naturally, science will show which models are the most likely and useful as additional facts are uncovered about the workings of visual system.

REFERENCES

Ames, A. (1955), *An Interpretative Manual*, Princeton University, Princeton.

Blank, A. A. (1959), "The Luneburg theory of binocular space perception," *Psychology: A study of a Science*, McGraw-Hill, New York, 395–426.

Bryant, A. (1956), "John Benson—2nd Lord Charnwood," *American Journal of Optometry*, 33, 663–668 (reprinted).

Charnwood, J. R. B. (1950), *An Essay on Binocular Vision*, Hatton, London, 89–110.

Dodwell, P. C. (1970), *Visual Pattern Perception*, Holt, New York, 151–154.

Fincham, W. G. A., and Freeman, M. H. (1974), *Optics*, Butterworth, London, 319–360.

Fry, G. A. (1950), "Visual perception of space," *American Journal of Optometry*, 27, 531–553.

Fry, G. A. (1953), *Binocular Space Perception*, The Ohio State University, Columbus.

Graham, C. H. (1965), "Visual space perception," *Vision and Visual Perception*, Wiley, New York, 504–547.

Julesz, B. (1963), "Towards the automation of binocular depth perception (automap-1)," *Proceedings of the IFIPS Congress*, North-Holland, Amsterdam.

Julesz, B. (1971), *Foundations of Cyclopean Perception*, University of Chicago Press, Chicago.

Julesz, B., and Spivack, G. J. (1967), "Stereopsis based on vernier cues alone," *Science*, 57, 563–565.

LeGrand, Y. (1967), *Form and Space Vision*, Indiana University, Bloomington, 303–313.

Luneburg, R. K. (1947), *Mathematical Analysis of Binocular Vision*, Princeton University, Princeton.

Luneburg, R. K. (1950), "The metric of binocular space," *Journal of the Optical Society of America*, 40, 627–642.

Marr, D., and Poggio, T. (1979), "A computational theory of human stereo vision," *Proceedings of the Royal Society of London*, series B, 204, 301–328.

Reading, R. W., and Woo, G. C. S. (1972), "Some of the time factors associated with stereopsis," *American Journal of Optometry*, 49, 20–28.

Schawlow, A. L. (1968), "Laser light," *Scientific American*, 219, 120–156.

Schor, C. M., and Tyler, C. W. (1980), "Spatio-temporal properties of Panum's fusional area," *Vision Research*, 21, 683–692.

Skavenski, A. A., and Hensen, R. M. (1978), "Role of eye position information in visual space perception," *Eye Movements and the Higher Psychological Functions*, Erlbaum, Hillsdale, N.J., 15–33.

Valyus, N. A. (1962), *Stereoscopy*, Focal, London.

Verhoeff, F. H. (1902), "A theory of binocular perspective," *American Journal of Physiological Optics*, 6, 416–448 (1924 reprint).

Wilson, H. R., and Bergen, J. R. (1979), "A four-mechanism model for threshold spatial vision," *Vision Research*, 19, 19–32.

Woo, G. C. S. (1974), "The effect of exposure time on the foveal size of Panum's area," *Vision Research*, 14, 473–480.

INDEX